DIAGNOSIS IN SPEECH-LANGUAGE PATHOLOGY

DIAGNOSIS IN SPEECH-LANGUAGE PATHOLOGY

Edited by
Irv J. Meitus, M.A.
Associate Professor and
Director of the Speech Clinic

and

Bernd Weinberg, Ph.D.
Professor and Head

Department of Audiology and Speech Sciences
Purdue University
West Lafayette, Indiana

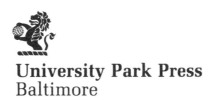

University Park Press
Baltimore

UNIVERSITY PARK PRESS
International Publishers in Medicine and Human Services
300 North Charles Street
Baltimore, Maryland 21201

Typeset by Maryland Composition Company
Manufactured in the United States of America by R. R. Donnelley & Sons Company
Designed by S. Stoneham, Studio 1812, Baltimore

Library of Congress Cataloging in Publication Data
Main entry under title

Diagnosis in speech-language pathology.

Includes index.
1. Speech, Disorders of—Diagnosis. 2. Language
disorders—Diagnosis. I. Meitus, Irv J. II. Weinberg,
Bernd. [DNLM: 1. Speech disorders—Diagnosis. 2. Language disorders—Diagnosis. WM 475 D536]
RC423.D47   1983   616.85′5075   83-5932
ISBN 0-8391-1810-4

CONTENTS

CONTRIBUTORS

John M. Hutchinson, Ph.D.
Professor and Director of Graduate Studies
Department of Speech Pathology and Audiology
Idaho State University
Pocatello, ID 83209

Laurence B. Leonard, Ph.D.
Professor
Department of Audiology and Speech Sciences
Purdue University
West Lafayette, IN 47907

Irv J. Meitus, M.A.
Associate Professor and Director of the Speech Clinic
Department of Audiology and Speech Sciences
Purdue University
West Lafayette, IN 47907

Marilyn Newhoff, Ph.D.
Associate Professor
Department of Communicative Disorders
San Diego State University
San Diego, CA 92184

J. Douglas Noll, Ph.D.
Professor
Department of Audiology and Speech Sciences
Purdue University
West Lafayette, IN 47907

Richard G. Schwartz, Ph.D.
Assistant Professor
Department of Audiology and Speech Sciences
Purdue University
West Lafayette, IN 47907

Bernd Weinberg, Ph.D.
Professor and Head
Department of Audiology and Speech Sciences
Purdue University
West Lafayette, IN 47907

PREFACE

We have prepared this text about diagnosis of speech and language disorders for use in teaching both upper-level undergraduate and graduate level university students and for use by practicing speech-language clinicians. Our intention is to provide a body of contemporary information essential to the understanding of diagnosis in speech-language pathology. In preparing individual chapters, we were aware that the amount of material available for inclusion might be very large, particularly when this volume is used to support single course offerings in diagnosis. We agreed at the outset that this text should be sufficiently comprehensive to have utility for readers with various levels of training and experience. From a teaching standpoint, sufficient information has been provided so that an instructor can vary the depth of study of the material in this text according to the level of student backgrounds.

We have prepared this text for three primary uses. First, we anticipate its use as a basic text for courses in speech-language diagnosis. Second, we have prepared this volume in such a manner that it can also be used in specialty area coursework (e.g., language disorders in children, voice disorders, stuttering, motor disorders of speech, aphasia, etc.). Hopefully, both students and instructors will find this text useful as a contemporary reference about diagnosis in specialty areas within the field of speech-language pathology. Third, we anticipate that practicing clinicians will refer to this book as a contemporary reference about diagnosis.

We believe that basic information about the nature of the diagnostic process and practical information about how this process gets implemented in actual clinical practice should be presented in a unitary manner. Learning *what* to observe about the patients, *how* to make these observations, and *why* such observations are necessary are essential prerequisites to clinical practice. Our teaching experience and contact with professional colleagues suggests that information about diagnosis is often not presented in a unitary manner. Rather, such information is often presented in a fragmented fashion. For example, information about diagnosis is often presented as part of a specific speech or language disorder course. In this case, material is frequently limited to only that which pertains to one particular disorder. As a second example, diagnostic information is sometimes organized into a course that deals with the administration and interpretation of specific tests, inventories, and so on. Here, emphasis is often placed upon the development of testing skills and appraisal of test strengths and liabilities. We do not equate test administration and interpretation with diagnosis.

In writing and editing this text, we have aimed toward achieving a balance between establishing a philosophy about diagnosis in speech-language pathology and describing practical approaches, strategies, and procedures that working clinicians use in their daily practice. We have consciously attempted to avoid being overly academic or pedantic. Likewise, we have avoided the manual or "cookbook" approach that tends to be overly simplistic. Building this type of balance into a multi-authored text that is broad in scope was no small undertaking. It is to the credit of the contributors that this balance could be achieved.

A few words about the contributors. Each writer was chosen for the following reasons. First, we wanted each contributor to be expert in his or her respective clinical area. Second, we felt it necessary for the contributors to be experienced university teachers, because this requirement would insure that they would understand the needs of clinical instructors. Third, we wanted contributors to be experienced clinicians, persons who have derived their knowledge about people with speech and language disorders from a sufficient base of clinical practice. Bringing these writers together has resulted in what we feel to be a contemporary description of diagnosis in speech-language pathology. Each of the contributors has dealt with specific areas of diagnosis of speech-language pathology in a manner consistent with the goals and approaches established for the preparation of this book.

This text has been organized in the following manner. We begin with a philosophical position about the role of diagnosis in rehabilitation. Our discussion of diagnosis is organized on a process level basis. The reader is lead through the assessment process from start to finish. Differential diagnosis is then defined. Here, we have attempted to make clear what a diagnosis is and what it is not. Emphasis is placed upon the parallels between scientific and clinical observation and data collection. After examining these more general issues, we discuss the kinds of information speech-language pathologists typically collect, how such information is gathered, and why we gather such information. Chapters dealing with diagnosis of specific types of speech and language disorders are then offered. Here, we review the nature of each of these disorders and consider contemporary diagnostic approaches and issues. Finally, the importance of professional communication from written and oral perspectives is considered. It is our hope that clinical instructors will find the information presented with sufficient clarity so that significant amounts of classroom time can be spent discussing actual clinical examples, rather than reviewing the text material exclusively.

It has been our intention to bring to the reader a usable text about diagnosis of speech and language disorders from a fresh perspective. We hope our readers will share the enthusiasm about diagnosis that has become a part of the preparation of this text.

Irv J. Meitus
Bernd Weinberg

ACKNOWLEDGMENTS

It is with a deep sense of appreciation that we acknowledge the people who have contributed significantly to the preparation of this book. In addition to the contributors who worked with us in a diligent and patient manner, we formally acknowledge Jeanette S. Swan who typed *all* preliminary drafts and the final version of the manuscript. In addition, we are extremely grateful for the contributions of Nancy P. Meitus for preparing the figures in Chapters 2, 7, and 10 and for her counsel regarding matters of graphic design. Arlene E. Carney of Purdue University provided special assistance in the preparation of the section on audition in Chapter 2. Janet S. Hankin, Senior Editor at University Park Press was especially helpful in encouraging us to undertake this project and in facilitating the rapid but careful completion of this text.

Our own students in the Department of Audiology and Speech Sciences at Purdue University merit special mention. In a broad sense, it has been our association with these students and their ever-present interest in our profession and work that fostered our desire to provide a text that would complement our teaching of diagnosis. In a more narrow perspective, we are grateful to these students for allowing us to evaluate versions of this material within our classes, thereby providing us with the opportunity to make necessary adjustments in the final product. Their comments and reactions were offered freely and openly. We are grateful to them.

Finally, the editors wish to share in the recognition of one another for the part each has taken in bringing this book to fruition. The concept of diagnosis and the format within which the content of this book is presented was derived largely from the clinical and teaching experience of Irv Meitus, while the eye for detail and the experience in professional writing of Bernd Weinberg provided what we hope is an even presentation. For both of us, the best part has been the shared learning that has taken place, both from our contributors and from one another.

DIAGNOSIS IN SPEECH-LANGUAGE PATHOLOGY

1

Approaching the Diagnostic Process

Irv J. Meitus

Outline

This is a book about the diagnostic process in speech-language pathology. This introduction to the process of diagnosis begins with a description of the rehabilitation process. We move from there to consider the role diagnosis plays in the rehabilitation of persons with disorders of communication. This introduction includes a discussion of the nature of clinical information and the scientific orientations common to diagnosis and appraisal. We conclude this chapter by specifying what a diagnosis is and make clear what it is not.

AN OPERATIONAL MODEL OF SPEECH-LANGUAGE REHABILITATION

Speech-language pathology is the helping profession concerned with rehabilitation of persons with disorders of human communication. As we shall see, the phrase *disorders of human communication* identifies a large number of disturbances, whereas the phrase *speech-language pathology* indicates that we will be concerned primarily with persons whose chief problems reflect disturbances in language, speech sound production, voice, or fluency. The process of rehabilitation typically begins with initial patient contact. It is here that specific complaints about communication problems are initially presented. Ideally, the rehabilitation process ends when the problem has been resolved or when additional professional help is no longer necessary. In the course of this process, speech-language pathologists provide two basic types of services: they diagnose and they provide therapy. Both of these types of services are part of a process: a continuous and systematic series of interdependent actions leading to the goal of problem resolution. As a first step toward understanding the meaning of diagnosis, we examine the rehabilitation process.

An operational model of the rehabilitation process is outlined in Figure 1.1. This model serves as a continuing reference for our discussion of diagnosis in speech-language pathology. Models do not, in themselves, necessarily constitute reality. In this sense, the description of rehabilitation reflected in Figure 1.1 represents a set of abstractions that identify significant or essential parts of the reality of clinical practice.

Clinical Services

The operational model of rehabilitation outlined in Figure 1.1 shows that speech-language pathologists provide two basic types of services. As we have said, they engage in diagnosis and they provide therapy (see right column, Figure 1.1).

Clinician Functions

A useful description of what is done as part of rehabilitation identifies what speech-language pathologists accomplish in clinical practice. Here (see left column, Figure 1.1), we identify the functions that are served by clinicians;

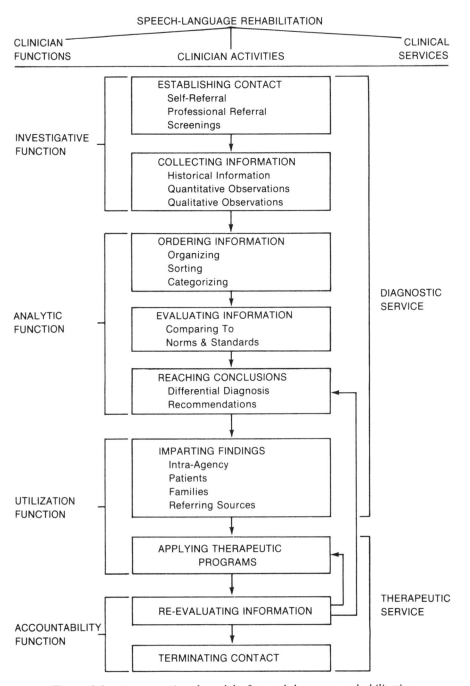

Figure 1.1.   An operational model of speech-language rehabilitation.

that is, the purposes to which clinical activities are directed. Four basic functions include:

1. the collection of clinical information and data (investigative function)
2. the analysis of information (analytic function)
3. the synthesis and use of information (utilization function)
4. the assessment of the effectiveness of clinical practices (accountability function)

The investigative function is undertaken to insure that sufficient information is collected. In this way, reasonable clinical judgments about the nature of communication problems, their severity, cause, and treatment can be made. You will learn that clinical information can be obtained from various sources and by various methods. Such information is obtained largely through interviewing and by direct observation and testing.

The analytic function represents the processing component of the rehabilitation process. Here, clinicians sift through, sort, evaluate, and classify information in order to identify precisely what the communication disorder is, and to rule out what the disorder is not. It is the analytic function that leads to what we will later elaborate upon as the "diagnosis."

After the patient's problem has been identified and differentiated from other problems, diagnostic information must be used to formulate treatment recommendations. The application of diagnostic information for the purpose of formulating treatment plans defines the third function served by speech-language clinicians: utilization.

The final clinician function is accountability. In this function, clinicians assess the effectiveness of rehabilitation. Clinical workers have a professional and ethical obligation to determine whether clinical treatment "makes a difference." Not only do clinicians want to know that they are helping people, they need to know how effective their treatment programs are to make the best use of both their own and their patient's time. Accountability for therapeutic services bears a reciprocal relationship to diagnostic accountability, for success in therapy should be highly dependent upon accurate diagnosis.

Clinician Activities

The process of rehabilitation can also be described by identifying the major activities in which clinicians engage as part of clinical practice. As illustrated in Figure 1.1, the two basic types of services and the four major functions clinicians fulfill during rehabilitation can be subdivided into a relatively small number of clinician activities (see middle column, Figure 1.1). These activities constitute the "doing" part of rehabilitation. They serve to define activities which would be readily recognized if we were to watch a clinician in the course of daily work.

Viewed sequentially, these activities capture what the clinician does from the beginning to the end of patient contact.

Establishing contact   Clinicians establish contact with patients through self, family, or professional referral and screening.

Collecting information   Clinicians collect clinical information by interviewing, observing, and testing.

Ordering information   Clinicians organize and prepare information for analysis.

Evaluating information   Clinicians evaluate clinical information and patient responses. Test performance is often compared to normative data and evaluated in terms of appropriate cultural standards.

Reaching conclusions   Clinicians often form an impression based upon diagnostic findings; they offer specific recommendations.

Imparting findings   Clinicians transmit diagnostic results to patients and families; diagnostic findings are summarized in the form of written reports, placed in clinical records, and communicated to referring sources.

Applying therapeutic programs   Clinicians use diagnostic information to formulate treatment plans.

Re-evaluating information   Clinicians continually re-evaluate patient status to determine the significance of behavioral change and to assess therapy effectiveness.

Terminating contact   Clinicians terminate patient contact when appropriate; provisions are made for follow-up contact as appropriate and necessary.

As we stated, operational models may not, in themselves, constitute reality. Students must not lose sight of the fact that the central focus of clinical practice is the patient. Thus, the operational model of rehabilitation offered in Figure 1.1 must be examined with a view toward highlighting our understanding of clinical relationships that develop between clinicians and patients. In addition, students must remember that rehabilitation is a process: a continuous and systematic series of interdependent actions leading to the goal of problem resolution. This definition of rehabilitation as a process highlights the ongoing and dynamic nature of professional activity in speech-language pathology and precludes viewing components of this process (clinician functions, behaviors, and services) as discrete or unrelated parts.

Rehabilitation as a Dynamic Process

Speech-language rehabilitation is a dynamically changing process. Clinicians become aware of change in many ways: patients' behaviors change; social and environmental circumstances surrounding a given disorder change; children grow, develop, and mature; and so on. Some changes are a product of what the clinician does with or for a patient; other changes are beyond the clinician's control. Some changes are positive, reflect improvement, and are often viewed as positive signs in rehabilitation. Other changes may be negative, may reflect regression, and may be viewed as negative signs in rehabilitation.

The dynamic nature of the process of speech rehabilitation is often evident in the fact that speech and language problems do not remain the same
when they are examined over time. Examples of this phenomenon abound
in clinical practice. The features of stuttering in adults are often quite different from those in school-age children. Developmental speech sound disorders reflect change as a function of childhood maturation and growth.
Language deficits of aphasic patients noted immediately after stroke are
often different from those observed several months later. Speech and language disorders are not static. In recognition of this fact, clinicians place
dates into clinical reports to inform the reader about when observations were
made and to distinguish these observations from those made at earlier or
later times.

The dynamic nature of the process of speech rehabilitation is also often
reflected by short-term changes. For example, voice disturbance may vary
significantly over the course of a day. Patients may capture the proper articulatory pattern during one moment only to lose it the next. Persons who
stutter may experience serious breakdown in fluency, followed by periods
of fluent speech production. Clinicians must constantly strive to understand
why these changes occur and develop therapy programs that lead to more
consistent production of more normal speech.

The dynamic nature of speech rehabilitation is highlighted further by
recognizing the influence of interactional effects. Speech-language pathology
is a helping profession that necessitates the development of relationships
and interactions between patients and clinicians. Behaviors, attitudes, and
appearances of clinicians and patients may influence the nature of clinical
interactions and relationships. Test performance may be altered significantly
by these factors. These interactional effects are always present in clinical
practice. Although the influence of these factors probably cannot be totally
eliminated, clinicians can learn to be aware of their presence and attempt
to minimize their influence.

Diagnostic Service in Relation to Therapeutic Service

The model of speech-language rehabilitation shown in Figure 1.1 illustrates
that the provision of therapy is preceded by diagnostic activity. This sequencing of services may seem rather obvious; however, such ordering of
clinical services does not always take place in actual practice. A fundamental
notion underlying our orientation to the diagnostic process is that sufficient
clinical diagnostic information and data must be obtained before treatment
is initiated.

Not only must diagnosis precede therapy, diagnostic activities also must
become an integral part of therapy. During the course of providing therapy,
clinicians often continue to engage in ongoing evaluation and diagnostic re-
finement. New and useful diagnostic information often stems from additional
testing, retesting, and additional observations of patient responses to ther-

apy. These types of information are carefully evaluated by perceptive clinicians and adjustments to the clinician's original impressions (tentative diagnosis) may be made. The reciprocity between diagnosis and therapy is highlighted further by the fact that therapeutic strategies are often adjusted in accordance with new diagnostic findings. In this manner, the flow of clinical activities and services is cyclical, continuous, reciprocal, and highly interdependent.

Clinicians also need to consider that the diagnostic process, in and of itself, can be therapeutic. Patients and family members often "feel better" after a speech-language diagnostic evaluation. This happens because the initial step toward obtaining assistance has been taken, the problem has been confronted and shared openly, and another human being has been found who is interested in helping. Most of us have experienced this effect at some time in our lives and this experience illustrates the fact that patients benefit from our services long before we actually begin to provide therapy.

Finally, an essential reason for viewing rehabilitation as a dynamic process is that clinical problems are multidimensional. For example, one approach to describing speech and language problems is to define the structural (anatomical) and functional (physiological) bases underlying such problems. Here, we often refer to physical dimensions of the speech act. As we have indicated earlier, the central focus of rehabilitation is directed to patients. Disturbances of human communication cannot be fully understood by merely describing the physical bases of dimensions of communication performance. Speech and language disorders must also be viewed in terms of psychosocial attributes or characteristics of the patient. For example, patients' attitudes about the significance, severity, and origins of their problems often play an important role in determining rehabilitative outcomes. Clinical problems must be understood in terms of environmental contexts. Here, we refer to an array of cultural standards, social attitudes, interpersonal relationships, and so on; all of which exert a significant influence upon communication behavior. These dimensions of clinical problems often interact in important ways and serve to emphasize the need to view rehabilitation as a dynamic process.

THE NATURE OF CLINICAL INFORMATION

Next we consider the sources and types of clinical information speech-language pathologists use in the diagnostic process. Clinicians' attitudes about these sources of information are also discussed. Emphasis is placed upon the clinical use of information, rather than upon specific strategies used in the collection of information.

Speech-language clinicians obtain patient-related information from various sources. Information about the presenting problem may be obtained in the form of a direct statement by the patient or may be obtained from family members. Information can be obtained before the examination when a preinterview questionnaire is used as part of the diagnostic protocol. Referring professionals constitute another possible source of information. Professional referrals are usually sent in the form of a brief letter which becomes part of the clinical record of the patient. When a referral is received via a telephone conversation, it is best to request that a written referral be sent in order to validate the clinical record. Such referrals come from medical, dental, educational, vocational, or mental health care professionals, or from other speech-language pathologists or audiologists.

Sources and Types of Clinical Information

Historical information represents another basis for diagnostic decisions. This type of information may come from interviews with the patient, from a parent, or from another responsible person. Historical information can also be drawn from preinterview questionnaires and from referral reports received before the evaluation. In obtaining a clinical history, 10 types of information are typically collected.

Conditions related to the onset of the problem
Conditions related to the development of the problem
Previous diagnostic findings
Previous rehabilitative services
General developmental status
Current health status
Educational/vocational status
Emotional/social adjustment
Pertinent family concerns
Other information volunteered by the respondent

A third major source of diagnostic information takes the form of examination findings. Here, clinical information is obtained in two basic ways: 1) from direct observation and testing of the patient without reliance upon formal test instruments; and 2) from the administration of tests, inventories, scales, and so on. Some tests have been standardized, indicating that there are data (norms) about the performance of "normal" speakers on such tests.

Direct forms of examination and testing enable clinicians to measure and observe specific aspects of speech and language performance. Speech-language pathologists obtain information about many aspects of communication behavior as part of the diagnostic process. Some major forms of assessment regularly used in the speech-language diagnosis are listed below:

General behavior observations
Examination of the speech mechanism
Evaluation of respiratory function

Linguistic characteristics
Speech sound production
Voice production
Fluency characteristics
Nonverbal aspects of communication
Audition and auditory perceptual skills
General developmental characteristics
Cognitive and intellectual functioning
Emotional and social status

Methods of Observation and Measurement

One primary goal of observation and measurement is to describe clinical events. As you know, observations and measurements may be reported in quantitative or qualitative terms. For example, a clinician's description that a patient's voice is hoarse represents a qualitative form of observation. On the other hand, a clinician's report indicating that the average rate of air flowing through this patient's larynx during the sustained production of vowel sounds is 100 cc/sec represents a quantitative form of observation.

Regardless of the terms in which observations are reported, clinicians should strive to obtain and report clinical information and data in an objective fashion. By objectivity, we refer to the ability of the clinician to observe and report findings without bias or influence of personal opinion or judgment. This is not to say that there is no room for opinion in the diagnostic process. There definitely is and the role of clinical judgment and opinion will be discussed later. For now, emphasis is placed upon what Nation and Aram (1977) refer to as "objectifying the data."

> The diagnostician objectifies the client's performance on the tools by whatever method of scoring he has available — numbers, descriptions, and qualitative judgments . . . He describes what clients said and did, rates the performance according to perceptual criteria, determines pass-fail responses, describes the type of errors made, counts the number of errors made, and records the consistency of the errors. He notes the situations that resulted in error responses, in better or normal responses, and in response variability, and he judges the extent of the errors — how many errors were made out of how many responses . . . All these analysis procedures are attempts to specify the degree and extent of the variation and not, at this time, to judge the presence or absence of a speech and language disorder (p. 295).

As we have said, clinical information may be obtained on either a qualitative or a quantitative basis. Clearly, some forms of behavior are easier to quantify than others. For example, the number of pronouns used in a language sample provided by a child is substantially easier to quantify than are the acoustic properties of the vocal productions of that child. Although the latter could be done, speech-language clinicians often have neither the time nor the instrumental devices necessary to make such measurements. Furthermore, many speech behavior attributes do not require quantification for diagnostic purposes. Carefully completed qualitative descriptions of speech and language behavior represent powerful sources of clinical information. Although quantified forms of data provide information about "how much" of a given behavior is occurring, such data often reveal few clues to the "how" or "means by which" certain behaviors occur. As we shall see, clinicians often use quantitative information to compare a given patient's behavior with that of comparable speakers from the general population. On the other hand, qualitative types of information are often indispensible to complete understanding of the nature of communication abnormality.

As part of our discussion of observation and measurement, the use of instrumentation in clinical data acquisition must also be considered. Various types of instruments have been developed for measuring speech and language behavior and attributes. Here, we refer to an array of "hardware" used in speech science research laboratories, in hospitals, and in some clinical settings. Much of this hardware was originally developed for basic research and has been adapted for use in clinical diagnosis. Except for a small number of clinical settings such as those just described, speech-language clinicians often depend primarily upon hearing, seeing, and feeling to obtain diagnostic information about speech-language function. Hearing, seeing, and feeling do represent powerful, instrumental forms of observation. The ability of clinicians to use their senses is often a sensitive, reliable, and valid form of clinical observation. Instrumental forms of assessment can often be used to help clinicians verify and quantify what they already suspect. In addition, various types of recording devices can be used to retain and provide permanent records of speech or language behaviors. Instrumental analysis may enable clinicians to divide speech behavior into components. Because rehabilitation decisions are rarely based solely upon quantitative forms of clinical data, clinicians are advised to develop keen personal observational skills essential to the careful and precise identification of abnormalities in communication behavior. Where needed, evaluation instruments can appropriately be used as extensions of the senses.

When considering the nature of clinical information, it is important to distinguish between fact and assumption. The ability to distinguish between clinical facts and assumptions is prerequisite to making careful diagnoses. Making explicit distinctions between facts and assumptions should be a natural part of the thinking process of the clinician and should be reflected in the writing of clinical records.

Clinical Fact versus Assumption

Clinical facts refer to events that actually take place and can be directly observed. Clinical assumptions refer to what clinicians judge to be true, although they may not observe or measure these events on a direct basis.

In general, descriptions of patient behaviors that have been observed on a direct basis can be regarded as factual. Historical information is factual, although such information is colored by the reliability of the provider of that information. In contrast, judgments or impressions formed by clinicians about the events or data can be regarded as assumption. Clinical assumptions are usually withheld until sufficient information has been collected and until the clinician is ready to formulate a clinical impression (diagnosis). As a rule, assumptions made on the basis of limited factual information are characterized by questionable validity.

The distinction between fact and assumption is not always clear. For example, labeling a child as "uncooperative," "shy," or "socially immature" represents assumptions a clinician might make in response to the failure of a child to respond in an expected fashion. In such an instance, it is a fact that the child did not respond in a given manner. There are various reasons why a child might not have responded in the expected manner, and these reasons may not be accessible to the clinician during the evaluation. In such instances, it is important to make the distinction between what is clearly known about the child and what has been interpreted or assumed. A further discussion of facts and assumptions, including several contrastive examples, can be found in the section in Chapter 9 entitled "Writing about Facts and Assumptions."

Clinical Bias

In ideal circumstances, clinical information will be free of bias. Clinical bias is defined as any distortion in information or observation. Bias may stem from several sources. For example, the personal characteristics of the clinician and the manner in which interpersonal communication is established represent two specific types of bias. Bias has not been addressed to a significant degree in the speech-language rehabilitation literature. Most references on this topic compare clinical bias to bias that occurs in research situations. The latter form is usually referred to as experimenter effect (Rosenthal, 1966). The work of Rosenthal (1966) and a summary of that work by Emmert and Brooks (1970) form the basis of our discussion of bias within the clinical diagnostic setting. We believe that the forms of research bias discussed by Rosenthal and Emmert and Brooks offer a helpful way of understanding the biasing factors that prevail in clinical work.

The factors that bias clinical information can be divided into two general categories: 1) factors that influence or bias the patient's behavior during the diagnostic process; and 2) bias caused by the manner in which clinicians deal with diagnostic information and data after it has been collected. First, let us consider some factors which may influence a patient's behavior during the diagnostic process. A potential source of bias are the biosocial characteristics of the clinician. The biasing effect of the clinician's age, sex, or race may serve to influence the quantity and quality of information obtained during clinical work. For example, parents in their middle years of life might be biased by the assumptions they make about the lack of clinical experience and expertise possessed by a young, inexperienced speech-language pathologist who is seeing their child. A second example is seen in the case of a black patient or parent who may feel that a Caucasian examiner is incapable of understanding the social ramifications of the presenting communication disturbance. A second source of bias is found in the psychosocial attributes of the clinician. For example, personal characteristics such as level of anxiety, need for approval, hostility, authoritarianism, dominance, warmth, openness, and so on can serve to bias patient responses.

A third general source of clinician bias arises from situational factors. Some forms of this type of bias include the effect of acquaintanceship between clinician and patient or family, and the degree of experience and expertise shown by the clinician conducting the evaluation. Additional situational factors include a variety of communication interruptors, for example, noise, incoming telephone calls, unintended interruptions such as door knocks, presence of children who may detract from efficient testing and interviewing, and insufficient time to conduct the interview or examination.

Clinician modeling, a fourth type of bias, occurs when the clinician demonstrates the task intended for the patient. Here, the clinician unwittingly teaches what is being assessed. An example of clinical modeling is seen in the behavior of a clinician who puts unusually strong stress or emphasis on a particular speech sound during the course of testing the patient's ability to say that sound correctly.

One additional form of bias is clinician expectancy. This form of bias has been referred to as the "Pygmalion effect" or the self-fulfilling prophecy (Rosenthal and Jacobson, 1968). Here, bias occurs because the patient knows what the clinician wants, and the patient behaves in such a manner as to please the clinician. In this situation, the examiner observes what is expected largely because of the manner in which the examiner relates to the patient. For example, a clinician who fails to examine significant factors that might contribute to a speech-language problem (because the pre-evaluation information "makes the problem evident") may be guilty of clinician expectancy. Likewise, an interviewer who asks questions in such a manner as to suggest or imply acceptable forms of behavior is also demonstrating expectancy (e.g., "How much time do you spend encouraging Johnny to name pictures?").

Next, let us discuss some sources of bias which come about due to the manner in which clinicians deal with diagnostic information after it has been collected. One source of influence of this type is clinician error during observation or testing. For example, failure to count the insertion of unnecessary sounds produced in spontaneous speech as moments of stuttering will invalidate any comparison with samples that include such sounds. Although such an error may be unintentional, it is usually not random and, therefore, leads to systematic bias.

Another type of clinical bias is incorrect interpretation of clinical information. Certain types of observation and information lend themselves to a variety of interpretations. For example, interpretation of the "psychological states" of patients is subject to considerable diversity of opinion. From another perspective, a strong theoretical point of view on the part of the clinician may serve to bias the manner in which a clinician interprets clinical findings. For example, a clinician with a strong psychoanalytic point of view might interpret clinical findings of dependency differently than would a clinician with a strong learning-based orientation. In this instance, the clinician might choose to interpret the clinical data in terms of the degree to which it is consistent with a particular theory. This latter form of bias, when coupled with clinician expectancy, often destroys the objectivity necessary to clinical activity.

A final type of bias arises from intentional fabrication of clinical data or information. Although this form of bias is rare, it must still be considered. This form of bias often arises out of the clinician's need to look good in the eyes of others. Fabrication can result from a failure to collect significant information or data, or from failure to record it properly and later attempt to reconstruct what was observed. Students-in-training are particularly vulnerable to this form of clinical bias. Needless to say, a frank statement that significant information was not obtained is absolutely essential.

Emmert and Brooks (1970) have suggested several strategies for controlling or minimizing bias in research. These strategies can be easily adapted to the clinical situation; they are summarized below:

1. Simple awareness of bias on the part of the clinician is a factor that can serve to objectify clinical behavior.
2. Use of recording devices (video and audio) and other instrumentation to quantify findings can promote clinical accuracy.
3. Errors in the interpretation of information are less likely when the clinician shares his or her findings with other professionals; scrutiny of data by others opens them to criticism.
4. Use more than one observer to validate findings.
5. Standardize, to some degree, the behavior of the clinician to promote consistency of interactions across patients and procedures.

SCIENTIFIC ORIENTATIONS TO
SPEECH AND LANGUAGE DIAGNOSIS

In this section, we discuss scientific orientations underlying speech and language diagnosis. A scientific orientation, when viewed as a general attitude toward problem solving, offers the clinician a broad framework that can be applied toward understanding and solving specific clinical problems. Perkins

(1977) has described speech pathology as an applied behavioral science responsible for habilitation and rehabilitation of speech-handicapped persons. Whether or not one views the practicing speech-language clinician as a "scientist," it is clear that the clinician must understand 1) the scientific basis upon which knowledge of speech and language performance and deviance is based; and 2) the necessity to ask significant questions that will foster meaningful solutions to speech and language problems. The philosophical attitudes associated with scientific orientations to clinical practice are emphasized in our discussion.

The use of the scientific method has been discussed by various writers in the field of speech and hearing as a natural approach to arriving at solutions to clinical questions. Perkins (1977) views the scientific method as helpful. This method may assist clinicians in understanding the nature of both normal and deviant speech or language behavior. Nation and Aram (1977) and Peterson and Marquardt (1981) have spoken directly about using the scientific method within the diagnostic process. Ringel (1972), Schultz (1972), and Schultz et al. (1972) have discussed the common features which exist between clinical work and scientific endeavor. Some of these common features are discussed below. They have been arranged on the basis of the order in which they are typically used in clinical practice.

The Contribution of the Scientific Method

1. *Defining the problem*   In both clinical work and scientific endeavor, the problem must be carefully defined and identified. (Clinical example: On the basis of information obtained in the preinterview questionnaire and from talking with Mary's mother, there is evidence that Mary has a language disorder.)
2. *Developing hypotheses*   In both clinical work and scientific endeavors, answerable questions or clinical hypotheses must be formulated. These questions might concern etiologic events (Clinical example: To what degree does a hearing deficit contribute to Mary's language behavior?) Questions might also be related to behavioral attributes. (Clinical example: To what degree does Mary show the ability to respond to spoken directions?) In general, hypothesis testing requires the clinician/investigator to ascertain the probability that certain factors are significant, or to determine the degree to which those factors can be discounted.
3. *Designing the inquiry*   Both clinical work and scientific endeavor require a planned program of inquiry. Research endeavors require the a priori development of a research design, whereas diagnostic activity requires the formulation of a careful plan of assessment activities. (Clinical example: Plan to question mother about Mary's early response to environmental sounds; plan a probe of Mary's ability to follow simple spoken commands; plan to administer an audiological examination.)

4. *Collecting data*   Both clinical work and scientific endeavor necessitate the collection of information and data. In both clinical work and research, observations must be made in a valid and reliable fashion and information must be collected and recorded accurately. (Clinical example: Mother reports that Mary is unresponsive to noises at home; Mary exhibits confusion when asked to perform simple tasks; the results of audiological testing indicate that Mary does have a hearing loss.)
5. *Analyzing data*   Both clinical and research data or information must be assembled in an orderly fashion so that they can be evaluated efficiently. Clinical findings are often compared to existing normative data bases and cultural standards. (Clinical examples: Mary's language is delayed by approximately 2 years in comparison with available normative measures. Historical reports of behavioral responses at home, responses to spoken communication during the examination, and findings during identification audiometry are consistent with known behaviors of children with significant hearing loss.)
6. *Accepting or rejecting hypotheses*   On the basis of differential findings, certain clinical or research hypotheses will be discarded, whereas others will be supported. The probability statements that are supported constitute what will later be referred to as the *clinical diagnosis*. Appropriate recommendations are made on the basis of this diagnosis. (Clinical example: Clinical findings suggest language delay associated with hearing impairment. Language delay not judged to be associated with cognitive-intellectual impairment. A hearing aid evaluation is recommended.)
7. *Generalizing from data*   On the basis of the results of a research problem or the study of a single patient, clinicians/investigators may make appropriate adjustments to their fund of knowledge or alter views about recognized theories or clinical issues. The findings of clinical inquiry and research may also confirm or enlarge understanding. Novel findings are shared with the professional community. (Clinical example: Mary's language delay has resulted from one or more of the known etiologies commonly associated with this communication disorder.)

Our discussion of scientific orientations to diagnosis makes it evident that the operational model of speech-language rehabilitation discussed in earlier sections of this chapter embrace major principles of the scientific method. This method of problem solving has its roots in the rational methodology of science. As we have seen, there are a number of similarities between the conduct of clinical work and scientific experimentation. There are also important differences. Schultz (1972) makes the important point that the clinician is largely oriented toward "people," whereas the researcher is often oriented toward "phenomena." If this statement is valid, we would expect the scientist/researcher to place greater emphasis on seeking solutions to important problems confronting speech-language pathology. The researcher would seek to more fully explain phenomena or questions and look for new issues to explore. On the other hand, the clinician would be more interested in ruling out alternative answers to very real and immediate questions about a patient, because the needs of that individual often necessitate immediate assistance and remediation.

Regardless of the difference in orientation that might exist between the clinician and scientist, both must be concerned with accountability. Both need to ask answerable questions that bear upon the problem that has been defined. Both need to sample behavior. Sampling must be sufficient, whether sampling is made across one patient or across many subjects. Both must verify their observations in a reliable manner and must recognize and state the limitations of their conclusions. Both must engage in activities that minimize bias and maximize objectivity. These statements are made in full recognition of the fact that clinical activity is often undertaken in such a manner as to preclude careful control of variables or biasing effects, whereas the essential nature of scientific investigation relies upon careful control of these influences.

Validity and Reliability in Clinical Practice

The two most frequently cited criteria used to determine objectivity in clinical or research observations are validity and reliability. Silverman (1977) describes validity in the following manner:

> The validity of observations refers to their *appropriateness* for answering the questions they are used to answer. If they are not appropriate, the answers they yield may be inaccurate and the interpretations made of them may be inappropriate (p. 218).

> The necessary question to answer when you wish to assess the validity of the observations used to answer a question is: *Were the observations made appropriate for answering the question asked?* That is, did the investigator observe and describe the attribute (or attributes) of the events that he wished to observe and describe? If the investigator did, the observations will be valid to some degree. If the investigator did not, they will be invalid (p. 222).

Silverman's description of validity makes it clear that the clinician must select or construct methods of observation that do, in fact, measure what the clinician intends to measure. Certain clinical phenomena are more readily measured in a valid way than are others. For example, the presence or absence of discrete perceptual phenomena (Was a part-word repetition present or not present?) lend themselves to valid observations when observers can readily agree upon what they are observing. Many articulation errors and moments of stuttering fall into this category of observation. There are also clinical phenomena that do not readily lend themselves to valid observation. Some examples might include judgments about the degree to which nasality is present, and judgments about psychological traits. In these examples, more elaborate means of establishing the validity of clinician observations must often be used, because it is inherently more difficult to define what is being measured.

In addition to being concerned about the validity of observations made by clinicians, there is a need to be concerned with the validity of measures used in the administration of formal test instruments. There are a number of indicators that can be used to assess the validity of measures used in formal tests. Three commonly used indicators are content validity, criterion-related validity, and construct validity. *Content validity* refers to the degree to which a test samples the specific types of behavior from which clinical inferences will be drawn. For example, tests of language comprehension in children should adequately sample a child's understanding of the various linguistic forms to which the child would be exposed in the natural environment. *Criterion-related validity* refers to the degree to which a particular test compares to other acceptable measures of the same behavior being tested. In this instance, the clinician might compare the results of the language comprehension test in question to the results of one or more other tests of language comprehension that have been proven to be accurate indicators of children's language comprehension ability. Another criterion-related reference would be found by comparing the results obtained using a particular test to the opinions of sophisticated observers. *Construct validity* refers to the degree to which a test measures the results of certain phenomena assumed to influence the test-taker. For example, if syntactic ability is a true or valid construct, then training the patient in syntax should be reflected in scores of tests designed to measure syntactic ability. Broader discussion of validity in test construction can be found in texts that describe mental measurement procedures. When using published tests in clinical examination, it is important for the clinician to inquire about the manner in which validity was established. This information is usually included in the literature that accompanies the test instrument.

Reliability has been described by Silverman (1977) as follows:

> The reliability of the observations used to answer questions refers to their *repeatability*. The more repeatable (or replicable) a set of observations, the greater will be their reliability.
>
> The extent to which observations can be repeated, or replicated, is a function of how similarly a *given observer* would describe them on *different* occasions, or how similarly a *group of observers* would describe them on a given occasion (or occasions). The description could be qualitative, quantitative, or a combination of the two. The more similar the descriptions, the more reliable the observations (p. 218–219).
>
> A necessary question to answer when accessing the reliability of observations is: *Were the observations made sufficiently free from random and systematic measurement error (including experimenter bias) to answer reliably the question asked?* (p. 223).

Lack of consistency in measurement can arise from several sources: questionable reliability on the part of the person being tested, the examiner, and of the test instruments or procedures used. Some examples might be helpful. In the case of the patient, questionable reliability might occur when what is being measured (e.g., moments of stuttering) is not consistent on a day-to-day or moment-by-moment basis. Questionable reliability might occur when clinicians do not sample sufficiently during data collection (e.g., failure to sample spontaneous speech in a child with a speech sound disorder). Examiner reliability is influenced by failure of clinicians to consistently apply the same criteria during repeated forms of testing (e.g., failing to consistently judge the same degree of hypernasality in a patient).

When necessary, the reliability of clinical observations and measurements can be statistically measured and tested. To increase the probability that the clinician's observations will be both valid and reliable, Darley and Spriestersbach (1978) urge clinicians to adhere to three important practices: 1) observe and report enough; 2) observe and report objectively; and 3) observe and report precisely.

Measured versus Functional Abilities

When a clinician describes the behavior of an individual, careful distinction should be made between how the patient performs on a given test, and how the patient would perform on similar tasks within the "real" world. Under ideal conditions, we would like to fully evaluate the patient in real world settings. For example, under ideal circumstances, it might be desirable to assess children's use of language as they interact with peers, parents, friends, etc. It might be desirable to evaluate the voice production of a minister by observing his actual voice problems during the course of a typical working day.

Unfortunately, most clinicians have neither the time nor the logistical means to gather "real world" diagnostic information. It is evident that the costs would be monumental from the standpoint of costs to both the consumer and the examiner. In addition, few persons in need of assistance would be served. The diagnostic process represents an alternative; it is a short-cut process used to accumulate information that hopefully is representative and predictive of patients' behavior in natural settings. The extent to which this is true depends upon the validity of the tests employed by the clinician, a concept discussed earlier. The clinician with only limited knowledge and experience quickly learns that test performance on evaluative instruments is neither necessarily representative nor predictive of functional skills or performance. An example of this point is shown in the aphasic woman who does remarkably well caring for herself within her familiar home environment, even though she cannot respond appropriately to simple clinical tasks ("Put the spoon in the coffee cup.") during clinical testing.

The intent is certainly not to make clinical observation and testing appear useless. On the contrary, the diagnostic evaluation represents the clinician's most useful tool in deriving information about people and their problems. As is the case for information in general, it can be properly used or it can be abused. People perform within a multidimensional context in natural settings. Tests are typically constructed in such a way as to reduce or minimize variables or influences. Knowing the assumptions under which tests have been developed and the assumptions underlying interpretations of test results should assist the clinician in understanding the predictive nature and the limitations of clinical data. Wendell Johnson (1946) made speech and hearing clinicians aware that "the map is not the territory." The interpretation of test results does not fully describe the patient.

The Role of Creativity   Thus far, we have discussed the manner by which clinicians collect and use clinical information and data in order to arrive at clinical diagnoses. We have seen that clinicians must collect adequate amounts of information and that such information must be both valid and reliable. These hallmarks of observation are deeply rooted in the basic scientific orientation to clinical activity we have been examining. A natural question which often arises in discussion about the nature of clinical practice concerns the role individual clinician differences might play in the execution of clinical procedures. As with any group of human beings, individual differences should be expected across a group of speech-language clinicians. It is expected that all clinicians will have certain minimal competencies. For example, they will all have an adequate fund of knowledge about the pathologies of communication and minimal knowledge and experience with diagnostic procedures and techniques. Beyond those basic competencies, clinicians should permit themselves to act with reasonable spontaneity and latitude.

Some clinicians are very good at allowing patients to lead, whereas other clinicians function better when they, more directly, lead the patient. In general, clinicians should not attempt to adopt a clinical style or image incompatible with their basic personality or style of personal interaction. Rather, they should be themselves, allowing their efforts to be directed toward the patient, rather than toward themselves. One clinician might favor test x over test y. Given that both tests yield the necessary information, clinicians should be willing to accept diversity. Motivating patients, especially young children, to comply and cooperate during evaluations frequently calls for the most creative aspects of the clinician's personality and clinical behavior to emerge. The clinician should feel confident to allow these personal attributes to emerge in clinical work.

In attending to "feelings" about patients and their families, clinicians often draw upon their knowledge of "people" as well as their knowledge of "patients" and "disorders." By the time one reaches the stage of professional training, hopefully the clinician-in-training has spent considerable time observing people. Although it is not always a conscious process, most of us mentally file away bits of information, forming a data base about "people and their problems." This file constitutes a broad form of empiricism which, when enlarged and refined objectively over time, can assist the clinician in using life experiences to better understand patients and their problems.

Finally, the role of opinion should be put into perspective. There is definitely room for the clinician's professional opinion in the diagnostic process. In fact, professional opinion is a necessary part of clinical practice. In the workaday world of diagnosis, the clinician is paid to have opinions. Without opinions, clinicians would merely be data collectors or information gatherers, unable to make the critical decisions regarding patient care. Naturally, opinions should be based upon objectively collected information and measurement. Subjectivity has limited value in information gathering and data acquisition. When clinical information is carefully interpreted by taking into account theoretical points of view, past experience, and knowledge (expertise), the clinician can influence the diagnostic process in a very personal manner. The clinician's opinion about the patient takes the form of the diagnostic statement, which is discussed in the following section.

THE DIAGNOSIS: DIFFERENTIAL FEATURES

In this section we consider what is meant by the term *diagnosis*. We specify what a diagnosis is and make clear what it is not. Finally, the utility of the diagnosis is considered.

A diagnosis represents the judgment of a clinician about patients and their presenting problems. Speech and language diagnoses are made on the basis of careful consideration of historical information and data gathered on the basis of direct observation and examination. The diagnosis is considered to be differential when it takes into consideration all significant variables that might contribute to the disorder and seeks to differentiate the patient's problem from related or dissimilar problems. The form in which the diagnosis is stated may vary; however, the content and structure of most diagnoses are organized as follows:

Components of a Diagnosis

1. Information specifying the classification of the disorder and its severity
2. A statement of the etiologic and/or behavioral factors which brought about and sustain the problem
3. Consideration of factors that may influence intervention
4. Recommendations
5. A prognostic statement

A diagnostic statement is not simply a summary of historical and examination findings. A diagnosis is also not simply a classification of a disorder. Although a very brief summary or statement of classification is an essential part of the diagnostic statement, diagnoses must give meaning to clinical information so that appropriate decisions about management can be made. Let us now examine the individual parts of the diagnosis.

1. Classification and Severity Statements

One major purpose of classification in diagnosis is to promote efficiency of communication among professionals. Imagine how difficult it would be to relate information to other persons if we did not have names (labels) for the many things experienced in life. Without names for disorders, the clinician would be left to describe each patient's problem using relatively long narrations. For example, stating that a patient exhibits part-word repetitions, sound prolongations, and silent intervals is certainly more cumbersome than stating that the patient has a fluency disorder, or that the patient stutters. Naturally, vital information is lost in reducing conditions, disorders, or behaviors to simplified labels. For example, the classification *language disorder* tells us nothing about whether the patient is experiencing difficulty understanding language, expressing language, or both. Furthermore, the classification language disorder neither tells us about the type of difficulty (phonological, syntactic, semantic, pragmatic), nor does it give insight into the scope of the problem (emotional and social components, intellectual features, etc.).

Classification statements should not attempt to relate too much information. At the same time, classification statements should not be so simplified that they fail to add knowledge about a patient over that which was evident at the onset of the examination. For example, it may not require extensive examination to determine that a child has a speech sound disorder. One value of classification is to provide increased understanding about the nature of the speech sound disorder, for example, is the disorder structurally based or learning based?

Clinicians will find a surprising amount of inconsistency in the terminology used by professionals to describe or classify speech and language disorders. Some classifications have been derived from medical orientations. In this case, the classification might focus on the etiology of the disorder (e.g., dysarthria and aphasia both imply neurologic impairment) or might even suggest a general site of abnormality (e.g., posterior aphasia indicates a lesion in the area of the brain which influences language comprehension). Another medical classification, dysphonia, merely indicates voice disturbance but gives no information regarding why the disturbance has occurred. Other classifications refer to disorders in terms of the processes used in producing speech (e.g., disorders of phonation, articulation, resonance, language, etc.). Finally, some classifications are simply labels that have come to be clinically accepted over time and offer no consistency with respect to their precise meaning (e.g., stuttering and voice disorder).

Within subsequent chapters in this text, the authors will use classification terminology with which they feel most comfortable in terms of their clinical experiences. Having read and heard other terminology used in various introductory texts and courses, clinicians-in-training may be confused. Students can gain knowledge about the sources of confusion by studying the historical bases of speech-language pathology with an eye toward understanding the origins and purposes of various classification terminology. Clinicians-in-training should compare various classification terms and use classifications that are most useful in clinical practice, rather than adhere inflexibly to a single classification system.

Severity statements are useful in diagnosis to the extent that they enlarge our understanding about the full impact of the disorder. Such statements are also useful in that they provide baseline information that can be used to assess the progress of the patient over time. Severity information is also often important in establishing priorities for the need, length, and type of clinical services provided. To some extent, the practicing clinician must make day-to-day decisions about the scheduling of patients. Questions such as "Who should be scheduled first?" and "Who should receive more time in therapy?" are often more easily answered if severity information is available. The clinician should keep in mind that some patients, children for example, might exhibit fairly good adjustment to their communication problem, although the parents express deep concern and frustration. Just how a clinician sets severity criteria will be a product of his or her philosophical attitude about speech and language problems and accumulated clinical experience.

Severity measures based solely upon counting the occurrence of speech or language errors in a given speech sample are of limited value in the diagnostic statement. Likewise, strict calculations (e.g., percent intelligibility), although empirically based and useful in specifying the degree to which listeners can understand highly structured speech utterances, often relate poorly with the larger concept of severity expressed earlier. In diagnosis, the clinician must consider the extent to which all significant variables contribute to the severity of the problem.

The next step in organizing the diagnosis is to consider etiologic (causal) factors and to specify behaviors that contribute to the ongoing nature of the speech or language disorder. Emerick and Hatten (1979) state that knowledge about predisposing, precipitating, and perpetuating factors will provide insight into the etiology of the disorder. It seems reasonable to assume that clinicians would want to identify causal and behavioral factors and specify those that are still operating so that their influence can, if possible, be altered. The interest of the speech-language pathologist in etiologic and behavioral features of communication disorders arises from two distinctly different orientations: the medical model of patient care (etiologic) and the educational model of training (behavioral). We will consider the impact that these two diverse ways of thinking about problems have upon speech-language diagnosis.

2. Etiologic and Behavioral Considerations

Basic to the etiologic orientation is the concept of cause and effect. In diagnosing an illness, physicians often view the patient's symptoms as an indication of some underlying disease or condition which their examination will hopefully identify. Under this model, proper treatment of the disease or disturbance results in elimination or improvement of symptoms. It is evident that this model of treatment depends heavily upon careful diagnosis; without it there is considerable risk.

An etiologic approach in speech language diagnosis raises some interesting questions. First, what is meant by *cause*? Are we referring to some original event that explains why a person speaks in a disordered manner? Or by cause, do we mean some contributing event(s) which sustain a disorder even though the original event is no longer present or active? Second, if we could agree on what cause means, can the cause(s) of speech and language disorders be treated in the same manner as the physician treats disease and disturbance? These are difficult questions, especially if one approaches them as a clinician-in-training with limited clinical experience. In clinical practice, certain disorders clearly should be considered on an etiologic basis to confirm or negate the presence of a disease process or a physical disability. In some cases the speech-language clinician can confirm the cause. In other cases, a medical specialist may be needed. We will consider some clinical examples to illustrate these concepts.

Phonatory disorders characterized wholly or in part by the presence of hoarseness are common in clinical practice. Hoarseness is known to result from a number of conditions affecting the vocal cords: allergies, localized inflammation due to infection or vocal abuse, nodules, polyps, malignant tumors, and so on. By being aware of the etiologic possibilities and including a laryngeal examination as part of the diagnostic protocol with voice-disordered patients, the efforts of the clinician are directed toward discovering the cause of the hoarseness. A second example illustrating our interest in cause concerns the clinician's need to differentiate between certain speech and language characteristics as an aid in determining the nature of neurologic impairment. Those clinicians working in medical settings will sometimes be requested to participate in differential neurologic diagnoses.

As a general rule, causes of speech and language disorders should be determined. This is particularly true to the extent that such information will bear upon the clinician's management of the patient. In many situations, however, causal factors for communication disorders cannot be determined with reasonable degrees of certainty. Furthermore, what is judged to be etiologic in many disorders is often no longer significant in the presenting problem. In this situation, the clinician is more concerned with understanding the behavior of the patient. Speech and language are products of both physical and mental behaviors. The ability of patients to control and alter behavior depends, in part, upon such factors as structural and functional adequacy of the speech mechanism, intellectual and cognitive factors, psychosocial influences, and so on. Using that belief as a general guideline, clinicians using behavioral approaches to diagnosis seek to determine the degree to which patients are able to modify or change behavior. Through the examination process, the clinician comes to understand the nature and predictability of the patient's behavior and the potential for change. In this manner, successful behavioral diagnosis is one that provides immediate information about the objectives and strategies for clinical intervention.

An example of the behavioral approach to diagnosis is typified by the child with a speech sound disorder. In the face of unremarkable physical and environmental findings, etiology is not clear. By determining the errors present in the speech of the child and the linguistic rules used in producing speech sound errors, the clinician comes to understand certain behavioral patterns. With this information, the clinician proceeds to determine the potential of the child to learn new rules of speech sound production by various evaluation and training strategies. Finally, a judgment is made regarding the most efficient way to help the child change speech behavior.

In some cases, etiologic and behavioral approaches have a circular and reciprocal diagnostic relationship. The behavioral effects of many original (causal) stimuli become the stimuli for new behavior, even though the original cause may no longer be present. Two types of clinical problems are interesting to consider in the context of this relationship. Vocal nodules (effect) most often occur in response to vocal abuse (cause). The presence of vocal nodules (cause) is responsible for vocal hoarseness (effect). Treatment options for patients with vocal nodules include voice therapy (behavioral management), removal of the growths (medical management), or some combination of the two. In the case of childhood stuttering, the clinician might judge some form of stress (cause) to be a precipitant in the onset of disfluency (effect). As the child begins to react to disfluencies (cause), new behaviors (effect) are used to cope with the frustration of disfluency. Is stress still a factor in the problem? Probably, but perhaps not in the original form. At any rate, the clinician needs to make that determination. As in the example of a patient with vocal nodules, two sets of circumstances require attention: the current condition and the original or precipitating influences, if they are still active. In summary, the clinician should realize that neither the etiologic nor the behavioral orientation is inherently better. Both are extremely useful.

The clinician is now ready to consider factors that may influence intervention. In addition to considering the etiologic and behavioral factors discussed in the preceding section, there are a number of factors that enhance or hinder the chances of changing communication patterns. These factors may be uncovered on the basis of historical information or direct examination. Some typical factors that may influence intervention are listed below.

3. Factors That May Influence Intervention

Typical Historical Factors
    Failure or success in altering behavior during previous rehabilitation efforts
    Health or physical limitations or assets
    Learning problems or disorders
    Vocational problems or support
    Familial, marital, sibling disturbance or support
    Interpersonal problems or support

Typical Examination Factors
    Social-emotional maturity or immaturity
    Motivation
    Presence or absence of developmental delay in areas other than speech and language
    Attention disturbance
    Psychological adjustment
    Orientation disturbances
    Hyperactivity
    Medication

The factors that may influence intervention may be viewed either as positive or negative influences. For example, familial or marital support is often viewed as a positive factor that may influence intervention; medication may be either a positive or negative influence, and poor motivation is generally regarded as a negative influence upon intervention. Clinicians must evaluate the potential influence these factors have upon intervention, and their opinion about these influences is typically reflected in the recommendations and statements about prognosis.

4. Recommendations   An essential part of diagnosis is the formulation of recommendations regarding patient management. Recommendations typically take the following form:

No need for concern or need for further contact
Re-evaluate at later date; no intervention needed now
Obtain further speech-language evaluative information
Obtain diagnostic information from other sources (medical, psychological, social services, etc.)
Speech-language therapy (individual, group, special programs, etc.)
Family involvement (education, counseling, training, etc.)
Coordinate speech-language intervention with other disciplines (academic, medical, psychological, etc.)

This list of recommendations is not exhaustive. The most important point concerning the formulation of a recommendation is that recommendations must be consistent within the diagnosis: the recommendations must follow logically from the diagnosis. In addition, information explaining the rationale for recommending particular forms of treatment and/or referrals should be offered as part of professional recommendations. For example, why should a patient with a tremor be seen by a neurologist? Detailed descriptions of therapeutic goals and strategies are not appropriate for inclusion in professional recommendations. The appropriate place for such information is discussed in Chapter 9, ''Clinical Report and Letter Writing.''

A prognosis is the clinician's statement concerning the likelihood of change (improvement or decline) of speech and language performance. It is a forecast of what is expected to develop in the future. Prognostic statements are often influenced by whether or not treatment (behavioral, medical, psychological, etc.) is being considered. Prognostic statements should include information about the time span over which predictions regarding change are being made. In every instance, prognoses are based upon all diagnostic considerations. Prognostic statements represent candid professional opinions. Overly optimistic and overly conservative prognostic statements may mislead patients and their families. Prognoses based upon insufficient clinical information are also professionally improper.

5. Prognostic Statements

Prognoses are important for at least two reasons. First, they provide patients and families with statements of expectations regarding communication improvement. Second, they force the clinician into a position of accountability. What is recommended for patients reflects our clinical predictions. Not all patients will profit from speech-language therapy. It is likely that some patients will improve without intervention. By comparing outcomes with predictions, clinicians can determine both the accuracy of their diagnoses and the appropriateness of their recommendations.

Experience with clinicians-in-training indicates that they generally do not like to make negative predictions or recommendations even when it is appropriate to do so. An altruistic attitude tends to prevail. This attitude often leads to the expectation that speech or language therapy is the only logical outcome of diagnosis. When this attitude prevails, prognoses will be strongly influenced by this form of clinical bias. Because prognostic statements represent candid professional opinions, clinicians-in-training must learn to make negative predictions when they are warranted. When the long-term prognosis for improvement in communication is poor, it is often helpful to focus upon short-term predictions. These short-term predictions are more likely to be accomplished. For example, some patients with degenerative neurological disease are likely to show significant deterioration in speech over time even with intensive speech therapy. The long-term prognosis is poor. If the prognosis for change is viewed in terms of short-range goals or predictions (e.g., what might be done for the patient to maintain nominal forms of communication such as single word productions, non-speech methods, etc.), the clinician can adopt a more positive attitude and be in a fully accountable position in the face of poor long-term expectations. More positive attitudes toward prognoses are also achievable when the standards for improvement are not based upon the achievement of "normal speech" objectives for patients who do not have that potential.

Utility of the Diagnosis

One way of summarizing the discussion that has been presented about diagnosis in speech-language pathology is to state what the diagnosis enables the clinician to achieve.

1. Diagnosis enables the clinician to establish a record of the clinical problem.
2. Diagnosis aids the clinician in understanding the cause of a communication problem from the perspective of onset, development, and maintenance.
3. Diagnosis differentiates one patient's problem from others which are related, similar, or dissimilar. Diagnosis distinguishes what is unique about the problem at hand. Diagnosis identifies what the patient has and rules out what the patient does not have.
4. Diagnosis can serve to chart a course of intervention.
5. Diagnosis may serve as a predictor of future status.
6. Diagnosis, when viewed as an ongoing function within the rehabilitation process, can establish a record of patient status, against which criteria for progress can be applied.

Study Guide

1. Identify and describe the major clinician activities that are a routine part of speech-language rehabilitation.

2. Describe the functions that are served by the clinician.

3. Describe the major sources of clinical information. What are methods by which the clinician obtain this information?

4. Why is it necessary to distinguish between clinical fact and assumption? Provide examples of what is meant by each.

5. Identify the basic forms of bias that are likely to influence clinical interaction.

6. Outline the essential parts of the diagnostic process.

7. Define what is meant by validity and reliability. Discuss the importance of these concepts to the clinical practice of speech-language pathology.

8. Specify what should be contained within a differential diagnosis. What uses can be made of the diagnosis?

REFERENCES

Darley, F., and Spriestersbach, D. 1978. Diagnostic Methods in Speech Pathology. 2nd Ed. Harper & Row Pubs., Inc., New York.

Emerick, L., and Hatten, J. 1979. Diagnosis and Evaluation in Speech Pathology. Prentice-Hall, Inc., Englewood Cliffs, NJ.

Emmert, P., and Brooks, W. 1970. Methods of Research in Communication. Houghton Mifflin Company, Boston.

Johnson, W. 1946. People in Quandries: The Semantics of Personal Adjustment. Harper & Row Pubs., Inc., New York.

Nation, J., and Aram, D. 1977. Diagnosis of Speech and Language Disorders. The C.V. Mosby Company, St. Louis.

Perkins, W. 1977. Speech Pathology An Applied Behavioral Science. 2nd Ed. The C.V. Mosby Company, St. Louis.

Peterson, H., and Marquardt, T. 1981. Appraisal and Diagnosis of Speech and Language Disorders. Prentice-Hall, Inc., Englewood Cliffs, NJ.

Ringel, R. 1972. The clinician and the researcher: An artificial dichotomy. Asha 14:351–353.

Rosenthal, R. 1966. Experimenter Effects in Behavioral Research. Appleton-Century-Crofts, New York.

Rosenthal, R., and Jacobson, L. 1968. Pygmalion in the Classroom. Holt, Rinehart & Winston, Inc., New York.

Schultz, M. 1972. An Analysis of Clinical Behavior in Speech and Hearing. Prentice-Hall, Inc., Englewood Cliffs, NJ.

Schultz, M., Roberts, W., and Yairi, E. 1972. The clinician and the researcher: Comments. Asha, 14:539–541.

Silverman, F. 1977. Research Design in Speech Pathology and Audiology. Prentice-Hall, Inc., Englewood Cliffs, NJ.

CHAPTER

2

Gathering Clinical Information

Irv J. Meitus and
Bernd Weinberg

Outline

Educational Aims

1. *To identify the major kinds of clinical information speech-language pathologists routinely gather as part of direct examination and interviewing*
2. *To make clear why these kinds of information should be gathered*
3. *To describe specific strategies or procedures commonly used to obtain such information*

In Chapter 1 we discussed the types and sources of clinical information speech-language pathologists use in the diagnostic process. They routinely acquire two primary types of clinical information: data which are historical in nature and data which are obtained on the basis of direct patient examination. These two basic types of information are common to diagnosis of virtually all disorders of human communication. In view of their importance, in this chapter we will define the specific nature and kinds of information speech-language pathologists should gather as they directly examine and interview patients. We will also make clear why these kinds of information should be gathered. Where appropriate, we define specific strategies or procedures commonly used to obtain such information.

HISTORICAL INFORMATION

Clinical information which is historical in nature can be gathered on the basis of direct interviewing or from preinterview questionnaires. Sample questionnaires we use to gather such information are provided for use and study in Appendices A and B. In Chapter 1 we learned that 10 types of information are typically collected in obtaining a clinical history. We now review these 10 types of information and make clear why such information should be gathered.

Careful identification of conditions related to the onset of speech and language problems often assists the speech-language pathologist in understanding the nature and causes of communication disorders. Some speech and language problems have clearly identifiable starting points. For example, some voice problems are characterized by sudden onset which can be related to important physical and/or psychological factors. Other speech and language problems, such as aphasia and dysarthria, are associated with physical difficulties (e.g., injury, trauma, disease, etc.) and are characterized by precipitous onset of communication difficulty. Still other problems do not have a clearly identifiable starting point that can be related to specific organic or psychological factors. For example, some voice problems are characterized by gradual onset which is difficult to relate to physical or psychosocial conditions. Developmental communication problems of childhood also often fall into this latter category.

Conditions Related to the Onset of the Problem

    Knowledge about conditions associated with the onset of communication problems is invaluable to the goal of identifying etiology or cause of speech-language disorders. In addition, such knowledge can assist the clinician in formulating treatment plans and making prognoses.

Conditions Related to the Development of the Problem

The manner in which speech-language problems develop often has particular diagnostic significance. Some patients have problems which are relatively constant in character and severity; others have problems which are variable. Still other problems (e.g., stuttering and some forms of dysarthria) are marked by periods of remission and exacerbation of symptoms. Careful monitoring of the manner in which speech-language problems develop can be used to establish a behavioral record. Clinicians often attempt to identify conditions related to the character and severity of speech and language behavior.

There are numerous factors responsible for change in the status of patients' behaviors. For example, change may be related to improvement in health status, administration of treatment (e.g., surgery, drugs, etc.), alterations in environmental circumstances, speech-language therapy, and so on. Knowledge about the development of communication impairment and conditions associated with these patterns is necessary to the formulation of treatment plans and the making of prognostic summaries.

Previous Diagnostic Findings

One principal reason for gathering information about previous diagnostic findings is to establish a comprehensive clinical record. Clinicians need to establish where or by whom the patient was seen and what significant findings emerged from these previous contacts. The clinician should request a written summary from professionals having previous contact with the patient. With this information, comparisons can be made between past professional opinions and current findings. Information about previous diagnostic findings can be used to determine congruence or disparity in clinical findings and/or opinions, and to identify changes that may occur over the course of time. Knowledge about previous diagnostic contacts also serves to alert the clinician to the extent to which the patient has been seeking professional assistance. In situations in which professional diagnostic contact has been frequent or excessive and opinions or findings have been congruent, counseling may be both appropriate and necessary.

Previous Rehabilitation Services

The reasons for gathering information about previous rehabilitation services are similar to those just discussed for previous diagnostic findings. Here, clinicians need to determine both the general therapeutic approaches and goals as well as the specific techniques used in previous treatment. It is important to determine whether the patient is currently receiving treatment from another clinician. Knowledge about therapeutic efforts or procedures that were considered either helpful or largely unproductive is often invaluable to the development of treatment plans and the formulation of a prognosis. Clinicians must ascertain the specific reasons for wanting to change therapy goals, approaches, therapists, or agencies when a change in therapeutic services is being sought.

Historical information is often gathered about early development. This is particularly important when children are being evaluated. Here, clinicians often solicit parental observations about the developmental status of their child in several areas: gross motor skills (e.g., support, balance, locomotion); fine motor skills (e.g., visual tracking, prehensile and manipulative skills); self-help skills (e.g., eating, dressing); and social skills (e.g., recognition of and interaction with others). These skills are considered by many to represent the foundation for cognitive learning and language development. Children's ability to explore their environment and realize interpersonal relationships often depends upon adequate maturation of these skills. Information of this type is often used to determine whether the communication problem is part of a larger developmental deficit, and may aid in determining the need for more comprehensive developmental evaluation (physical and psychological) by other professionals.

General Developmental Status

When developmental information is interpreted together with information about communication skills, clinicians can often recognize patterns. Several major patterns may exist. For example, some communication problems exist in the absence of developmental delays. In other cases, performance varies (i.e., there are peaks and valleys) across a variety of developmental skills. Finally, there may be significant deficits across a broad range of developmental skills. Knowledge about developmental patterns prior to direct examination can be especially helpful in determining the types of behavioral probes and tests to be used during the examination. In addition, such information can validate a clinician's impression about a child formed on the basis of assessing communication behavior.

Knowledge about early development often will not play a significant role in the diagnosis and treatment of the adult patient. For this reason, the focus of attention is typically directed toward gathering information about the current status of the adult patient.

Knowledge about the current health status of a patient can serve to 1) establish constraints that may be present during the examination; 2) highlight the need for a medical referral; and 3) serve as a prognostic indicator. In the first situation, we provide the example of a neurologically impaired patient with aphasia and a history of right homonymous hemianopsia. The presence of this visual field deficit should alert the clinician to place all visual materials within the patient's field of vision during the examination. In the second situation, we offer the example of a child whose parents report a history of chronic ear problems which have not been evaluated or treated. Identification of these problems alerts the clinician to the potential need for otolaryngological referral. In the third situation, clinicians can often expect speech- and language-impaired patients with complicating health problems (paralysis, vascular disorders, psychological disorders, etc.) to have poorer prognoses than those without such problems.

Current Health Status

**Educational/
Vocational Status**

Historical information about the educational status of a patient can serve a variety of purposes. Speech and language problems may be directly related to more general types of learning problems or may, in some cases, actually impede learning. Knowledge of the presence and extent of such problems is critical to the planning of interdisciplinary programs for children with communication disability. In addition, educational data about capacity for learning and achievement often provides the clinician with useful information which may bear directly on treatment planning. Gathering information about patients' level of educational aspiration may provide additional indications about their ability and desire to overcome a deficit or handicapping condition. In some instances, communication problems limit a person's educational opportunities. The degree to which the patient is aware of these limitations is often clinically important. Finally, the clinician will want to determine the extent to which the speech or language problem directly or indirectly influences educational progress.

Strong parallels can be drawn between the educational factors and those having to do with employment. Information about a patient's employment status can often be useful. Here, clinicians may identify problems that are technical in nature (e.g., difficulties hearing or speaking on the telephone) or problems of an interpersonal nature. Vocational achievement level and aspirational level should be examined to identify constraints that might be imposed by either the speech or language deficit (e.g., laryngectomy, aphasia), the vocation, or the vocational environment. Again, the extent to which patients are realistic about these limitations often provide prognostic indications that merit clinical consideration.

**Emotional/Social
Adjustment**

Information about emotional and social adjustment is often important. Such information is used to determine the patient's readiness to accept a diagnosis and to define the patient's motivation for therapy. Such information is generally divided into two broad categories: intrapersonal and interpersonal adjustment. Clinical opinions about a patient's intrapersonal adjustment are derived from information about feelings or attitudes which relate to the speech or language disorder, expressions of self-concept, levels of self-acceptance, and related psychological states (e.g, depression, denial, etc.). Interpersonal adjustment can be assessed by obtaining information about the manner in which the patient responds to and deals with other persons in the environment. To illustrate these broad categories, consider an adolescent who stutters. He may express rather negative feelings about himself and his disorder, and may be depressed about his failure to respond positively to therapeutic experiences (intrapersonal behaviors). When faced with the necessity to speak with people, this young man might react by avoiding certain situations or by getting his peers to talk for him (interpersonal behaviors).

Information about issues related to emotional and social adjustment may be difficult to obtain from a parent or responsible caregiver, because it is extremely difficult to interpret intrapersonal and interpersonal behaviors solely on the basis of historical reporting. As a result, much of this type of information will stem from direct examination of the patient. We will consider this topic again later.

When a patient is brought to a diagnostic evaluation by a parent or responsible family member, a clinician might naturally expect that the main concern is the speech or language deficit. Although this is most often the case, clinicians need to be sensitive to the other concerns that parents, spouses, and other responsible caregivers have about the patients they bring to speech and language professionals. For example, parents of developmentally delayed children will sometimes focus on the child's language deficits, although this emphasis may mask their real concern or guilt about the possibility of retardation. In another example, wives of husbands who have suddenly suffered brain injury have many concerns about matters such as the physical care of the patient, family management, finances, and so on. It is important to realize that these concerns can influence the manner in which people approach the diagnostic session. This topic is discussed more fully in Chapter 10, where interviewing and counseling relationships between clinicians and families are considered.

Pertinent Family Concerns

This category of information is included to point out that respondents often volunteer all sorts of information during the course of historical reporting. Some of this unsolicited information may be irrelevant, although often such information may be highly significant. For example, information about marital problems, problems with siblings, economic issues, parental health problems, and so on may have a significant bearing upon the speech or language disorder being evaluated. The degree to which these types of unsolicited information will be considered or reported in the written record will depend upon the judgment of the examining clinician regarding the relevance of such information to diagnosis or rehabilitation.

Other Information Volunteered by the Respondent

DIRECT PATIENT EXAMINATION

As we have indicated, clinicians also gather first-hand knowledge about patients and their communication problems. This knowledge is gathered chiefly on the basis of direct examination. In Chapter 1, we learned that several major forms of assessment are regularly used in diagnosis and assessment of communication disorders. We now review these forms of assessment and make clear why they are undertaken.

**General Behavior
Observations**

Clinicians routinely gather first-hand knowledge about patients and their communication problems by keenly observing general behavior. These observations often establish the overall behavioral context within which diagnosis is undertaken. Observations about such general behavioral attributes as the level of responsiveness, degree of cooperation, and ability to follow instructions and complete tasks merit attention, because such behavioral influences may exert a profound effect of both diagnostic and remediation outcomes. Observation of patients' interactional styles with the examiner and family members often provides useful diagnostic information. Notations of behavioral characteristics made in conjunction with general conversation with patients enable clinicians to obtain information about speech-language deviance and level of social communication competence. These early, general observations also enable clinicians to establish a style of interpersonal communication that is mutually productive. For example, when early, general observations reveal that a patient is unintelligible and is anxious and uncertain about the examination, initial interviewing techniques that elicit yes-no responses might be more productive than open-ended questioning techniques. Obviously, general behavioral observations are made within a relatively constrained social context and do not depend upon the administration of formal tests.

**Examination of the
Speech Mechanism**

An essential part of the diagnostic process is an examination of the integrity of the organs and systems used to produce speech, voice, and language. We have emphasized that the formulation of effective therapy depends upon accurate diagnosis. Thus, physical examination of the speech mechanism forms a vital part of diagnosis in speech-language pathology. Some primary goals of this examination are:

1. To identify structural (anatomical) and/or functional (physiological) differences and abnormalities
2. To specify whether the differences or abnormalities that have been identified influence or cause disturbance in speech, voice, or language
3. To determine whether the differences or abnormalities that have been identified warrant referral and additional evaluation by other professionals (e.g., physicians and dentists)
4. To determine whether the speech mechanism needs to be modified

This examination should be brief and be conducted in a planned fashion. We will provide specific information about how to conduct an examination of the speech mechanism. In addition, you are encouraged to read the materials of Dworkin and Culatta (1980), Mason and Simon (1977), and St. Louis and Ruscello (1981) to obtain additional information about completing the speech mechanism examination. The heart of this form of appraisal is the oral-facial examination.

Physical examination of the oral-facial region is completed largely by relying on the senses: seeing, feeling (palpation), and hearing. The initial task is to complete an orderly examination of the organs and systems used to support speech, voice, and language for the purpose of identifying differences and abnormalities. For most of this examination additional equipment is not needed; however, a flashlight and tongue depressors are often useful. The bulk of examination can be accomplished if the clinician is seated directly in front of the patient with the clinician's eye level parallel to the mouth of the patient.

The Oral-Facial Examination

We often begin the examination by visually inspecting the external features of the face and head. Here we may seek to identify facial asymmetry, disproportion among various parts of the face, discolorations and conditions (scars, etc.), deviant resting postures of the head, face, and lips, predominant manner (nasal versus oral) of breathing, deviation in facial expression, and so on. Both full-face (frontal) and lateral profile visualization should be undertaken.

Examination of External Features of the Face and Head

From a frontal view, the midline of the nose, philtrum of the upper lip, space between the central incisors and the midline of the chin should be aligned at rest and when the lower jaw is opened and closed. The eyes should be aligned along the horizontal plane, should be properly spaced, and should move normally. A general rule clinicians might use to assess upper facial proportion is to consider the face as five eyes wide. There should be room for about one eye width between the bony structures that separate the two eyes. Excessive space between the eyes is seen in patients with various craniofacial syndromes.

In the vertical dimension, the face extends from the bridge of the nose to the chin. The area of the forehead is part of the neurocranium, rather than the face. Vertical facial dimension is often divided into two parts: upper versus lower facial height. Upper facial height extends from the bridge of the nose to the base of the nose, whereas lower facial height extends from the base of the nose to the base of the chin (Figure 2.1). Again, the general rule is that lower facial height is greater (about 20% for adults; 10% for children) than upper facial height. This can be verified by placing the index finger on the bridge of the nose and the thumb on the base of the nose. Next, rotate these fingers 180 degrees by keeping the thumb on the base of the nose and rotating the index finger 180 degrees. Now, the index finger should be on the chin; some facial tissue (about 10% to 20%) should be below the index finger.

Rapid estimation of facial profiles can be made by visualizing patients in a lateral profile (Figure 2.1). Three landmarks are used for this estimation: the bridge of the nose, the base of the nose, and the most prominent point of the chin. As a general rule, these three points should be on a straight or slightly protruded line (i.e., Class I or normal facial profile). If they are not,

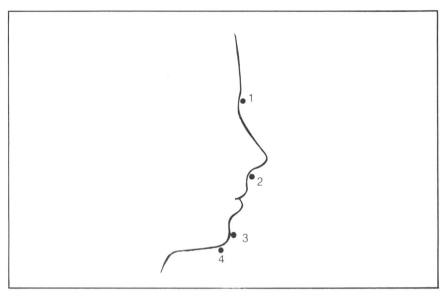

Figure 2.1.   Lateral view of the face. Important landmarks include: 1) the bridge of the nose; 2) the base of the nose; 3) the most prominent point on the chin; and 4) the lowest point on the chin.

it means that the upper jaw is protruded in relation to the lower jaw (Class II tendency), the lower jaw is protruded in relation to the upper jaw (Class III tendency) or both are somehow dimensionally disproportionate. Another useful technique is to place an index card so that it is touching the front of the nose and the front of the chin. In this situation, the card should touch the lower lip and the upper lip should be about 2–3 mm behind the card or finger.

The functional integrity of upper face can be examined by noting whether the patient can raise the eyebrows or close the eyes tightly against resistance. Functional integrity of the face can be examined by observing facial expressions and resting postures.

This phase of the examination should also include appraisal of the external features of the nose, the lips (see Figure 2.2), and the mandible. Frontal visualization can be used to identify nasal septal deviations. Palpation can often be used to identify bony spurs or other septal deviations. Visual inspection of the nares can be accomplished using both frontal and inferior views. By tilting the patient's head back slightly, the clinician can assess the relative size and symmetry of the nares and deviations in the columella. The patient's nostrils should be open or patent upon visualization. Using a flashlight and gently displacing a nostril to the side, the clinician should be able to see the inferior nasal turbinates. They should appear deep red. If they are pale, the patient may have an upper respiratory problem, nasal allergy, irritation, or rhinitis. Finally, the clinician should determine whether patients can breathe without appreciable resistance through both nostrils. This determination can be made several ways. First, ask the patient. Second, determine whether there are any inequalities between the nostrils in nasal resistance during resting (tidal) breathing. The clinician can alternately occlude each nostril during tidal exhalation and note apparent discrepancies in air flow rate, respiratory effort, or production of noise or turbulence. In a similar fashion, patients should be able to sustain an effortless hum through both nostrils. Nostril discrepancies in humming which occur when the nostrils are alternately occluded should be noted.

Frontal visualization of the face can also be used to evaluate the lips. The philtrum (vertical, midline indentation of the upper lip) and cupid's bow of the upper lip should appear normal. At rest, the lips should be approximated or nearly so and the patient should be breathing through the nose. Movements of the lips should be bilaterally symmetrical during protrusion ("say /i/") and retrusion ("say /u/") and during various facial expressions (smile, laugh, etc.). Functional integrity of the lips can be assessed using labial diadochokinetic activities which require patients to produce rapidly alternating syllables (*pah*). Rate, pattern, and consistency of movements should be used as criteria for determining functional integrity.

Important clinical observations can also be made about the lower jaw, or *mandible*. First, the mandible should be capable of being lowered widely and should not deviate from the midline during depression or elevation. A

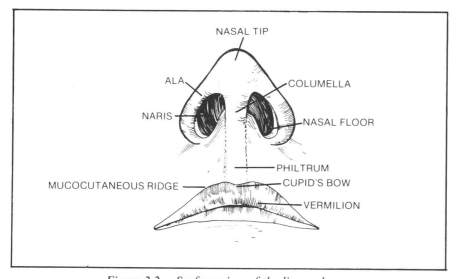

Figure 2.2.   Surface view of the lips and nose.

useful clinical technique to detect midline deviations is to place the index finger of each hand on the top of the patient's mandibular condyles. To locate the condyles, the clinician's fingers are placed opposite the tragus of each ear. With the fingers in this location, the clinician asks the patient to open the mouth widely. The clinician's finger will fall into the fossa of the temporal-mandibular joint and the clinician will feel whether or not the movement of the condyles is equal bilaterally.

Visualization and palpation can also be used to form impressions about the structural adequacy of the mandible. As a general rule, the ramus of the mandible is shorter (about one-third) than the body or corpus. This can be verified by placing the thumbs on the angles of the mandible and the index fingers on the top of the condyles (i.e., at the ear tragus). This distance defines the length of the ramus. Keeping your thumbs at the angles, rotate the index fingers to the planes of the mandible. There should be some portion (about one-third) of the body of the mandible lying in front of the index fingers. Discrepancies in this relationship may help to explain problems in facial profile and dentition identified in other parts of this examination.

Finally, appraisal of external features should include visualization of the ears. Identification of irregularities, such as microtia, pre-auricular tags, ear canal deformities, and so on, are readily made by simply looking at the ears.

Intraoral Examination   Intraoral examination is completed to evaluate the dentition, the hard and soft palate, the lining of the mouth and pharynx, the faucial isthmus, and the tongue (see Figure 2.3). Examination of the status of the dentition (type of occlusion, absence of teeth, presence of large spacing between teeth, tooth rotations, quality of dental hygiene, etc.) is essential. Examination of occlusal relationships is relatively simple to accomplish. The general rule is to ask the patient to "bite on the back teeth and show your gums." In this position, the clinician can move one cheek aside with a finger or tongue depressor and look at the relationship between the upper and lower first permanent molars. Normally the mandibular (lower) molar is one-half tooth or cusp ahead of the maxillary (upper) molar. This normal relationship is referred to as Class I occlusion. In some people, the lower molar is one-half tooth or more behind the upper molar. This relationship specifies what is known as Class II occlusion. Here, there is a tendency for the maxillary arch to be protruded in relation to the mandible. In other people, the lower molar may be more than one-half tooth ahead of the upper molar. In this situation, we have a Class III relationship and there is a tendency for the lower jaw to be protruded in relation to the upper jaw. This classification system is consistent with the one used for specifying facial profile characteristics, described earlier. This appraisal of molar relationships must be completed for both sides of the mouth. When this has been done, the clinician can specify the posterior occlusal relationships of dentition.

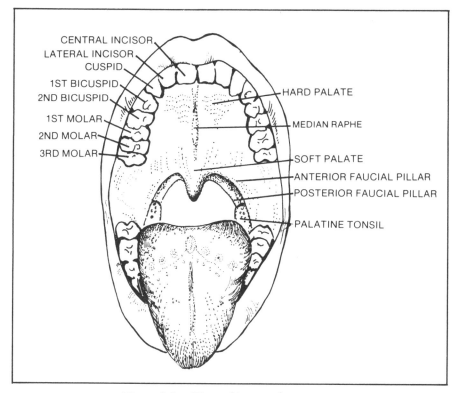

CENTRAL INCISOR
LATERAL INCISOR
CUSPID
1ST BICUSPID
2ND BICUSPID
1ST MOLAR
2ND MOLAR
3RD MOLAR
HARD PALATE
MEDIAN RAPHE
SOFT PALATE
ANTERIOR FAUCIAL PILLAR
POSTERIOR FAUCIAL PILLAR
PALATINE TONSIL

Figure 2.3.   View of intraoral structures.

Younger children being evaluated may not have permanent molars. The best clinical approach is to focus on the canines (the "eye" teeth). Normally the mandibular canine should be one-half tooth ahead of the maxillary canine. If it is ahead by more, there is a Class III tendency; if it is behind there is a Class II tendency. If the canines are not present, look at the back (most posterior) teeth and specify occlusal relationships in the same manner as outlined above.

In addition, clinicians need to examine the front of the mouth. Here attention is directed to anterior dental relationships. Again, these observations are made with the patient "biting on the back teeth and showing the gums." In this situation, about one-half to one-third of the crown of the lower central incisors should be covered by the upper incisor. This degree of overlap between the incisors in the vertical plane specifies a normal amount of *overbite* or the vertical relationship between the upper and lower arches and dentition. There is an excessive degree of overbite if more than one-half of the crown of the lower incisors is covered by the upper incisors. Conversely, if the degree of overbite is reduced, the edges of the incisors may be aligned vertically or there may be a space between the edges (i.e., an anterior open bite is present).

In addition to specifying overbite, the clinician needs to specify *overjet*. Overjet refers to the relationship between the upper and lower incisors in a horizontal plane. Normally, the upper incisors are 1–3 mm ahead of the lower incisors. If the degree of horizontal separation between the upper and lower incisors is great, there is an excessive overjet. If it is reduced, there is insufficient overjet.

Appraisal of the status of the dentition should be concluded by identifying missing teeth, deviations in spacing between teeth, disturbances in axial inclination of teeth, tooth rotations, cross-bite and quality of general dental hygiene.

Intraoral examination should next be directed to structures located deeper in the mouth. The patient should be instructed to open the mouth moderately, but not completely. In this position, note should be made of the condition of the mucous lining of the mouth and pharynx, because alterations in the color and topography of this lining provide important clues about the patient's history and existing conditions (e.g., smoking, allergic response, upper respiratory problems, anemia, etc.). Inspection of the faucial isthmus should be made to identify tonsil enlargement and airway encroachment.

Appraisal can be made of the tongue during this phase of the examination. From a structural perspective, any anatomical differences or abnormalities (e.g., lesions, scars, fissures, missing tissue, etc.) must be identified. Obvious disproportionality between the size of the tongue in relation to the size of the oral cavity should be noted. Restrictions in the length of the lingual frenulum should be identified. From a functional perspective, evaluations should be made of strength, range, speed, symmetry, tone, and accuracy of tongue movements. Basically, patients are examined as they engage in a variety of speech or speech-like (e.g., diadochokinetic) movements and nonspeech (stick tongue out, lateralize tongue, etc.) movements. Specific tasks and procedures which can be used to assess these attributes of tongue motions are outlined by Noll in Chapter 8. Finally, clinicians must examine the tongue at rest to identify functional problems (e.g., resting deviations of the tongue, presence of fasciculations, etc.) and to determine whether the tongue functions normally during the act of swallowing.

From here, the hard and soft palate should be examined (see Figure 2.4). The hard palate is the bony platform onto which the soft palate is based. General estimation of palatal vault adequacy can be made by comparing vault height and vault width. On a structural basis, a midline raphe should be visually apparent. If a raphe is not present, a palatal torus may be seen. Palatal torii are fairly common and represent benign exostoses or extra growths of bone. Examination should also be directed to identify palatal fistula, present in some children with a history of palatal clefting. Finally, appraisal should be made of the posterior boundary of the hard palate. Two

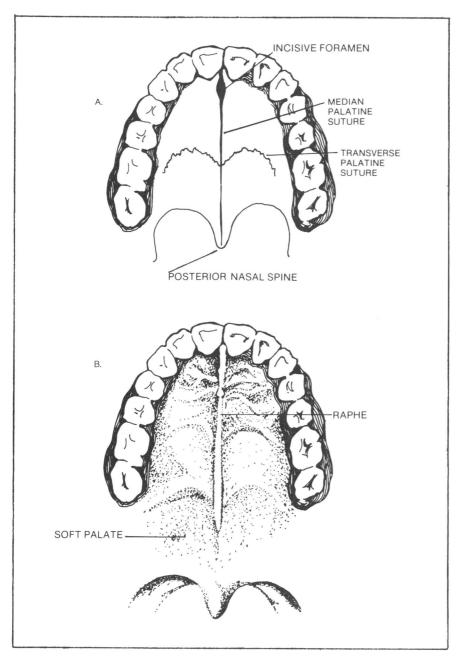

Figure 2.4.   The hard palate (A) and surface view of hard and soft palate (B).

important things must be identified in this region. First, the posterior boundary should be scalloped in appearance. Second, the boundary must be continuous. This can be verified by visual inspection, palpation, or transillumination. The nasal spine (mid-line peak) should be present.

The normal coloration of the hard palate in the region of the posterior nasal spine is pink-white. In some patients, the coloration in this region has a blue tint. Identification of such a tint is generally a strong indication that there is a problem in the bony structure in this region of the palate (Figure 2.5). The blue tint merely reflects the fact that the blood supply is close to the surface. In such patients, there is often a bony defect in midline portion of the posterior boundary of the hard palate. This defect is heralded by the presence of a V-shaped bony notch or absence of the peak. Here, the normal scalloped appearance of the posterior border of the hard palate is altered. Such defects can readily be identified by visual examination, finger palpation, and nasal transillumination. Identification of these defects is important because they mark the characteristic signs of submucous cleft palate.

The soft palate should be examined with the patient sitting in an upright position, head postured normally (i.e., eyes focused straight ahead), mouth moderately open (about three-fourths maximal opening), and the tongue at

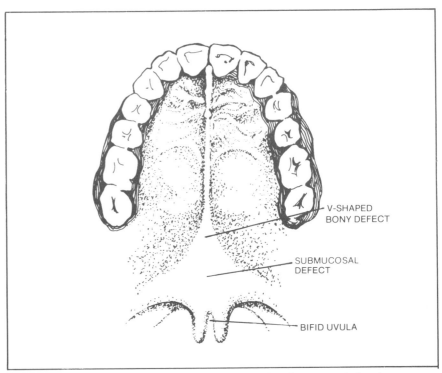

Figure 2.5.   Intraoral view of patient with submucous cleft palate.

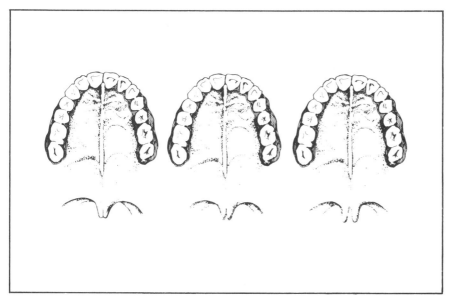

Figure 2.6.   Examples of bifid uvula.

rest (i.e., not protruded). From a structural perspective, attention should initially be directed to assess the adequacy of midline, muscular union of the soft palate. The normal coloration of the midline of the velum is pink-white. The presence of a blue-purple tint heralds abnormal muscular union, another cardinal feature of submucous cleft palate. In submucous cleft palate a primary defect is the failure of velar muscles to unite in the midline. This defect is reflected by the abnormal coloration and the thin or hypoplastic appearance of midline soft palate tissue. Again, the submucosal defect is readily identified by visual examination or nasal transillumination.

The uvula is examined next. The uvula should appear as a single midline structure acting as the most posterior part of the soft palate (see Figure 2.3). From a structural perspective, efforts should be made to identify any indentation or split (bifidity) in the uvula (Figure 2.6). Bifid uvula is fairly common (1 in every 75 adults) and may occur as an isolated phenomenon or may be associated with other problems such as submucous cleft palate. Bifid uvula can often be identified by visual examination. It is obviously important to obtain a full view of the uvula. In some cases, the bifid portions of the uvula stick together and can simply be pulled apart by gentle stroking with a tongue blade.

From a functional perspective, the adequacy of velopharyngeal port function for speech cannot be determined on the basis of visual, intraoral examination. Although this statement is made, intraoral examination forms a vital part of the diagnostic process used to evaluate palate (velopharyngeal) function in relation to speech. As we have seen, intraoral examination findings are often used to identify conditions associated with velopharyngeal impairment (signs of submucous cleft palate, signs of oral-facial syndromes or genetic predisposition to clefting, presence of oronasal or labio-oral fistulae, scarring, etc.) In addition, intraoral examination can be used to identify gross problems in velar elevation and asymmetry in velar elevation. This is accomplished by noting the degree and symmetry of palatal movements achieved during the production of sustained vowels.

Examination of Velopharyngeal Port Function in Relation to Speech

As we have stated, adequacy of velopharyngeal port function for speech cannot be determined on the basis of visual, intraoral examination. This is true because the velopharyngeal port cannot be seen on an intraoral basis. We will now consider how speech-language pathologists can evaluate velopharyngeal adequacy in relation to speech. We have chosen to discuss this topic at this place in the text for several reasons. First, the velopharyngeal mechanism is an integral part of the speech mechanism. Second, assessment of the structural and functional adequacy of this mechanism forms a vital part of examination of the speech mechanism.

For most patients, clinical judgments about the adequacy of velopharyngeal function for speech can be made quickly by noting an absence of historical information compatible with velopharyngeal impairment, an absence of clinical signs during intraoral examination, and an absence of speech characteristics compatible with velopharyngeal inadequacy. For patients with cleft palate and some neuromotor disturbances, velopharyngeal function might be expected to be impaired. From a diagnostic perspective, the cause of the problem in these patients is often largely, although not wholly, determined by the presence of the palatal cleft or definition of the specific type of neuromotor disturbance. Thus, the diagnostic goals are to determine "what part" or "how much" of the speech disturbance is related to velopharyngeal impairment in comparison to other contributing factors, to determine whether the functional problems uncovered warrant referral to other professionals, to determine whether the speech mechanism may need to be modified, and to formulate a plan of remediation. Finally, there are patients referred for evaluation of velopharyngeal function who do not have overt cleft palate or neuromuscular problems. Here, the diagnostic goals include specification of the etiology as well as those just specified.

Regardless of the cause of impairment, four main evaluation techniques can be used to provide information about adequacy for velopharyngeal function for speech. These four techniques include: 1) obtaining a thorough history; 2) completing an examination of the speech mechanism; 3) completing a reasonably thorough perceptual analysis of articulation proficiency and voice quality; and 4) verifying tentative impressions made on the basis of these three techniques through evaluation by more complex, instrumental methods. No single technique or form of observation can be used to determine the adequacy of velopharyngeal function for speech.

As is the case for other kinds of disturbances, evaluation of velopharyngeal function in relation to speech must include the gathering of comprehensive historical information. Particular effort should be made to uncover evidence compatible with velopharyngeal impairment. Some specific forms of evidence include:

1.   History of nasal regurgitation
2.   Familial history of clefting or oral-facial syndromes
3.   History of speech disturbance following tonsillectomy or adenoidectomy
4.   History of speech disturbance compatible with velopharyngeal problems
5.   History of oral-facial myoneural disorder

As we have indicated, evaluation of velopharyngeal function in relation to speech must also include an examination of the speech mechanism. One main goal of this phase of examination is to identify conditions known to be associated with velopharyngeal impairment. Particular efforts should be made to identify:

1.   Clinical signs of oral-facial syndromes associated with palatal clefting
2.   Signs reflecting genetic predisposition to clefting (e.g., submucous cleft palate, congenital lip pits, etc.)
3.   Oro-nasal or labio-oral fistula
4.   Additional physical irregularities (e.g., scarring, motor disturbance, etc.)

Other routine parts of speech mechanism examination have been discussed earlier in this chapter.

A third, vital part of evaluation of velopharyngeal function is the assessment of speech. There is universal agreement that impairment of velopharyngeal function is associated with two major forms of speech disturbance: 1) errors in the production of speech sounds; and 2) inappropriate nasalization. In view of this fact, thorough evaluation of speech sound production proficiency is required. When possible, testing should incorporate articulation tests which permit assessment and differentiation of speech sound errors unrelated to velopharyngeal incompetence (e.g., cognitive and developmental factors) from those related to velopharyngeal incompetence. The Iowa Pressure Test of Articulation (Morris et al., 1961) and the /p/-/b/ test described by Van DeMark and Swickard (1980) are particularly useful for the latter purpose. In addition, clinicians should elicit sentence repetitions to determine whether production of speech sounds is altered during the production of more complex discourse. Finally, they should engage the patient in conversation to determine whether speech sound production deteriorates during connected discourse.

During all forms of speech sound testing, clinicians should attempt to determine whether:

1. Nasal emission of air is present during the production of fully oralized stops, fricatives or affricates. Techniques which may be used to determine the presence of nasal emission are: a) listening in free air, through a stethescope or nasal catheter; b) use of a p-paddle, a mirror, or finger placed under the nostrils; or c) actually measuring the presence and magnitude of nasal air flow (Thompson and Hixon, 1979)
2. Unusual types of errors (pharyngeal fricatives and glottal stops) are present
3. Nasal turbulence or obvious nasal alae constriction is present

Although it is generally agreed that velopharyngeal insufficiency is frequently associated with excessive nasalization of speech (hypernasality) in addition to speech sound disturbance, we do not recommend the use of ratings of the severity of nasality for evaluation. This decision is based upon the fact that individual raters' judgments of the severity of nasalization of speech are known to be characterized by questionable reliability and unknown validity, are biased by the presence and severity of other primary speech attributes, and are not linearly related to the size of the velopharyngeal orifice or gap (Bradford et al., 1964; Counihan and Cullinan, 1970; Curtis, 1970; Sherman, 1954; and Spriestersbach, 1955). For these reasons, clinical decisions about adequacy of velopharyngeal function for speech should be based upon attributes other than the severity of speech nasalization. Finally, a brief perceptual assessment must be completed to identify phonatory based voice problems (hoarseness, breathiness) present in some individuals with velopharyngeal incompetence.

Strong inferences about the adequacy of velopharyngeal function for speech can be made on the basis of data synthesized from historical information, examination of the speech mechanism, and the speech assessment procedures just described. In cases in which the inference is that there is evidence supporting inadequacy of velopharyngeal function for speech, additional evaluation is recommended. Definitive conclusions about the adequacy or inadequacy of velopharyngeal function for speech should not be made until the inferentially-based data is verified with clinical information gained from additional evaluations using more complex, instrumental forms of assessment. The major forms of instrumental assessment currently used include:

1. Video and cinefluorographic evaluation of velopharyngeal port function
2. Aerodynamic assessment of velopharyngeal port function
3. Nasopharyngoscopy or nasoendoscopy

Persons involved with the management of patients with potential velopharyngeal incompetency should either have access to these forms of instrumental evaluation or refer to centers where such evaluations can be undertaken.

Contemporary discussion of speech production typically embraces respiratory considerations, whereas description of human voice production typically embraces aerodynamic-myoelastic principles. Such descriptions highlight the fact that critical aspects of speech and voice production are mediated by interactions between respiratory drive and upstream (laryngeal and vocal tract) adjustments. Thus, examination of respiratory adequacy for speech and voice production represents an essential part of the diagnostic process. For most patients, estimations about respiratory adequacy for speech and voice production can simply be made through judicious observation and listening. Specific procedures and issues to consider in more detailed evaluation of respiratory function are discussed in Chapter 5 (see "Evaluation of Respiratory Function").

Examination of Respiratory Function

Detailed information about the content of the examination of linguistic behavior is presented in Chapters 3, 4, and 7.

Linguistic Characteristics

Detailed information about the content of the speech sound production examination is presented in Chapter 4.

Speech Sound Production

Detailed information about the content of the voice examination is presented in Chapter 5.

Voice Production

Detailed information about the content of the examination of fluency is presented in Chapter 6.

Fluency Characteristics

Direct examination of nonverbal communication behaviors often provide the examining clinician with additional information about the patient and the speech or language problem. There are a number of nonverbal dimensions of human communication that can be examined: body motions (kinesic behaviors), touching behaviors, paralanguage, and proxemics (Knapp, 1972). Kinesic behaviors can be divided into facial expressions, head movements, hand/arm movements, and body movements or postures. Careful, direct observation of kinesic behavior often aids the clinician in determining how "comfortable" or "at ease" the patient is with the clinical situation, both in relation to the clinician and to the discussion of presenting problems. Clinicians will want to observe the degree to which there is congruence between what a patient says and what the body "says" on a nonverbal basis during the process of interviewing and direct examination.

Nonverbal Aspects of Communication

Patients' touching behavior and proxemics (use of personal space) often also provide information about the relationship that patients are willing to establish within both personal and clinical situations. Such observations often provide important clues to understanding significant features of interpersonal relationships. With children, these relationships can be observed in the context of parent-child and clinician-child interactions.

Paralanguage deals with various types of vocalizations sometimes referred to as vocal characterizers (sighing, yawning, throat clearing, etc.), vocal qualifiers (pitch, intensity, duration), and vocal segregates (intrusive use of "uh-huh," "um," "uh," "ah," etc.). These types of vocalizations should be carefully examined from the perspective of understanding the meaning they give to spoken communication. These types of speech vocalizations must be distinguished from the specific features of some speech disorders that will be addressed in other chapters of this text.

It is also important for the clinician to define the extent to which patients use nonverbal communication as a substitute for speaking. For example, children who are delayed in language development and adults who have suffered language loss due to stroke may develop highly organized gesture systems to aid in communication. In some cases, gestures may be appropriately used to enhance communication, whereas in other cases, the patient's skill with nonverbal communication may serve to hinder the development of speech and language.

Clinicians must remember that many nonverbal characteristics are culturally bound or may reflect highly individualized, idiosyncratic, personal aspects of behavior. Hence, judgments about the meaning and/or appropriateness of nonverbal behaviors should always be interpreted in these contexts and with caution.

Audition and Auditory Perceptual Skills

Securing first-hand information about the hearing status of patients is basic to most speech-language evaluations. Traditionally, hearing screening or identification audiometry, has consisted of completing a short pure-tone test procedure. A number of pure-tone stimuli are presented at a fixed hearing level through headphones. The examiner records whether the patient heard the pure tones that were presented. The purpose of this screening test is to identify patients whose hearing is not normal, that is, those patients who have a hearing loss sufficient to interfere with communication. Once the identification of hearing loss is made, the patient is then referred to an audiologist for an audiologic assessment. During this process, the patient receives hearing threshold testing to determine the exact nature and extent of the hearing loss.

A set of guidelines for identification audiometry has been published by the American Speech-Language-Hearing Association (ASHA, Committee on Audiometric Evaluation, 1975). These guidelines recommend that patients be screened individually under headphones with pure tone stimuli at frequencies of 1000, 2000, and 4000 Hz. Testing at 500 Hz is not recommended because of the interference of low-frequency ambient noise. The recommended screening levels are 20 dB hearing level (HL) (American National Standards Institute, 1970: ANSI-1969) at 1000 and 2000 Hz and 25 dB HL at 4000 Hz. Patients fail the screening when they fail to respond at any frequency in either ear at the recommended levels. The guidelines also stipulate that all patients who fail an initial screening must be re-screened, either during the same session or within one week. Those patients who fail a re-screening should then be referred for an audiological assessment. The guidelines further suggest that screening programs which involve large numbers should be supervised by an audiologist. The actual screening may be done by an audiologist, a speech-language pathologist, or personnel trained and supervised by these professionals.

Since the publication of these guidelines in 1975, there has been increasing concern on the part of audiologists and speech pathologists about the frequency of middle ear dysfunction, particularly in children. Estimates have been made that a large portion of children, possibly as high as one-third, have had multiple episodes of otitis media. The incidence appears greatest in children 6 to 24 months of age (Klein, 1978). Many professionals now believe that the mild, fluctuating hearing loss caused by repeated episodes of otitis media may have effects on language development and auditory perceptual abilities. (See Ventry (1980) for a complete discussion of this issue.) For this reason, a second set of guidelines for acoustic immitance screening of middle ear function was developed by ASHA in 1979 (ASHA Committee on Audiometric Evaluation, 1979). These guidelines recommend the assessment of middle-ear status by both tympanometry (a measure of the change in stiffness of the tympanic membrane with changes in ear canal air pressure) and acoustic reflex testing (the bilateral contraction of the stapedius muscle in response to loud sound). Screening is recommended annually for children from nursery-school age through grade five.

The stimulus for acoustic reflex testing should be a pure tone of 1000 Hz presented contralaterally at 100 dB HL (re: ANSI-1969). For tympanometry, ear canal pressure should be varied from $+100$ to -300 mm H_2O. A patient fails the screening if their middle ear pressure exceeds $+100$ mm H_2O or is less than -200 mm H_2O *and* if the acoustic reflex is absent. A referral is then made for audiological and medical followup.

Pure tone screening and immitance screening can not be substituted for each other. In the former, hearing acuity is assessed; in the latter, middle ear function is evaluated on a physiological basis. In selecting a screening procedure, consideration must be given to the purpose of the examination. It has frequently been shown that significant middle ear dysfunction can exist in the absence of a communicatively significant hearing loss, that is, a hearing loss less than 20 dB. Many professionals have now chosen to do both pure tone and immitance screening. (For a complete discussion of this topic, see Wilson and Walton, 1978).

A number of children pass both the screenings for pure tones and for middle ear dysfunction, and yet seem to demonstrate some type of "auditory processing disorder" or "auditory perceptual disorder." It is extremely difficult to screen for these problems. The stimuli used are often meaningful words or sentences, and the tasks generally are also sample aspects of auditory memory and linguistic abilities. If a child passes pure tone and middle ear screenings, and yet has some receptive difficulties that appear to be auditory in nature, he or she should be referred for "auditory processing" testing either by an audiologist or a speech-language pathologist (refer to discussions of auditory processing by Newhoff in Chapter 3 and by Schwartz in Chapter 4).

In addition to the forms of audiometric screening and testing just described, a number of clues about the hearing status of young children who do not respond well to testing can be derived from the history, and from the interpersonal behavior of the child during the examination. During history taking, parents sometimes report that children act as though they do not hear specific parental requests, instructions, and so on. This, of course, needs to be differentiated from the possibility that the child chooses not to respond in contrast to not actually hearing. Another historical example might be evident in the report of a child who consistently turns the television or radio to an inappropriate loudness level.

During the examination, the clinician needs to note instances in which a child fails to react to environmental noises with curiosity, acts confused or incorrectly carries out instructions. Responses that result from the presence of a hearing problem must be differentiated from those related to a lack of language comprehension. Children who frequently say "huh?," ask for statements to be repeated, or indicate some physical discomfort with their ears (pulling at the outer ear) should be carefully evaluated on an audiological/otological basis.

We have emphasized the need to identify hearing problems in children because of the important role hearing plays in the development of speech and language. Naturally, adults can also have problems associated with hearing loss and should be examined clinically from that perspective. As a general rule, it is prudent to administer a hearing screening to all adults who come for examination. When adult patients are seen after any trauma or disease, or when the patient has reached the fifth decade of life, it is essential to include audiometric screening as part of the diagnostic evaluation.

General Developmental Characteristics

Speech-language pathologists may need to directly examine general aspects of development in children seen for evaluation. Direct examination may be used to verify information obtained through history.

Parents who bring children for speech and language evaluations are often unaware of other subtle developmental delays or deficiencies. As stated earlier, the speech-language clinician may be the first to recognize or identify a particular developmental pattern which may later merit further attention by other professionals. In general, the clinician will want to observe a child's level of development in the following areas:

1. *Gross motor skills*   Control of muscular activity necessary for bodily support, balance and locomotion. Included are behaviors such as head posture, sitting, walking, stair climbing, and running.
2. *Fine motor skills*   Control of muscular activity necessary for appropriate timing, force, range, and direction during activities such as reaching, grasping, release, throwing, and manipulation of objects and writing tools.
3. *Visual-motor perceptual skills*   Ability to integrate visual stimuli with an organized motor response appropriate to the completion of a specific task, such as puzzle completion or copying geometric patterns using pencil and paper.
4. *Self-help skills*   Ability to execute behaviors associated with eating, dressing, toileting, safety, and so on.
5. *Social-skills*   Skills related to recognition of others in the environment and interaction with parents, other adults, and peers within the environment.

Information about these general aspects of development can often simply be collected by asking patients to perform various nonstandardized tasks and by observing patients during their natural interaction with the examiner. In a more formal manner, the clinician can elect to use instruments designed to measure such skills. These instruments may take the form of tests or scales, or may simply be check-off forms which list the developmental milestones in a chronological sequence. The following instruments are representative of those commonly used in clinical practice.

Revised Denver Developmental Screening Test (Frankenburg et al., 1970)
Vineland Social Maturity Scale (Doll, 1965)
Portage Guide to Early Education (Bluma et al., 1976)
Inventory of Early Development (Brigance, 1978)
Developmental Test of Visual Perception (Frostig, 1963)
Motor-Free Visual Perception Test (Colarusso and Hammill, 1972)

When examining adults with acquired neurological impairments, observations of motor, self-help, and social skills can also provide valuable information. Deficits in these areas should be noted before the administration of speech and language testing and other forms of direct examination so that the clinician will know how to adjust testing procedures to meet the physical needs of the disabled patient. Such information will also have prognostic significance in relation to functional communication opportunities.

Cognitive and Intellectual Functioning

Cognitive and intellectual function may be intimately related to the cause and remediation of speech and language problems. Cognitive and intellectual ability may determine the facility with which patients are able to learn tasks and utilize knowledge to solve practical problems related to everyday living. Cognitive and intellectual adequacy is a prerequisite to normal speech and language development in children, and is necessary for the maintenance of normal speech and language function in adults. Abnormalities in communication patterns due to cognitive and intellectual deficits in children and adults will be discussed further in Chapters 3, 4, and 7.

Speech-language clinicians will be in a position to make direct observations about the manner in which patients approach specific diagnostic tasks and about the adequacy of patients' responses. When patient responses require adaptive functioning, the clinician may be in a position to derive some feeling about the general intellectual ability of the patient. Beyond this general level, clinicians may need to administer specific tests to assess the patient's intellectual capacity, or refer the patient to a clinical psychologist for the necessary assessment. The degree to which the speech-language clinician is able to administer specific tests of intellectual behavior will be a function of academic and practical training. Performance on certain tests of language function (e.g., tests of receptive vocabulary such as the Peabody Picture Vocabulary Test, Dunn 1965, 1980) do correlate positively with the more general tests of intelligence (e.g., Wechsler Intelligence Scale for Children—Revised Edition, Wechsler, 1974). However, decisions about a patient's intellectual abilities should never be made solely on the basis of test instruments which do not sample a wide range of skills. The prudent clinician will seek out the assistance of a clinical psychologist where expertise is necessary.

Emotional and Social Status

As indicated earlier, speech-language pathologists often gather information about emotional and social adjustment. Information about emotional and social adjustment is usually gathered by means of direct interview with the patient. In addition, there are a number of questionnaire-type instruments that can be used to survey emotional adjustment patterns. Interpretation of responses to these more general type of adjustment instruments usually requires training in psychology. There are some questionnaires, however, which are very narrow in design and which focus on the patients' specific reactions to a specific speech disorder. This type of questionnaire is often used in assessing stuttering in adults (See Chapter 6 for a discussion of questionnaires surveying attitudes toward stuttering).

The extent to which the speech-language clinician is able to explore the emotional and social attributes of the patient is also discussed broadly in Chapter 5 and in detail in Chapter 10. Careful attention should be given to the ethical issues associated with information gathering in this area by the speech-language clinician.

Study Guide

1. a. List the ten types of information typically gathered as a part of obtaining a clinical history.
    b. Briefly clarify why such information is gathered.

2. a. What are the primary goals speech-language pathologists seek to achieve when they complete examination of the speech mechanism?
    b. Briefly review the organs and systems to be evaluated as part of:
        1) The examination of the external features of the face and head
        2) The intraoral examination
    c. Describe how velopharyngeal port function is assessed.

3. List the types of direct examinations speech-language pathologists commonly complete as part of diagnosis of communication disturbance.

4. Review how audition and auditory perceptual skills are evaluated.

5. Define the following terms or concepts.

syndrome	mandible
upper facial height	maxilla
lower facial height	frontal view
ramus	turbulence
Class I, II and III occlusion	overbite
	overjet
nares	diadochokinetic
velopharyngeal port	fistula
velum	kinesic behaviors
cleft	paralanguage
proxemics	fine motor skills
tympanometry	
gross motor skills	

REFERENCES

American National Standards Institute. 1970. American National Standards Specifications for Audiometers, ANSI-53.6-1969. American National Standards Institute, Inc., New York.

ASHA Committee on Adudiometric Evaluation. 1975. Guidelines for identification audiometry. Asha 17:94–98.

ASHA Committee on Audiometric Evaluation. 1979. Guidelines for acoustic immittance screening of middle-ear function. Asha 21:283–288.

Bluma, S., Shearer, M., Frohman, A., and Hilliard, J. 1976. Portage Guide to Early Education. Cooperative Educational Service Agency 12, Portage, WI.

Bradford, L. J., Brooks, A. R., and Shelton, R. L. 1964. Clinical judgment of hypernasality in cleft palate children. Cleft Palate J. 3:329–335.

Brigance, A. 1978. Inventory of Early Development. Curriculum Associated, Inc., North Billerica, MA.

Colarrusso, R., and Hammill, D. 1972. Motor-Free Visual Perception Test. Academic Therapy Publications, San Rafael, CA.

Counihan, D. T., and Cullinan, W. L. 1970. Reliability and dispersion of nasality ratings. Cleft Palate J. 7:261–270.

Curtis, J. F. 1970. The acoustics of nasalized speech. Cleft Palate J. 7:380–396.

Doll, E. A. 1965. Vineland Social Maturity Scale. American Guidance Service, Minneapolis, MN.

Dunn, L. M. 1965, 1980. Peabody Picture Vocabulary Test. American Guidance Service, Circle Pines, MN.

Dworkin, J., and R. Culatta. 1980. Dworkin-Culatta Oral Mechanism Examination. Edgewood Press, Inc., Nicholasville, KY.

Frankenburg, W., Dodds, J., and Fandal, A. 1970. The Revised Denver Developmental Screening Test. B. F. Stolinsky Laboratories, Department of Pediatrics, University of Colorado Medical Center, Denver.

Frostig, M. 1961. Developmental Test of Visual Perception. Consulting Psychologists Press, Palo Alto, CA.

Klein, J. 1978. Epidemiology of otitis media. In: E. Harford, F. Bess, C. Bluestone, and J. Klein (eds.), Impedance Screening for Middle Ear Disease in Children. Grune & Stratton, New York.

Knapp, M. L. 1972. Nonverbal Communication in Human Interaction. Holt, Rinehart & Winston, Inc., New York.

Mason, R., and Simon, C. 1977. The orofacial examination checklist. Lang. Speech Hear. Serv. Schools 8:155–163.

Morris, H. L., Spriestersbach, D. C., and Darley, F. L. 1961. An articulation test for assessing competency of velopharyngeal closure. J. Speech Hear. Res. 4:48–55.

Sherman, D. 1954. The merits of backward playing of connected speech in the scaling of voice quality disorders. J. Speech Hear. Disord. 19:312–321.

Spriestersbach, D. C. 1955. Assessing nasal quality in cleft palate speech of children. J. Speech Hear. Disord. 20:266–270.

St. Louis, K., and Ruscello, D. 1981. The Oral Speech Mechanism Screening Examination. University Park Press, Baltimore.

Thompson, A. E., and Hixon, T. J. 1979. Nasal air flow during normal speech production. Cleft Palate J. 16:412–420.

VanDemark, D. R., and Swickard, S. L. 1980. A pre-school articulation test to assess velopharyngeal competency: Normative data. Cleft Palate J. 17:175–179.

Ventry, I. 1980. Effects of conductive hearing loss: Fact or fiction. J. Speech Hear. Disord. 45:143–156.

Wechsler, D. 1974. Wechsler Intelligence Scale for Children (WISC) (Revised). Psychological Corporation, New York.

Wilson, W., and Walton, W. 1978. Public school audiometry. In: F. N. Martin (ed.), Pediatric Audiology. Prentice-Hall, Inc., Englewood Cliffs, NJ.

APPENDICES

A. Speech and Language Case History—Child Form

Date _____

I. IDENTIFYING INFORMATION

Name of Child_____ Birthdate _____
        (First)   (Middle)   (Last)

Name by which your child is called _____ Age _____
Address _____ Telephone _____
City _____ County _____ State _____ Zip _____

Parents: Name   Age   Occupation   Education

Father _____ _____ _____ _____
Mother _____ _____ _____ _____

If the address of either parent is different from that of the child, please indicate:

_____

Children in the family:

Name	Sex	Age	School-Grade
_____	_____	_____	_____
_____	_____	_____	_____
_____	_____	_____	_____

Who referred you to the speech clinic? _____
Address (if professional) _____
Child's Doctor: Name: _____ Address: _____

Do you want a copy of our report sent to your child's doctor? _____ Yes _____ No
To what other professional persons or agencies do you want a report sent? _____
_____
_____

Name of person filling out this questionnaire: _____
Relationship to Child: _____

II. STATEMENT OF THE PROBLEM:

Describe in your own words what problem your child is having with speech, language, and/or hearing: _____
_____
_____

When was the problem first noticed? _____
Who noticed the problem? _____

What changes in your child's language and/or speech have you noticed since that time?
_____
_____

What reactions does the child, parent, sibling, relative, and/or friend have towards the problem? _____
_____
_____

Do you have any thoughts on the cause of the problem? If so, please describe: _____
_____
_____
_____

What have you done to help your child's speech? _____
_____
_____

Has this helped? _____
If your child's speech varies, under what circumstances does it become
1. better: _____
2. worse: _____
If you ever sought professional advice about your child's speech or language problem before,
Was it for an evaluation? Yes _____ No _____ Therapy? Yes _____ No _____
Whom did you see? _____ Address: _____
_____ When? _____
For how long? _____ Results: _____
_____

What recommendations were given? _____
_____

What has been done since then? _____
_____

How does your child feel about his or her speaking ability? _____
_____

Check the items that your child seems to do more than other children the same age:
_____ 1. Avoids speaking at school.
_____ 2. Avoids speaking in play situations.
_____ 3. Avoids speaking at home.
_____ 4. Avoids speaking to children (male _____, female _____)
_____ 5. Avoids speaking to adults (male _____, female _____)
_____ 6. Avoids saying certain words.
_____ 7. Cries when unable to communicate.
_____ 8. Becomes aggressive when unable to communicate.
Have any relatives had speech and/or language problems? _____ Yes _____ No
If yes, relationship to child: _____
Type of problem _____
Results of any therapy: _____
_____
_____

SPEECH, LANGUAGE, AND HEARING DEVELOPMENT

Did the child make babbling or cooing sounds during the first 6 months of life? _____

At what age did the child say his or her first word? _____

What were the child's first words? _____

Did the child keep adding words once he started to talk? _____ At what age did the child begin using 2- and 3-word sentences? _____ Examples: _____

_____

Did speech learning ever seem to stop for a period of time? _____ Does the child talk frequently? _____ Occasionally? _____ Never? _____ Does the child prefer to talk _____ gesture _____ both talk and gesture _____ Does the child most frequently use sounds _____ single words _____ 2-word sentences _____ 3-word sentences _____ more than 3-word sentences _____ For example: _____

_____

Does your child make sounds incorrectly? _____ If so, which ones? _____

Does your child hesitate, "get stuck", repeat or stutter on sounds or words? _____

If so, describe: _____

Describe any recent changes in the child's speech: _____

_____

Can the child say a nursery rhyme? _____ Tell a simple story? _____

How well can he or she be understood by his or her parents? _____ Sisters and brothers? _____

Strangers and relatives _____ Friends _____

Does the child understand what you say to him or her? _____ Can he or she follow simple commands? _____ Will he get common objects when he or she is asked to do so? _____

Please describe: _____

Does your child ever have trouble remembering what you have told him or her? _____ If so, when does this seem to happen? _____

Does your child use any books or records? _____ How often do you read to your child? _____

DEVELOPMENTAL HISTORY

Check which is applicable: This is our biological _____, foster _____, adopted _____ child.

How many pregnancies has the mother had? _____ Which pregnancy was this child? _____

Has the mother had any miscarriages? _____ Which pregnancy? _____ Stillbirths? _____

Which pregnancy? _____ Mother's age at the time of this pregnancy? _____ Any medical problems before this pregnancy? Yes _____ No _____ Describe: _____

Did the mother have any of the following during the pregnancy? German measles _____ Toxemia _____

Accidents, injuries _____ Kidney infection _____ Anemia _____

Please describe, including medical attention: _____

_____

Did the mother take any prescription and/or nonprescription medication during this pregnancy? _____

What kinds? _____

Was the child full term? _____ Premature? _____ Months _____ Was the delivery normal? _____ Length of hard labor? _____ Were forceps used? _____

Comments: _____ Caesarian? _____ Comments: _____ Breech? _____

Comments: _____ Was the mother given any drugs during labor and delivery? _____

Describe: _____

How long were the mother and child in the hospital? _____ Give the name of physician and hospital: _____
Child's weight at birth? _____ Any birth injuries? _____ Was the child an Rh baby? _____ Was the child a blue baby? _____ Did the child require oxygen? _____
What special medication or treatment did the child receive at birth, if any? _____
_____ Breast or bottle fed? _____ If breast fed, for how long? _____ Did the infant have feeding problems? _____ Seizures? _____
Convulsions? _____ Weight after one year: _____ Present weight: _____
Give ages at which the following first occurred: Held head up _____ Sat up unsupported _____
Crawled _____ Reached for an object _____ Stood _____ Walked un-aided _____ Ran _____ First tooth erupted _____
Bladder trained _____ Bowel trained _____ Night trained _____
Which hand does the child use most frequently? Right _____ Left _____ No preference _____
Has any attempt been made to change which hand the child uses? Yes _____ No _____

MEDICAL HISTORY

	Age	Mild	Mod.	Severe		Age	Mild	Mod.	Severe
Adenoidectomy					Heart problems				
Allergies					High fevers				
Asthma					Influenza				
Blood disease					Mastoidectomy				
Cataracts					Measles				
Chickenpox					Meningitis				
Chronic colds					Mumps				
Convulsions					Muscle disorder				
Cross-eyed					Nerve disorder				
Croup					Orthodontia				
Dental Problems					Pneumonia				
Diphtheria					Polio				
Earaches					Rheumatic fever				
Ear infections					Scarlet fever				
Encephalitis					Tonsillectomy				
Headaches					Tonsillitis				
Head injuries					Whooping cough				

Describe any other illnesses, accidents, injuries, operations, and hospitalizations of the child. Include the age of child: _____
_____

Is the child's health good? _____ Fair _____ Poor? _____ Is the child now under medical treatment or on medication? Yes _____ No _____ Please describe any treatment or medication: _____

MEDICAL EXAMINATION HISTORY
Month/year of last physical exam _____ Doctor _____
Results: _____
Month/year of last vision test _____ Doctor _____
Results: _____
Month/year of last hearing test _____ Doctor _____
Results: _____
Did/does the child wear a hearing aid? _____ Glasses? _____ Explain: _____
_____

Dates of other medical examinations? _____
Doctor _____ Results: _____

EDUCATIONAL HISTORY
Does your child attend? Day care _____ Nursery _____ Kindergarten _____ Grade School _____

School	Grade/Level
_____	_____
_____	_____
_____	_____

Does he or she do average _____ below average _____ or above average _____ work in school? What are the child's best subjects? _____
His or her poorest subjects? _____ Does the child receive any special assistance or help at school? _____ Describe: _____
_____ Has he or she repeated a grade? _____
If so, which one(s)? _____ What is your impression of your child's learning abilities? ___

Describe any speech, language, hearing, psychological, and special education services that have been performed including where this was done. How often was your child seen in this service? _____
_____
_____

DAILY BEHAVIOR

How does your child get along with other children? _____

Does your child prefer to play alone? _____ Does your child play alone as well as play with other children?
_____ What games and toys does your child prefer? _____
_____

How many hours each day does the child watch television? _____ Which programs does he or she watch
the most? _____

Check these as they apply to your child:

	Yes	No	Explain: give ages if possible.
Eating problems			
Sleeping problems			
Toilet training problems			
Difficulty concentrating			
Needed a lot of discipline			
Underactive			
Excitable			
Laughs easily			
Cried a lot			
Difficult to manage			
Overactive			
Sensitive			
Personality problem			
Gets along with children			
Gets along with adults			
Emotional			
Stays with an activity			
Makes friends easily			
Happy			
Irritable			
Prefers to play alone			

Describe any other type of behavior you consider to be a problem: _____

FAMILY

Who disciplines the child the most? _____ What are the usual types of discipline? _____ What types are most effective? _____ _____ What is the child's reaction to discipline? _____ Which parent spends the most time in activities with the child? _____ How does the child get along with brothers and sisters? _____ Is there ever any parental disagreement with regard to money, religion, discipline, child up-bringing, etc? Please describe: _____ _____ If parents are divorced, describe any problem with your child in relation to this _____ _____ What kinds of activities are engaged in by the whole family? _____ What things does the child do particularly well? _____

B. Speech and Language Case History—Adult Form

Date _____

Name _____ Date of Birth _____ Age _____

Home Address: _____
          Street   City   State   Zip   Phone

Campus Address: _____
          Street   City   State   Zip   Phone

Referred by _____ _____ Reports to be sent _____
      Name   Address

to _____

Name (and relationship) of person filling out form _____

Address _____
      Name   City   County   Zip   Phone

EMPLOYMENT HISTORY (most recent)

	Place	Date	Position
1.			
2.			
3.			
4.			

PHYSICIAN(S)

	Name	Address	Phone
1.			
2.			
3.			

MARITAL STATUS _____ Spouse _____ Age _____

Children: Name _____ Age ____ Name_____ Age ____

               _____ ____ _____ ____

               _____ ____ _____ ____

               _____ ____ _____ ____

Other persons living in home and relation to family: _____

EDUCATIONAL HISTORY:

	School	Location	Highest grade completed or degree	Date
1.				
2.				
3.				

DESCRIBE YOUR PRESENT HEALTH: _____

Is there a history of:

	YES	NO		YES	NO		YES	NO
Allergies	___	___	Glandular imbalance	___	___	Retarded sexual		
Sinus infection	___	___	Hyperthyroidism	___	___	development	___	___
Anemia	___	___	Hypothyroidism	___	___	Syphilis	___	___
Asthma	___	___	Hormone therapy	___	___	Typhoid fever	___	___
Broken nose	___	___	Heart trouble	___	___	Tremor/twitching	___	___
Bronchitis	___	___	Numbness	___	___	Ulcers	___	___
Chronic colds	___	___	Paralysis/paresis	___	___	Visual problem	___	___
Chronic laryngitis	___	___	Incoordination of			Glasses	___	___
Chronic rhinitis	___	___	face or tongue			Whooping cough	___	___
Cleft palate	___	___	muscles	___	___	Poor dentition	___	___
Diabetes	___	___	Influenza	___	___	Other: _____		
Diphtheria	___	___	Mouth-breathing	___	___	_____	___	___
Ear disease	___	___	Mumps	___	___	_____	___	___
Hearing problem	___	___	Pneumonia	___	___	_____	___	___
Hearing aid	___	___	Physical defect	___	___	_____	___	___
Emotional difficulty	___	___	Poliomyelitis	___	___	_____	___	___
Psychological			Rheumatic fever	___	___	_____	___	___
counseling	___	___	Scarlet fever	___	___	_____	___	___
Smoking	___	___	How much per day?	_____				
Drinking	___	___	How much per day?	_____				

If the answer to any of the above items is "yes," give the relevant details (e.g., how frequent are these episodes, how severe are these episodes): _____

_____

List periods of hospitalization or medical treatment:

	Hospital/City/State	Date	Reason
1.	_____	_____	_____
2.	_____	_____	_____
3.	_____	_____	_____

List all surgical procedures: _____

List all prescription and nonprescription medication used over the past year (name the type if you can not remember the generic name, i.e.: aspirin, allergy pills).

_____

Have you had a neurological examination? _____ If so, by whom, when, and where?

_____

If you speak a language other than English, please state the language _____

Are you bilingual? Yes _____ No _____

Please describe in your own words the nature of your communication problems. _____

_____

_____

What do you think caused the problem? _____

When did you first notice its presence? _____ What were the circumstances?

_____

Have any members of your family had hearing or speech problems? _____

_____

How do you feel your speech problem has affected your social life? _____

_____

_____

How do you feel your speech problem has affected your occupation? _____

_____

_____

If you didn't have a speech problem, how would your life be different? _____

_____

_____

Describe the reaction of people, including your immediate family, to your speech problem.

_____

_____

_____

Do any specific communication situations present difficulty for you? _____Explain:_____

_____

_____

Do you avoid any communication situations? _____ Explain: _____

_____

List interests you have or activities you engage in (clubs, hobbies, organizations, etc.):

_____

_____

What, if anything, have you tried to do to correct the speech problem? _____

_____

_____

Are you coming to the Speech & Hearing Clinic on your own? _____ On the advice of another? _____

Have you ever received any prior speech or hearing evaluation? _____ Therapy?_____

Agency: _____ Agency: _____

Address: _____ Address: _____

Dates: _____ Dates: _____

Results: _____ Results: _____

Did prior evaluation or therapy relate to the present problem? _____ How effective has prior therapy been in helping you with your problem (what helped the most/least)?

_____

_____

_____

If therapy was terminated, describe why: _____

How long has the present problem existed? _____ Has the nature of the problem

changed at any time? _____ Explain: _____

_____

List any additional sources of information which may be helpful to us in assisting with your problem: _____

_____

3

Diagnosis of Developmental Language Disorders

Marilyn Newhoff and
Laurence B. Leonard

Outline

Educational Aims

1. *To define what is meant by the term language*
2. *To define and describe the four components (phonology, syntax, semantics, and pragmatics) of the English language*
3. *To describe the process of normal language acquisition during childhood*
4. *To clarify how language disordered children are classified*
5. *To identify the goals of language examination*
6. *To define strategies and procedures used in diagnosis of children with developmental language disorders*

Throughout the past 20 years numerous advances have been made in the area of normal language acquisition. From the professions of field linguistics, psycholinguistics, and, more recently, speech-language pathology, our knowledge base has grown and the impact of this knowledge explosion has been profound and far reaching. The approaches we take to language assessment and remediation have been specifically influenced. Today, children who come for language assessment must be judged on the basis of their entire language system. That is, we must concern ourselves with both comprehension and production of language, the meaning of language, the grammatical form of language, and the use of language in the environment; and all of these must be viewed in relation to children's cognitive status. How we have evolved to this more complete language perspective is the direct result of hundreds of studies of young children acquiring language. And although certain issues have temporarily been laid to rest, other issues still leave us somewhat perplexed and confused. All of these issues, however, must be given due consideration as we learn about diagnosis of developmental language disorders. One purpose of this chapter is to acquaint you with a number of the concerns to be considered in diagnosis. Although it would be impossible to provide an exhaustive review of the data surrounding each issue, we will provide at least a brief reflection of current thinking in the area.

Our approach is not without its biases and you should be aware of these from the outset. Based on currently available information, we proceed from certain underlying assumptions. First, each clinician should have a thorough understanding of how language is normally acquired. Second, diagnostic procedures should be based on a developmental model and should insure representativeness of significant dimensions of language. Finally, assessment of language is incomplete without a judgment of the relationship between performance in language areas and cognitive capacity.

Let us assume that tomorrow you will be responsible for conducting an evaluation of Kent. Kent is a "language" case. You check Kent's file and find only a form his parents completed as a precursor to the evaluation. From their report you learn that Kent is 3 years of age, the product of a normal pregnancy and delivery. Furthermore, he seems to have walked on time (14 months), has never presented unusual behavioral problems, has had no prolonged illness, was "potty trained" at 2;6 years of age, and "understands almost everything we say to him." So why are the parents concerned? "Kent doesn't talk like his brother did at this age. We can understand him, but his sentences aren't very long."

Now it is up to you to determine if the concerns of Kent's parents are well founded. Is there a language problem? If so, is Kent's *understanding* of language impaired or does his primary difficulty center around *expressing* language? What aspects of language are involved? Are there potential explanations for a language deficit? Might he benefit from a language intervention program? What should be the goals for such a program? What seems to be the best method to achieve these goals?

These questions represent some of the major issues that must be addressed during the diagnostic process; and by their nature they will govern your language examination plan. Your choices will be governed not only by the individual characteristics of the patient, but also by your personal philosophies regarding how children normally acquire language, what can lead to breakdown in normal acquisition, and what you believe to be the most strategic avenues to intervention.

LANGUAGE DEFINED

Although we may not recall how we learned to talk or use language, we would agree that language is quite a complex behavior. Taken a step further, therefore, it may be easy to understand why it is such a difficult term to define. Part of the reason has to do with interpretation of ''language'' based on one's perspective. For example, variation in definitions occurs based on one's interest: the history of words, dialectical usage, cultural influences on language, the formal properties of language systems, or language as an art medium (Halliday, 1975). Our interest, however, is focused on language acquisition, diagnosis, and remediation. From our perspective, then, what is language? For the purposes of this discussion we have chosen the definition set forth by Bloom and Lahey (1978): ''. . . language is a code whereby ideas about the world are represented through a conventional system of arbitrary signals for communication'' (p. 4).

The English language code can be divided into four components: phonology, semantics, syntax, and pragmatics.[1] Although these components are not easily separated in language analysis, for purposes of presentation we will examine each of them individually.

Phonology

Phonology is generally defined as the study of the sound system of our language. We are able to recognize a word because of the particular sequence of sounds we hear (for example, the sounds that make up the word *pen*), and because we learned long ago to associate this particular sound sequence with its referent (a long, thin object used for writing). As children acquire new words they are associating particular sound sequences with their re-

---

[1] It should be noted that whereas most authors use the terms phonology, syntax, semantics, and pragmatics to differentiate the components of language, the characterization set forth by Bloom and Lahey (1978) is unique. These authors use the term *content* to represent the semantic component, *form* to represent the phonological, syntactic, and suprasegmental areas, and *use* to represent the pragmatic component. For a more complete discussion of this concept, refer to Bloom and Lahey (1978).

ferents. Children must also learn that changing a sound in a sequence can change the referential meaning. For example, a change in the initial phoneme of *pen* can result in *hen* or *den,* quite dissimilar referents. The phonological dimension is discussed by Schwartz in Chapter 4. For the remainder of our discussion we will confine ourselves to the other components of language.

When we think of semantics, we are concerned with the meaning of a word **Semantics** or group of words. As children begin to identify words, to understand their meaning, and to produce them, they begin to represent their knowledge of the world through language. Each word is referred to as a lexical item and the number of vocabulary words understood and produced make up the child's lexicon. Children also combine words to produce meaningful relationships which again reflect their worldly knowledge. For example, children learn that certain things that are frequently in the presence of an individual can be possessed by that person. The semantic relationship of possession may be expressed as "Daddy car," for example, as the child points to his or her father's automobile. The same utterance, "Daddy car," might also express another relationship for the child. For example, the child may look out the window and see his or her father sitting in the car. In this instance, the child's utterance "Daddy car" may express a locative relationship. Determination of semantic relationships reflected in children's speech is often difficult and, for very young children, requires careful consideration of the situational context in which the utterance was produced.

The semantic component of language has received much attention by researchers interested in both normal and disordered aspects of language development. Numerous semantic relationships have been identified and some of these are included in Table 3.1.

Children also learn that rules apply to the ordering of words for meaning to **Syntax** be understood and conveyed. Further, they must recognize that the organization must be such that one understands what was done to, or by, whom. A child might understand individual lexical items (words) of an utterance, but without an understanding of word ordering, will not be able to send or receive messages adequately. For example, in the utterance "Steven hit Gina" it is necessary to know that the word before the action usually is the agent, that is, the person doing the act. The recipient of the act, on the other hand, will usually follow the action word. The rules governing the word order of language is one aspect of syntax.

Greater specificity is seen, however, as children gain insights into another aspect of syntax, morphology. The development of the inflectional system of English, that is, the prefixes and suffixes we add to words to effect changes in meaning, is yet another language skill to be acquired. These inflections clarify the time of events through verb tenses, number of objects

Table 3.1. Some semantic relationships expressed in early child language

Relationship	Definition	Context	Utterance
Existence	The knowledge that an object exists; frequently expressed through naming or requesting the name of an item while touching it or pointing towards it.	(Pointing to kitchen chair) (Holding up a cucumber)	That a chair. What this?
Nonexistence	The knowledge that something has disappeared or that an object is not where it is expected to be.	(Finished drinking and puts down cup) (Dickie looks at his one bare foot)	All gone juice. No shoe.
Recurrence	The knowledge that something can reappear or that an action can occur again.	(Finishes drinking and holds up cup) (After a push in the swing) (After hitting a bell)	More milk. More push. Hit 'gin.
Rejection	The opposition to an object or cessation of an activity.	(Daddy hands Beth a cup of milk) (After Dickie hits Beth)	No milk! No hit.
Denial	The rejection of a proposition or truth of an immediately preceding utterance.	(Mom says: "You're a little boy") (Dad says: "Did you hit the kitty")	No little boy. Me no hit.
Attribution	The recognition of particular properties of an object that distinguish it from other objects in the same class.	(Mom: "Do you want the big ball?") (Dad: "Is this a funny hat?") (Requesting favorite shoes)	Want little ball. Funny hat. Sneaker shoes.
Possession	The recognition that an object may belong to, or is frequently in the presence of, a particular person.	(Looking at a sack of Purina Dog Chow) (Beth grabs her bear from Dickie)	Fifi food. It my teddy.
Action	The knowledge that an object may be affected by movement.	(Jumping up and down) (Watching Beth push a truck) (Asking Beth to pull him in a wagon)	Me jump. Beth push truck. You pull me?
Location	The knowledge that two objects may be related spatially.	(Seeing a ball on a chair) (Beth sees her brother in a wagon) (Dickie asks Beth to climb off the table)	Ball chair. Dickie in wagon. Get off table.

and/or events through pluralization, and the like. The contribution of inflections to our language system is obvious in the following: Twelve mad dogs chased the policeman as he was running down the streets of Birmingham's red light district. From this example, we see inflectional markers to indicate plural, regular past, present progressive, and possessive constructions.

An area of language which recently has enjoyed great research popularity   **Pragmatics**
is that of pragmatics, or language use in its social context. Language use is generally governed by the particular function we want to serve when we speak, as well as by the linguistic and nonlinguistic context.

Recently a set of 5-year-old twins was overheard as they played in the clinic waiting area, well within earshot of their parents. One of the twins, Jason, had received a "peel and stick" book during his evaluation and was engaged in removing various stickers from one page and placing them in the appropriate, empty spaces on the next. Joshua, waiting for his turn with the clinician, had not yet received such a token and was anxious to share in Jason's activity.

(Joshua reaches toward Jason's book and a sticker)	Does that one go here?
(Jason, pulling the book away)	Leave that alone!
(Joshua, looking at Jason) (Jason does not look up and makes no response)	Can I have one please?
(Joshua, grabbing the book from Jason and running to another corner)	Gimme that!
(Jason running to his parents)	Joshua took my book away.
(Jason's mother, looking at him and then at Joshua)	Joshua, did you take Jason's book?
(Joshua stops his activity)	Yes, but I asked him nice first.

Learning to "ask nice" is a pragmatic skill. It requires development of an ability to move from direct to more indirect requesting behavior. In the above example, "Gimme that" is a direct request, the question form "Can I have one please?" is less direct and is also marked by the addition of *please*, thus appearing to be more polite by societal standards. The request "Does that one go here?" is the most subtle type of requesting behavior, used solely for politeness, and perhaps unrecognizable as a request at all were it not for the additional information provided by context. In this vein, note that both "Can I have one please?" and "Does that one go here?" function syntactically as yes-no question forms, a piece of information of interest in language diagnosis. The pragmatic component, however, allows a perspective on analysis which is far more representative of a child's language abilities than the simpler capacity to formulate a yes-no question.

Language serves a variety of functions other than to request permission or action. Language is used to obtain information (Where is the nearest bar?); to give information (Down on the corner.); to make a comment (It's a pretty nice bar, too.); to warn (Be careful, it gets raided periodically.); to threaten (I'll punch your face if you say I sent you.); to promise (I'll meet you there at six.); and so forth.

Both linguistic and nonlinguistic contexts of utterances govern language use. For example, children must learn turn-taking behavior in conversation. They also must learn to address different people in different ways. A 5-year-old must learn to simplify his language somewhat to be understood by his 2-year-old brother. Likewise, interactions with peers call for one language code, with one's parents another, and with a stranger still another. Consider, for example, a 5-year-old saying "I don't like this. Give me another." to a stranger. The stranger would probably think the child ill-bred or spoiled. The same utterance spoken to a parent might result in a verbal reprimand. To a peer, however, the politeness factor of this utterance might never be considered. The simplified language used when speaking to the younger brother, however, if directed to a peer, might receive a strange glance and a response such as "Why are you talking like a baby?"

Judgments based on the immediately preceding utterance of conversational partners must also be made. If I ask you "When are you going home?" you might respond "In about 10 minutes." Now your response is only four words long and is not a complete sentence, yet it is totally appropriate in discourse. To say "I am going to go home in about 10 minutes" is to include redundant and unnecessary information. The ability to recognize and exclude redundant information in this way is referred to as *ellipsis*. Sometimes we use a referential pronoun in much the same way. If I said to you, "Howard and Shirley are coming for a visit," you might query "When are they coming?" but not "When are Howard and Shirley coming?" as an immediate response to my statement.

These are only a few of the ways in which the linguistic and nonlinguistic contexts contribute to our language choices. The important thing to remember is that children must learn to apply rules in the pragmatic domain of language just as to the phonological, semantic, and syntactic domains. Even with such a cursory and brief review of the components of language, the task confronting the language learning child can be seen to be quite a complex one indeed. We now turn our attention to a few of the language developmental milestones typically achieved by children as this task is undertaken.

LANGUAGE ACQUISITION

Semantic Acquisition   Somewhere around their first birthday, children begin to use single-word utterances meaningfully. Although these utterances are used to express a variety of meanings, there seems to be a degree of similarity among children's early lexicons. For example, approximately half of children's first 50 lexical items (words) consist of common nouns (*juice, shoe, ball, doggie,* etc.). Proper nouns, such as *Daddy, Fifi, Gretchen,* etc., make up about 14 percent of the earliest vocabulary. Lexemes which describe or request actions (*up, more, byebye,* etc.) make up about 12 percent; modifiers (*red, mine,* etc.), 9 percent; personal-social items (*please, no, yes*), 8 percent; and function words (*what, for*) only 4 percent. This early, single-word lexicon represents the period just before children begin to combine words for production (somewhere between 18 and 24 months of age). During this period, however, children may comprehend up to four times as many words as they produce and most of these will be object names. Lexical production continues at a rapid pace such that between the ages of 3 and 4 years children may produce up to 900 different items, and by 6 years of age vocabulary may include 2,500 words.

Obviously lexical growth is an important aspect of semantic acquisition. It is only one part of the semantic picture, however, and for accurate examination of this dimension clinicians must also be concerned with the semantic relations expressed by children.

At about 2 years of age, after the acquisition of approximately 50 words, children begin to produce two-word utterances. The meanings expressed in the single-word period (e.g., *more* to indicate recurrence) continue to be expressed, but now the meaning is somewhat clearer (e.g., *more juice* to indicate what is to recur). When the meanings of children's two-word utterances are examined without regard for whether the utterances are expressed by a particular syntactic rule for word combining, the earliest semantic relations appear in a relatively consistent order. For example, expressions of existence, recurrence, and rejection appear in children's speech before those such as attribution, possession, action, and location. However, one of the obstacles confronting young children is the problem of arriving at a syntactic means of coding these relations. For this reason, authors such as Bloom and Lahey (1978) describe them as semantic-syntactic relations.

Syntactic Acquisition

The earliest multiword utterances used by children consist of content words. Morphological inflections and function words are notably absent. When children exhibit a mean length of utterance of approximately 2.5 words (somewhere around 2;6 years), however, function words such as *in* and *on* appear. Likewise inflections such as *-ing* begin to emerge. Within a few months articles such as *the* and *a* are apparent, as well as the possessive marker *-s* and past tense *-ed*. At about 3 years of age, the "to be" form *is* appears, first as a main verb (He is happy) and later as an auxiliary verb (Sandie is running).

The ability to use inflections and function words allows the child to communicate new meaning. For example, the use of the present progressive marker *-ing* or the past tense marker *-ed* and irregular past tense verbs (e.g., *ran*), allow the child to express notions concerning time. Through the use of the plural marker *-s* the child can express quantity, and so on.

Between 3;6 and 4;0 years of age, children's syntactic skills reflect new acquisitions. Verbs such as *can* and *may,* prepositions such as *behind* and *beside,* and reflexive pronouns such as *myself* and *herself* are evident. A very important milestone of this period is the ability to add syntactic complexity to utterances. No longer are children bound to the simple active-declarative sentences of their earlier development. For example, children at this age can use conjunctions such as *and, but,* and *if* to join two propositions sharing *coordinate* (Pat is going and Merrill is going, too), *antithetic* (Pat is going but Merrill must stay), and *epistemic* relations (I know that Pat is going if Merrill does).

Children also learn to correctly deny propositions during this period as well. For example, whereas earlier development reflected utterances such as "No him go," and later, "He not go," children between 3;6 and 4;0 years can produce syntactically appropriate negation such as "He isn't going" or "He will not go." Further syntactic development is also obvious in this period through children's use of question forms. Whereas earlier questions were expressed with statements followed by rising intonation (You pick me up ↑), and later by a WH-form preceding a statement (Why you do that?), at this stage children are capable of producing appropriate question forms (Why did you do that?).

While syntactic complexity continues to develop into the school years, with the acquisition of more complex structures such as the passive form (Marc was hit by Sandy), most children are able to produce all the frequently cited semantic-syntactic relations by their fourth year. That is, although increasingly complex forms are used, the basic meanings expressed in these do not undergo further change.

When children reach school age, they demonstrate an ability to determine the correctness of sentence forms, and to judge reversible and non-reversible utterances as appropriate or not. For example, "The girl, who ate the cookie John baked, chased the dog" is a reversible, syntactically complex sentence. It is reversible because the words *girl* and *dog* can exchange places in the sentence and the sentence will make sense. On the other hand, "The bee, who landed on the cookie John baked, stung the girl" is nonreversible. If the words *girl* and *bee* are positionally exchanged, the sentence is silly, or nonsensical. Recognition of such forms is a skill not normally acquired by children until their fifth year or later. Performance on tasks of this type represent *metalinguistic awareness,* or the ability to use language to talk about language. Not until the school years are children able to explain why something does or does not make sense, to explain the meanings of words or sentences, and so on.

Even before children begin to talk they are capable of communicating a variety of functions through gestures and/or through vocalization. For example, if an 11-month-old child walked over to you, lifted her arms, and looked up at you, you would probably assume she wishes to be picked up, and most likely you would be correct. Such a child would have effectively communicated to you a request for action, that is, to pick her up. Now imagine that you have placed this child's blanket on a tabletop such that she could see it but not reach it. Were she to walk to the table and hold one hand up, outstretched toward the blanket, you might rightly assume she wanted the blanket. She has indicated another communicative function, a request for an object. This child is probably also capable of other functions, for example, request for information. This might be demonstrated as she walked around a room pointing to things she wants you to name. Or she might acknowledge your message was understood by withdrawing her hand from a plant as you said "Don't touch."

Children continue to communicate such intents as they begin to talk so that in the period from 12 to 18 months such functions are accompanied by spoken language. Children may request an object's name, for example, by pointing to it and saying "dis" (for *this*), or they might name an object in response to your request "What's this?" (acknowledgment). By 3 years of age, other communicative intents are expressed by children. They can be humorous, they may qualify their statements and/or protest prior utterances or occurrences.

During the single-word period, children also demonstrate their acquisition of rules for participating in conversation. For example, children seem to be able to choose a single word based on the amount of information it will convey to the listener. Reaching for a truck a child might name it, "truck." Once in his grasp, however, he is more likely to name the appropriate action which accompanies it, "push," than to name the object again. As development continues, children are able to make greater distinctions about what needs to be said based on their perception of their conversational partner. This ability, termed *presupposition,* reflects the knowledge that certain elements of a situation are shared by both conversational participants.

Children early on demonstrate that they are aware conversation is composed of a series of turns by its participants. However, their ability to continue a topic increases with age. In response to an adult's verbalization, children at 21 months of age remain on topic only 39 percent of the time; whereas at 36 months of age, their ability has increased to 48 percent. (For a more complete account of the development of intent and discourse skills, refer to Chapman, 1981.)

Children's abilities to modify their language based on their listener's needs for comprehension represent yet another skill to be developed. For example, 4-year-old children are capable of simplifying their utterances syntactically when addressing younger children. Furthermore, 5-year-old children have the ability to choose earlier developmental forms of semantic relations as well as earlier conversational forms when they talk to children younger than they.

Cognitive Development

As mentioned at the outset, understanding language behavior is incomplete without a feel for the relationship between cognitive status and performance in all language dimensions. Why is this so important? Primarily because children's language development is thought to be guided by, or at least intricately related to their cognitive attainments. Researchers and theoreticians alike have disagreed on the exact nature of this relationship, and although resolution awaits a great deal more scientific study, enough is currently known to command our attention to the area.

There are two commonly held views of the relationship between cognition and language. The first, the *cognition hypothesis*, holds that a certain cognitive attainment is a prerequisite ability for development of its related language skill. For example, object permanence is a cognitive skill acquired by normally developing children during their first year of life. This skill reflects the child's knowledge that something can exist even though it is not immediately present. Those who support the cognition hypothesis believe that knowing an object has permanence is a prerequisite skill to being able to use its linguistic symbol—that is, its name—meaningfully. Some researchers, however, have demonstrated that children may use single words meaningfully before demonstrating a fully developed concept of object permanence. Such a finding provides support for an alternative to the cognition hypothesis, the *correlational hypothesis*.

According to the correlational hypothesis, common maturational or cognitive factors underlie development in both the language and cognitive areas (Bates et al., 1979). Thus, although the two are strongly associated, it is not assumed that in all cases a certain cognitive skill must precede its related language attainment. It may well be the case that certain cognitive skills do precede certain language skills, whereas other cognitive skills may follow the development of related language capabilities (Camarata et al., 1981; Folger and Leonard, 1978).

The model of Piaget (1963) is often applied in studies of cognitive development. Piaget has described four stages of cognitive development. Speech-language researchers and clinicians are most often concerned with the first two stages: the sensorimotor period (birth to approximately 2;0) and the preoperational period (2;0 to 4;0 years, approximately). These periods parallel children's most rapid and varied language development.

During the sensorimotor period, children learn about the world through their own physical interactions with the objects and people in the immediate environment. We say children need to be able to act on their environments for cognitive growth to progress. During this period, children move from crying when an object disappears (fearing it is lost forever), to crude searching behaviors (usually unsuccessful), to the ability to go to the place an object was last seen to locate it. You may recall that these behaviors are quite consistent with early lexical development as children note the disappearance of items (shoe?), the locations of things (shoe!), the possessor of things (Mommy) and the things acted on (shoe, juice, car, baby, etc.).

As the preoperational period begins, children become able to pretend, to let one object represent another. The child no longer has to recall where the baby's bottle was last seen, find it, and then feed the baby. The child now can pick up a pencil, pretend it is a bottle and feed the baby. This ability to participate in *symbolic play* is quite consistent with the ability to symbolize through language. Children at this stage are using mental means to solve problems rather than acting on objects to learn. (For a nice overview of cognitive behaviors consistent with Piaget's developmental theory, refer to Ault (1977) or Wadsworth (1971).)

Other Contributions to Language Acquisition

We have advocated that language acquisition will be somewhat guided by cognitive growth. Obviously, other factors are involved for potential in one or both areas to be realized. Children must possess central nervous systems of sufficient integrity to allow for physical and mental growth. Perception through hearing and visual modalities must be of a certain capacity for beneficial interactions with the environment. The oral mechanism must be functionally and structurally sound for language learning to progress unimpeded. And, of course, children must have individuals within the environment with whom to interact, although the exact type and degree of interactions that are necessary for language to be acquired normally remains open to question.

RELATED ISSUES

Choosing the most efficient avenue to examine language depends on more than just knowledge of developmental language milestones. Clinicians must also be aware of how certain other factors impinge on language learning. For example, on what basis will speech-language pathologists determine that a child is fully competent in language? What roles do imitation, comprehension, and production play in the overall scheme of language acquisition, or lack thereof? And what might account for variation within a given child or among children? In this section we briefly discuss such concerns, for they must be considered in a valid interpretation of the observations clinicians make.

Communicative Competence

In recent years, those concerned with describing language behavior have sought to more clearly differentiate language competence and language performance. *Competence* refers to knowledge about language. Children's ability to use various syntactic structures to communicate similar meanings or intents is, therefore, a reflection of language competence. But it is through performance—that is, production or comprehension of these various structures—that we are able to make inferences about competence. Until recently, researchers and clinicians have focused their attention largely on the syntactic domain of children's language, and were concerned primarily with what was termed *linguistic competence*. However, we have become aware that competence involves more than knowledge of syntax alone. Children must also be able to apply rules for the expression of semantic relations as well as appropriate discourse structure and other pragmatic skills. Thus, linguistic competence is more broadly defined today. The term *communicative competence* is used to reflect the child's knowledge of all components of language. In diagnosis, therefore, we want to be able to address the child's competence in semantics, syntax, and pragmatics. We will base judgments of communicative competence, however, on performance in various language situations; and these will include evidence of comprehension as well as production.

Determination of the underlying knowledge children have, based on what they do with language, is not as easy as it may at first seem. Getting even a partial impression of any child's communicative competence is a task which cannot be accomplished using any currently available test. Tests are obviously limited by the number and types of items included to sample a given language ability. Clinicians can do somewhat better by assessing competence through a variety of measures, both formal and informal. Clinicians are limited with regard to obtaining a complete picture of communicative competence.

Imitation, Comprehension, and Production

In earlier studies of language learning, researchers attempted to document the relationships between the imitation, comprehension, and spontaneous production of a language structure. One viewpoint held that the ability to imitate preceded the ability to comprehend which, in turn, preceded the ability to produce language spontaneously (Fraser et al., 1963). More recent evidence supports the notion that children comprehend a language principle first and then begin to imitate it. Each of these events is then viewed as precedent to production. Still other data are available to suggest that the ability of normal children to both comprehend and produce a specific language principle is similar. Children with language difficulties, however, may do somewhat better in comprehension than in production (Lucas, 1980).

Each of these viewpoints is reflected in available diagnostic procedures. Each is supportable to a degree by available information, yet each must be carefully studied to determine how it operates in any particular test. For example, Rees (1975) has differentiated *elicited imitation* from *spontaneous imitation*. During assessment using elicited imitation the child is required to imitate a model immediately after it has been presented ("Johnny, say, 'The girl chased the boy.'"). The rationale for such an approach is based on the notion that children's imitations reflect their knowledge of a particular rule. Thus, a child whose morphological development has not yet begun might be expected to reduce the utterance "The girl chased the boy" to "Girl chase boy." This might be considered meaningful imitation which, in turn, is thought to imply comprehension. Spontaneous imitation, on the other hand, occurs after the fact, with no prompting, and may or may not reflect comprehension by the child who is producing the imitation.

Available information regarding elicited imitation is in conflict. A child may process a stimulus and imitate it in some correct or reduced form. What process or processes are activated? Comprehension? Production? Or is there an interaction between the two? A great deal more information regarding normal children's performance on such tasks is needed to answer these questions. And information about the processing strategies of language-disordered children during elicited imitation is seriously lacking. Both formal and informal measures of elicited imitation can be useful, particularly when used to supplement direct measures of comprehension and/or production. One formal measure currently in preparation, which can also be used as an elicited imitation procedure, is the Miller-Yoder Test of Grammatical Comprehension (Miller and Yoder, 1972). The number of words per stimulus item is always five. Complexity varies when syntactic elements such as negation, possession, verb inflections, and the passive construction are measured. The total number of different words is small and only a single proposition is used in each stimulus. Clinicians frequently design their own elicited imitation tasks to examine a child's ability to imitate infrequently occurring constructions, constructions which did not appear during assessment, and/or to determine progress in remediation. If elicited imitation tests are constructed so that the stimuli isolate the language features of concern, and if scoring is designed so that clear decisions can be made, implementing such tasks is worthwhile.

Tests to measure comprehension ability are designed to determine the child's understanding of various lexical items or various linguistic rules. Children are usually asked to point to one of several objects or pictures, or to perform an action based on the input stimulus. For example, a child may be shown a picture of a girl chasing a boy and another of a boy chasing a girl. He or she might then be told: "Show me, 'The girl is chasing the boy.'" The Northwestern Syntax Screening Test (Lee, 1971) utilizes this approach. Alternatively, the child may be asked to respond to a request such as "Put the doll *behind* the house," by manipulating toys to reflect the spatial relationship specified in the stimulus utterance. The Vocabulary Comprehension Scale (Bangs, 1975) uses this type of approach.

Comprehension tests have been criticized from a number of standpoints. For example, the linguistic cues provided by the examiner frequently confound the rule being tested. Situational cues may also provide additional information and influence response choice. Stimuli are limited, especially in view of the fact that some language structures are quite difficult to place into a picture (consider, for example, "The boy knew the rock broke the window"). Finally, on comprehension tasks it is somewhat difficult to know when a child is just guessing.

As previously mentioned, there is disagreement about whether production lags behind comprehension and to what degree. The bulk of evaluation is, however, accomplished through language production analysis. Procedures available for measuring production vary in terms of the amount of structures imposed on the child as well as the nature of the task.

We have discussed elicited imitation tasks as one procedure for measuring production. *Delayed imitation* tasks also are implemented for production assessment. For example, the Northwestern Syntax Screening Test (Lee, 1971) includes a type of delayed imitation task. A child is shown, for example, two pictures. Without pointing, the examiner says, "The baby is sleeping. The baby is not sleeping." Then, based on the instructions, the examiner points to one of the pictures and says, "Now what's this picture?" The child is then expected to produce the appropriate utterance. Unlike a "pure" delayed imitation task, here the child must also select the appropriate stimulus to imitate. Question-answer formats, modeling, and sentence completion tasks represent other strategies which have been applied for production analysis. In some instances, nonsense words are used to determine whether children can apply certain linguistic rules ("Here is a deek. Now, here are two _____."). More recently, analyses of spontaneous language samples have been used to obtain representative measures of children's production abilities. We will return to the issues involved in evaluation of production elsewhere.

Variation in Child Language

An issue of critical importance to the understanding of language performance is that there is variability. Variability occurs among children as well as within a given child. Inexperienced clinicians may be more comfortable with an examination task that results in a specific score that translates into an age equivalency. For example, Kenn, age 3;6 years, may perform at the 3;0-year level on a particular test. The clinician might then be likely to say that Kenn is 6 months delayed on a particular dimension. This approach, however, is not without serious problems. Studies of normal children have indicated that although regularity exists, there is definite variation among children.

For example, Brown (1973) reported the order in which morphological inflections are likely to emerge, based on a longitudinal study of three children, Adam, Eve, and Sarah. Within these three children the order was not rigid. Children's language learning patterns seem to vary in other ways. Some children, in expressing early two- and three-word relationships, use an abundance of nouns as agents and locations. Their utterances are represented in examples such as "Box go chair" or "Put ball table." Other children use a different strategy to communicate similar meaning. They more often use pronouns in the positions where nouns might occur; for example, "This go here" or "Put that there." Such variation does not appear to be related to size of lexicon, and each type of child seems capable of using the opposite strategy on occasion. It is just that some children indicate a preference for one type of strategy or the other (Bloom et al., 1975). Such reports have led to the recognition that even at similar language levels, variation exists among children; variation which is systematic and unrelated to language adequacy.

Further consideration involving variation in child language can be illustrated with an example. As an examining clinician, you may observe Erica for a period of time and note that most of the time her utterances, although not grammatically complete, are four or five words long. You have heard utterances such as "Put big boy in chair" or "He push truck on bridge." Now you are interested in Erica's use of specific forms. You decide to try some elicited imitation to determine her ability to use certain function words and inflectional markings. Because she has four- and five-word utterances, you feel justified in presenting items of that length. Here is what might happen:

Your Stimulus	Erica's Response
The boy is fishing.	The boy fishing.
The baby is eating dinner.	Baby eating dinner.
Sue eats cereal.	Sue eats cereal.
Sue puts some bread on the table.	Sue put bread on table.

Study of Erica's responses reveals that articles and third person singular (-s) inflections are used in some sentences, but not others. What is going on here? You obviously have not violated her language abilities in terms of length, so what is different? The explanation may be found, at least in part, in the notion of linguistic constraints. And this notion serves as the basis for at least some variation we observe in individual children. As children begin to learn a new language rule, its use may first be observed at the expense of another language rule. Thus, whereas Erica could produce four- and five-word utterances, she did so with few function words or inflectional markings. As these forms begin to appear in her language, we might expect they would do so in utterances that are shorter than four words in length. It is as if the language system cannot simultaneously deal with both length and greater complexity. It is constrained. This notion is sometimes explained as follows: new forms will first be expressed through old content; or conversely, old forms will be used to express new content. Given this premise, clinicians will want to look at a given child fully expecting variation, to examine this variation for systematicity, and to explain variation through the emerging language system.

With the knowledge that variation may be logical and expected both within and between children, it is easier to see why the use of age equivalency scores alone must be viewed as a practice replete with limitations. It just is not an easy task to paint a picture of the semantic, syntactic, and pragmatic abilities at any given age. The continuum of "normalcy" is probably far greater than a few months deviation. Of course, one task in diagnosis is to determine when deviation from normal is sufficient to warrant attention.

CLASSIFYING THE LANGUAGE-DISORDERED CHILD

Various labels have been applied to the child with developmental delays in the language areas. The choice of a label frequently reflects the clinician's orientation to language difficulties; and these orientations may be classified under two rather broad categories. First, children may be classified on the basis of etiologic considerations. Second, they may be classified according to descriptions of the language behaviors they exhibit. There does not appear to be general consensus about the most appropriate classification terminology.

Etiologic Considerations

Descriptions of children based on etiologic considerations are concerned with the possible cause of the language disorder. For example, mental retardation, neurological impairment, hearing loss, emotional disturbance, and autism can interfere with the normal acquisition of language. When behaviors in areas additional to the language impairment are consistent with one of these labels, the particular term may be used to categorize the child. Labels applied to children based on these precipitating factors are used to categorize the whole child, and therefore, do not apply exclusively to the language impairment itself. The primary difficulty with this approach lies in the fact that language behaviors within any one category can vary considerably. At the same time, the language characteristics of children given different clinical labels can sometimes be more similar than their separate labels would lead one to expect. For example, to say that a child is language disordered secondary to mental retardation may be accurate; it is not, however, descriptive of the particular child's difficulties with the language system. Even with the same "degree" of retardation, individual children do not necessarily exhibit the same comprehension and production abilities in any of the language components. The same holds true for other etiologic labels such as hearing loss, neurological impairment, emotional disturbance, and autism.

Another categorical label based on etiologic factors is that most often termed *auditory processing disturbance* (or *specific abilities orientation,* Bloom and Lahey, 1978). The orientation of clinicians who use this label to refer to the language-disordered child is based on an attempt to identify those behaviors thought to be necessary for language learning. Within this framework, such behaviors include aspects of processing such as auditory memory, discrimination, and association. Clinicians with this orientation diagnose children's language difficulties through measures included in such instruments as the Revised Illinois Test of Psycholinguistic Abilities (Kirk et al., 1968) and portions of the Clinical Evaluation of Language Functions (Semel and Wiig, 1980). From such evaluations, strengths and weaknesses of a child's processing abilities are identified. Intervention then focuses on remediation of the weak areas.

The "auditory processing" approach to diagnosis of language disorders is shrouded in controversy. Obviously, children must use processes such as discrimination, memory, association, an so on in language learning. The precise contribution of these to the language disorder remains unclear. For example, deficits in auditory memory, processing of multisensory inputs and processing of rapid auditory signals have been reported to exist in language-disordered children. These findings then have been viewed as causative factors for the language disorder. In fact, these deficits may be due to the language disorder itself, and may not be the cause. In other words, children may perform poorly on these tasks because of a higher order language disturbance, rather than the reverse. The literature supports neither the contention that these processing abilities are entirely separate behaviors, nor the contention that they are prerequisites for language learning.

Etiologic categories may be difficult to avoid altogether, particularly when they may have a bearing on whether or not a child qualifies for state or federally funded services. For the purposes of diagnosis, however, it would seem that clinicians should focus on measures that will allow them to determine what children know about language and what they are ready to learn. Intervention programs can then be based on this information.

More recently, clinicians have moved from a search for etiologic factors to a concern for the knowledge a child has about language and how this knowledge functions in comprehension and production. In diagnosis, therefore, one focus is on obtaining as complete a description as is possible of the child's language system. This description then lends itself to specific intervention goals based on the child's meaningful use of language. Even within such descriptions, however, various labels come to be applied to the child

Descriptions of Language Behaviors

with language learning difficulties. These include language impairment, language delay, language disorder, language disability, and language deviance.[2] Although some professionals may apply these terms selectively to indicate a distinction between qualitative and quantitative differences in language development, most often the terms are used interchangeably. For our purposes we have elected to use the term *language disorder* as a descriptive term to encompass those language behaviors which are different from those expected at a given chronological age. It should be noted that the term is descriptive, not based on etiologic considerations.

LANGUAGE EXAMINATION

Goals of Language Examination

There are three reasons we conduct an evaluation of a child's language abilities. First, clinicians want to determine that a problem in language learning exists. Second, given difficulties in language learning, clinicians want to insure that diagnostic procedures provide specific goals for language intervention and a certain amount of insight into the remediation techniques which might facilitate achievement of these goals. Finally, clinicians use diagnostic procedures to determine the progress being made in intervention, to determine if the remediation approach is effective, and/or to obtain possible suggestions for modifications of goals or implementation techniques. The concern in the present chapter is primarily with the first two of these goals.

General Considerations in Diagnosis

Hearing Screening

All children who are evaluated for language problems must have a screening test for hearing acuity. Because middle ear pathology is so frequent in children, they need additional testing to evaluate middle ear function (see Audition and Auditory Perceptual Skills in Chapter 2 for details). Although the exact degree of hearing loss that can inhibit normal language learning is not known, there is a professional responsibility to identify the presence of hearing loss and to make referral to the appropriate professional(s) when children fail screening tests.

---

[2] It should be noted that the terms *childhood aphasia* and *congenital aphasia* are sometimes used as well. These terms can be misleading for two reasons. First, aphasia is a term implying loss of language sometime after a period of normal acquisition. However, this term has often been applied to children who experience language learning difficulties at the outset. Second, the condition of aphasia is the result of demonstrable brain damage. Yet, when applied to children who show language learning difficulties, such damage has sometimes only been suspected, not documented. For these reasons, use of the term congenital aphasia should probably be avoided, and the label childhood aphasia should be reserved for the child who incurs head trauma at some point in his or her development and is left with residual language disturbance. These children do not represent developmental language problems and therefore will not be considered individually in our discussion.

Clinicians must also determine that children have an adequate speech mech- *Examination of the*
anism. As in the case of hearing loss, the exact degree to which structural *Speech Mechanism*
and functional deviations of the speech mechanism contribute to language
acquisition is not explicitly known. Clinicians must be cognizant of these
factors, however, for necessary referral and possible remediation (see Chapter 2 for details).

As previously mentioned, diagnosis of language disorders in children is not *Cognitive Assessment*
complete without information about the child's level of cognitive function-
ing. Such information is often obtained through informal observations of the
child's play behavior. For example, if during play the child made Pla-Doh
cookies and then pretended to eat one, the clinician would have one observation of his or her readiness for two word combinations; that is, the child
demonstrated a nonlinguistic ability, symbolic play, that has been found to
be correlated with two-word utterance usage.

Sometimes it is necessary to construct specific cognitive tasks in order
to obtain appropriate data. The Scales of Infant Psychological Development
(Uzgiris and Hunt, 1975) provide specific procedures for examination of
children in the sensorimotor period of cognitive development (see also
Dunst, 1980). However, assessment of the cognitive abilities commensurate
with the preoperational period might require the clinician to examine the
child's spontaneous play behaviors, using as a basis the clinician's knowledge of this developmental period. Play analysis scales such as those developed by Nicolich (1977) and Lowe and Costello (1976) are also useful.

Children with language learning problems may also exhibit sensorimotor
and play behaviors that fall below age level. In these cases it seems best to
refer the child to a clinical psychologist for formal assessment of intellectual
ability. Because these children have known deficits in the language area it
is most often recommended that they be given nonverbal intelligence tests
such as the Leiter International Performance Scale (Arthur, 1952).

Interestingly enough, a number of children with developmental delays
in language may perform quite well on formal, nonverbal intelligence tests,
but exhibit difficulties when confronted with specific Piagetian tasks. Such
varied performance may be related to the nature of the tasks involved in
each. For example, a language-impaired child may do quite well with visual
tasks such as matching shapes and colors, tasks frequently used in nonverbal
assessment of quite young children, yet demonstrate difficulty with tasks
requiring symbolic representation (as in pretending to eat a Pla-Doh cookie).

Speech-language pathologists are also responsible for addressing other as- *Assessing Other*
pects of the child's performance. These include the phonological system of *Abilities*
the child (as discussed by Schwartz in Chapter 4) as well as suprasegmental
components.

Many clinicians, especially during evaluation of preschool age children, are interested in performance in other areas as well. For example, assessment of gross and fine motor skills, personal and social skills, and visual perception abilities are often included (see Chapter 2 for additional details). Tests designed to measure such skills include the Revised Denver Developmental Screening Test (Frankenburg et al., 1970), Developmental Test of Visual Perception (Frostig, 1961), the Motor-Free Visual Perception Test (Colarusso and Hammill, 1972), and the Inventory of Early Development (Brigance, 1978). The decision to include examination procedures such as these may be based on information provided in the case history, observations made during the actual evaluation, and/or on the need for data to substantiate referral to other professionals.

Avoiding Overassessment

It may seem paradoxical now to offer a word of caution regarding overassessment. Both comprehension and production should be evaluated with a concern for all language components, and peripheral components such as hearing, the oral structure, and cognition must be considered. However, it is imperative to approach the diagnostic task with clearly delineated objectives. To administer a number of tests to a child without a specific reason for each can result in excessive redundancy and/or unusable information.

Setting and Context

The setting in which observations of children occur is of critical importance. For example, it is logical to assume that children might use a greater range of their language capabilities in a setting familiar to them. Therefore, ideally, examination of language would occur in both clinical and home environments. Given that home visits are frequently impossible, clinicians might want to spend at least a portion of examination time observing the child interacting with people who are familiar; (e.g., a parent, a sibling, a friend). For our own time with the child we would want to insure a play environment with toys appropriate to the child's age and likely interest. These situations, created to allow for as natural and relaxed communication as possible, impose less structure than do settings in which a child is seated and administered standardized tests. There are advantages to each.

A setting with minimal structure is created for the purpose of evaluating language behaviors which might naturally occur. The child has the opportunity, if able, to verbally interact, to choose topics of conversation which are easiest to retrieve from memory, to initiate as well as respond, and to direct activities as well as to follow the lead of others. With such minimal structure, certain infrequent language behaviors may not occur and the information obtained may need to be supplemented through other means. The language that is observed has occurred within a social context, however, permitting an observation of the child's pragmatic skills as well as his or her command over the semantic and syntactic components of language. Such a setting is currently recommended as the optimal one for obtaining a complete language picture by numerous researchers (see, for example, Bloom and Lahey, 1978; Crystal et al., 1976; Miller, 1981; Tyack and Gottsleben, 1974). 1974).

Settings with greater structure imposed include those used for formal testing. Although clinicians lose flexibility for interpretation of results, they gain information regarding a child's performance in a formalized setting and can determine whether the child's responses are similar to those of other children who have been tested under the same circumstances. Formal observations have been criticized for the lack of information they provide. Some of the criticism is misplaced. For example, most formal tests have taken years to develop and thus focus on features of language that, according to more recent research, no longer seem to be the most appropriate features to assess. However, this is not a weakness of the formal test format itself. A more valid criticism is that the structure imposed by a formal test provides less opportunity to observe how the child puts language to use in everyday communication.

Time

How much time is provided? — two hours on one day, several hours over several days, or is the clinician perhaps unlimited in the time needed? The allotted time will be yet another consideration as you approach the diagnostic process. In the time available, what observations under what conditions will provide the greatest amount of pertinent data?

Case History

In many clinical settings parents are required to complete questionnaires before their child is seen. From these questionnaires clinicians may gain certain insights that might influence their diagnostic protocols. For example, if the clinician knows Peter is being followed by the audiological service, appropriate reports can be requested and audiological screening can be bypassed. If Peter is 3;2 and using only 12 to 15 words, the clinician might opt to plan cognitive tasks appropriate to the sensorimotor period, no formal production measures, but several informal and formal comprehension tasks.

Some diagnosticians like to make a parent contact by telephone after receipt of the questionnaire and before the child's appointment. The purpose of these contacts may vary. Perhaps the clinician has noted in the questionnaire that Peter has been previously seen by a neurologist. In this case, the clinician would want to request a copy of the report. At times information supplemental to the questionnaire is desired. Still other contacts are made to request the parent to bring in a list of specific language output, (e.g., items in Peter's lexicon, or to allow Peter to bring several of his favorite toys for play). Finally, at times the contact is made to explain the procedures in which the child will be engaged. This can serve two purposes: 1) to reduce the time that is needed at the outset for such explanations; and 2) to reduce any parental anxiety regarding the unknown procedures.

SELECTION OF LANGUAGE MEASURES

As we have indicated, certain general considerations and prior information will help to determine the appropriate examination protocol. Each child is unique and speech-language pathologists must approach the diagnostic process with this in mind. This will promote diagnostic efficiency, eliminate redundancy, and prevent administering the same language battery to all children. Examination procedures are generally divided into those which are standardized and those which are not. We have alluded to these in our prior discussion on setting considerations, but let us take a closer look now.

Norm-Referenced Measures

Examination procedures which allow a direct comparison of one child's behaviors to those of other children are norm-referenced measures. The comparison may be based on age, where a particular child's behaviors are assessed and the score received represents the average age at which most children demonstrate similar behaviors. For example, the Peabody Picture Vocabulary Test (PPVT), (Dunn, 1965, 1980) yields a raw score which is then converted into a mental age equivalent. If the child you are testing is 4;8, and the score on this measure yields a mental age of 3;6, it would mean that this child's ability to function on this particular measure is more like the average performance of children 3;6 years of age.

Norm-referenced measures may also include a percentile rank which indicates how the child you are assessing ranks in comparison to age-equivalent peers. If, for example, a child's PPVT raw score converts to the 30th percentile, it would indicate that 70 percent of the children at the same age would perform at a higher level on this particular measure. Other examples of norm-referenced tests are included in Table 3.2.

Norm-referenced scores must be considered in light of the sample of children on whom the normative data were obtained. In other words, you must be sure that the normative data were obtained on children from the same socioeconomic and cultural background as the child you are testing. If not, the interpretation of results is questionable. When tests are appropriately normed, however, the age-equivalent and/or percentile rankings of norm-referenced measures provide a rich source of information for meeting one goal of diagnosis—to identify the existence of a problem. These two factors, normative comparison and determining the existence of a problem, are the major strengths of standardized, norm-referenced tests.

Norm-referenced measures may have certain weaknesses. By their very nature, standardized language measures typically violate the normal flow of linguistic interchange. The rules of face-to-face conversation (i.e., discourse) are not in play, and there is a gross lack of contextually based information. Therefore, the nonlinguistic and linguistic cues typically available to children are missing and standardized measures are not thought to yield the most representative sample of a child's language abilities. Another weakness of

Table 3.2. Examples of norm-referenced examination procedures

Norm-referenced measure	Type of task(s)	Normative ages	Dimension(s) examined
Test for Auditory Comprehension of Language (Carrow, 1973)	Comprehension	3–6	Semantics, syntax
Peabody Picture Vocabulary Test (Dunn, 1965/1980)	Comprehension	2;6–18;0	Semantics
Full Range Picture Vocabulary Test (Ammons and Ammons, 1948)	Comprehension	2;0–35;0	Semantics
Boehm Test of Basic Concepts (Boehm, 1969)	Comprehension	Grade Levels K–2nd	Semantics
Miller-Yoder Test of Grammatical Comprehension (Miller and Yoder, 1972)	Comprehension	5;6–21;5[a]	Syntax
Assessment of Children's Language Comprehension (Foster, Giddan, and Stark, 1973)	Comprehension	3;0–6;5	Syntax
Northwestern Syntax Screening Test (Lee, 1971)	Comprehension, production (delayed imitation)	3;0–7;11	Syntax
ITPA Verbal Expression Subtest (Kirk, McCarthy, and Kirk, 1968)	Elicited imitation	2;7–10;1	Semantics
Stephens Oral Language Screening Test (Stephens, 1977)	Elicited imitation	4;4–7;0	Semantics, syntax
Carrow Elicited Language Inventory (Carrow, 1974)	Elicited imitation	3;0–7;11	Syntax
Developmental Sentence Scoring (Lee, 1974)	Production	2;0–6;11	Syntax
Michigan Picture Language Inventory (Wolski and Lerea, 1962)	Comprehension, production	4;0–6;0	Semantics, syntax
Sequenced Inventory of Communication Development (Hedrick, Prather, and Tobin, 1975)	Comprehension, production	0;4–4;0	Semantics, syntax
Test of Language Development (Newcomer and Hammill, 1977)	Comprehension, production, elicited imitation	4;0–8;11	Semantics, syntax
Test of Adolescent Language (Hammill, et al., 1980)	Comprehension production	Grade Levels 7–12	Semantics, syntax

[a] Experimental data based on mentally retarded subjects.

these measures rests in the fact that standardized procedures typically are not designed with language intervention specifically in mind. Through inspection of the child's performance on a standardized test, it will be possible to identify several features with which the child may be having difficulty. However, few if any of these features will have been tested in sufficient detail to allow you to determine the specific degree of difficulty the child is experiencing. Therefore, choosing the feature that should serve as the initial focus of intervention can be a problem. Nonstandardized, criterion-referenced observations assist us in this regard.

Criterion-Referenced Measures

Criterion-referenced measures are used to gain information about a child's ability to perform specific language functions or tasks. Thus, they provide information about the nature of the child's language system relative to certain specified skills. The purpose of criterion-referenced measures is not to compare a given child with other children. Rather, it is to determine how well a particular language behavior is established based on a preestablished standard. For example, Bloom (1970) used the frequency of occurrence of a particular semantic-syntactic relation as a criterion. Her determination of productivity of such a rule was five occurrences of the particular relation by a child during 5 or more hours of observation. Brown (1973), in a study of inflectional acquisition, set 90 percent use of a particular marker in contexts where the marker is required in adult language as his criterion for acquisition.

In day-to-day clinical activities, clinicians frequently set a criterion of productivity for various communicative behaviors to determine when they have succeeded in remediating a particular behavior and to determine when it is time to move on to another goal. For example, it might be decided that when James is using /t/ in his spontaneous speech with 80 percent accuracy, he has demonstrated an adequate level of usage. Any criterion-referenced observation, therefore, compares observations of a particular child with preset quantitative criteria. Two frequently used procedures which are criterion-referenced are *nonstandardized elicitation* and *language sampling*.

Elicitation involves constructing situations in which a child is most likely to exhibit or demonstrate comprehension of a linguistic feature of interest. At times, this feature may be one which occurs infrequently in normal communication and that the clinician has not had the opportunity to observe. At other times, elicitation procedures may be used to assess intervention progress. Elicitation tasks allow clinicians to determine if given rules are productive in a short period of time. Specific situations may be devised to check a child's ability to use questions, negation, specific semantic-syntactic relations, etc. For example, if interested in a child's use of recurrence in two-word utterances, the clinician might set up a tea party situation in which the child might be expected to request "More tea" or "More cookie." (For a more complete discussion of elicitation procedures, see Miller, 1981, Chapter 5.)

Obtaining a sample of a child's spontaneous language is another non-standardized, criterion-referenced procedure. Explicit approaches to language sampling have been put forth by Miller (1981), Bloom and Lahey (1978), and others. In language sampling, clinicians generally construct situations which closely resemble natural settings. They follow the child's lead in both conversation and activity. The clinician's own dialogue is kept to a minimum to provide the child maximum opportunity to use the full range of his or her language system. Whenever possible, the sample is obtained in a variety of settings, such as in the waiting room with a parent, walking down the hall, during play, etc. Language sampling is tape recorded. Generally, a sample of 100 spontaneous utterances is considered the minimum number needed to obtain a representative picture of a child's speech. With less verbal children, this level of sampling may not be possible in the time allotted. The minimum period of interaction with the child is 30 minutes (Bloom and Lahey, 1978).

Utterances are transcribed from the tape recording immediately following the assessment time. Utterances transcribed from a portion of a language sample are reported in Table 3.3. Note that in the left hand column the input to the child is tabulated together with the context in which utterances occur. The child's utterances are in the right column.

There are a number of procedures available for analyzing language samples. The choice of procedures will be based on the general level of language development reflected in the sample as well as the linguistic features which

Table 3.3.   Portion of a transcription obtained from spontaneous language sampling procedures

Clinician utterances and nonlinguistic context (in parentheses)	Child utterances
(Kevin places car by the gas pumps)	This needs gas.
Joyce: It must be empty.	
(K trying to stick the gas nozzle in the car)	This can't go in.
J: Maybe you could pretend.	
(K picking up another car)	I gonna use another one.
J: That's a good idea.	
(K putting car in gas station)	It goes in here.
(K gets up and moves to the doll house; holding up a toy chair)	I found a chair.
J: There are lots of things in there.	
(K sorting through the furniture)	This a bed.
	This a potty.
(K holding up a doll)	Look at the daddy.
J: I wonder where the mommy is?	The mommy in the bedroom.
(K pointing in the house)	See.
J: Yeah. There she is.	
(K moving mommy and daddy to the table)	They gonna eat supper.
(K moving a cup to the table)	I make a good supper.

Child: Kevin, age 3;9. Clinician: Joyce.

Table 3.4. Examples of locative action utterances analyzed according to the procedures of Bloom and Lahey (1978).

Content category: Locative action   Child's name: Jeanette   Age: 3;4   Date of sample: 3/2/82

	Form analysis								Use analysis	
	Subject-verb-complement constituents				Expected constituent omitted					
	Included		Expected		S	V	C	Comments	Context	Function
Utterances	2	3+	2	3+						
4 baby go in here		3		3					CH-i[a]	Comment
16 put it on	2		2						CH-I	Demand
21 my daddy go work		3		3					RQ+	
30 not go in car	2		2		0				RS+	
37 he going doctor		3		3					CH-I	Comment
53 it not come off	2			3					CH-I	Comment
62 mommy in school	2			3		0		−Verb	CH-I	Comment
69 put baby in bed		3		3					CH-I	Demand
83 I fall down	2		2						CH-I	Comment
102 potty in here	2			3		0		−Verb	CH-I	Comment
Frequency of utterances (productivity)	6	4	3	7						

Proportion of utterances with expected constituent included (achievement) $4 \div 7 = 0.57$

Coordinated categories (utterances that include two constituents plus another content category)

Nonexistence	Rejection	Denial	Recurrence	Attribution	Possession	Quantity	Time	Mood	Dative	Specification	Causality	Conjunction	Wh-Question	Place	"a"	Verb plus preposition
		$\frac{not}{30}$			$\frac{my}{21}$		$\frac{ing}{37}$									$\frac{in}{4}$ $\frac{on}{16}$ 30 62 69 102

[a] CH-I, Child-initiated utterance; RQ, response to a question; RS, response to a statement. Appropriateness (+) and Inappropriateness (−) of comments also indicated.

are of primary interest. A sample work sheet used in language sampling set forth by Bloom and Lahey (1978) is presented in Table 3.4. This example demonstrates the analysis of 10 utterances, placed in the locative action content category, which were part of the 100 utterances obtained from Jeannette. Form (syntactic) and use (pragmatic) analysis is also possible. Syntax is examined with regard to the number of subject-verb-complement structures included by the child in comparison to how many are expected in adult usage. The semantic categories that are reflected or deleted in the child's speech are also noted. Context is reported as child-initiated (CH-I), response to a question (RQ), or response to a statement (RS). The appropriateness, or lack thereof, is indicated with plus (+) and minus (−) designations, respectively. Finally, the function of the child's utterance is indicated (request, comment, command, etc.).

The strengths of such a criterion-referenced procedure include the facts that context can be considered (linguistic and nonlinguistic information), and that analysis of the semantic, syntactic, and pragmatic components of language is possible, yielding a more representative picture of the child's language system. This information, in turn, leads to a specific intervention plan, thus meeting a second goal of diagnosis. Weaknesses of this type of criterion-referenced procedure are that it can be time consuming and generally requires a high degree of clinical skill. The nature of the information obtained, however, generally offsets such weaknesses. In the hands of an experienced clinician, language sampling is well worth the time expended and can be used in lieu of, or in combination with, standardized norm-referenced measures.

Language sampling and analysis procedures are not necessarily criterion referenced. Some procedures do not offer the precision necessary to assess the degree to which the child has attained a particular linguistic skill. Other procedures, such as Developmental Sentence Scoring (Lee, 1974), actually serve as norm-referenced measures.

Whether a clinician decides to use norm-referenced measures, criterion-referenced measures, or a combination of both will depend, in part, on the age of the child as well as the information obtained from the parent questionnaire. Although the information derived may be similar using any of these measures, sufficient variation in language behavior exists to warrant some special consideration based on age.

EXAMINATION STRATEGIES

We are, fortunately, in an era in which there is a great deal of emphasis on early identification of language-disordered children. It is not unusual, therefore, for speech-language pathologists to be asked to examine children 2 years of age or younger. Clinicians are also referred older children who are

Examining the Very Young or Prelinguistic Child

only minimally verbal, if at all. Examination of these children requires that we determine the prelinguistic behaviors children exhibit which are related to later language learning.

Based on our earlier discussion, one important determiner of language acquisition for children in this age group are the cognitive attainments of the sensorimotor period of development. Examination of very young or minimally verbal children is, therefore, dependent on a measure of these skills.

Before meaningful linguistic communication, children use gestures, which may or may not be accompanied by vocalization, to direct and control their environments. That is, they use gestural behavior to request or reject an object, to request information (e.g., pointing to an object which the adult then names), to get attention, and so on. These early prelinguistic behaviors are viewed as precursors to later language abilities when such intents are expressed through verbalization (Bates et al., 1975). Consequently, the intent to communicate through gestural behavior will be an important observation to be made in prelinguistic children. Such behaviors should not be observed out of context.

Toys appropriate to the child's age, as well as toys which are broken, out of reach, and/or hard to open should be included. Interactional style will be important as well. The clinician will want to allow the child to direct the activities. Clinicians may be tempted to ask many questions, in the hope of eliciting responses. Questions are appropriate at times, particularly when looking for signs of comprehension (e.g., Where's the *truck*, Jack?). Generally, however, questions should be kept to a minimum. By their very nature, questions take the lead away from the child.

Standardized measures of prelinguistic development frequently depend on an interview with the parent or guardian. The Receptive-Expressive Emergent Language Scale (REEL), (Bzoch and League, 1971) uses such a technique in an attempt to sample communicative behaviors between birth and 3 years of age. The Sequenced Inventory of Communicative Development (SICD), (Hendrick et al., 1975) samples similar behaviors through 4 years of age, through a combination of parental interview and clinical observation. The Vineland Social Maturity Scale (Doll, 1965) and the Verbal Language Development Scale (Mecham, 1958, 1971) are two other measures based on parental interview. A promising measure of the communicative behaviors relevant to the sensorimotor period has become available. This is the Initial Communication Processes Scale (ICPS), (Schery and Glover, 1982). Snyder (1981) has suggested that these procedures be evaluated with the following questions in mind:

1. Does the measure sample those prelinguistic and early linguistic behaviors which are basic to communicative development?
2. Does the measure consider the communicative efficiency of the child's efforts?

3. Does the measure distinguish between signals and early symbols?
4. Does the measure look for changes in the use of single-word utterances?

It is most likely that after a standardized measure is chosen, informal strategies will be needed to supplement your findings. For example, for the child producing single-word utterances, the category system of McShane (1980) might be employed to determine whether a child's sample reflects a variety of communicative functions.

Preschool children suspected of having a language disorder are frequently examined when they are talking, but are doing so at a level more like that of younger normal children. In a review of the literature comparing normal and language-disordered children, Leonard (1979) found that language-disordered children often follow the same developmental pattern as normal children in the semantic, syntactic, and pragmatic components of language. They do so at a slower rate, and the degree to which each component is delayed may vary. For example, language-disordered children may show a greater lag in the syntactic area than the semantic and pragmatic areas. Clinicians will also want to determine the degree of delay in each language component through both comprehension and production measures.

Examining the Verbal, Preschool Age Child

   The language abilities of these children lend themselves to numerous formal examination procedures. For example, comprehension of vocabulary can be assessed through measures such as the Peabody Picture Vocabulary Test (Dunn, 1965, 1980) and the Vocabulary Comprehension Scale (Bangs, 1975), of syntax through the Miller-Yoder Test of Grammatical Comprehension (Miller and Yoder, 1972), of semantics and syntax through the Test for Auditory Comprehension of Language (Carrow, 1973), as well as other available measures.

   Formal production measures include the Carrow Elicited Language Inventory (Carrow, 1974) for assessing syntax, the Grammatic Completion subtest of the Test of Language Development (Newcomer and Hammill, 1977) for morphology, the Environmental Language Inventory (MacDonald and Horstmeier, 1978) for semantic relations, and the Expressive One-Word Picture Vocabulary Test (Gardner, 1979) for vocabulary. Language sampling procedures also are quite appropriate for the preschool age, verbal child. Formal procedures include the Developmental Sentence Scoring of Lee (1974); the Language Sampling, Analysis and Training, by Tyack and Gottsleben (1974); and the Language, Assessment, Remediation and Training Procedure (LARSP) of Crystal et al. (1976). With the exception of the LARSP, which includes some assessment of the pragmatic area, these sampling procedures focus solely on the syntactic domain. In order to assess other components of language, clinicians often apply analyses employed by normal-child language researchers to the language samples of their patients. For example, the communicative act categories of Dore (1978) have been used by some clinicians as one measure of a child's pragmatic abilities.

Bloom and Lahey's (1978) procedures for analysis allow for a thorough view of a child's semantic-syntactic relations and certain pragmatic skills. As previously mentioned, their procedures result in well-defined intervention goals as well. Prutting and Kirchner (1982) have compiled a checklist of pragmatic skills which can also be observed during language sampling to provide for a more thorough look at this language dimension. Their list of observations include specific pragmatic behaviors with expected age ranges for normal performance. Finally, an interesting and uncomplicated approach to pragmatic assessment is contained in the "peanut butter" procedures outlined by Creaghead et al. (1980). Their procedures, based on an interaction focusing on a jar of peanut butter, knife, and crackers, allow for observation of a number of pragmatic behaviors such as requesting an object or action, commenting, initiating, maintaining, and changing conversational topic, requesting clarification, and protesting. In all, they provide a checklist of 20 such behaviors which may be observed in this activity centering around peanut butter.

Informal assessment of cognitive skills for this age group requires observation of those behaviors consistent with Piaget's preoperational period (2;0 to 4;0 years). These may include certain conservation, perspective taking, and classification tasks. Children at this age level are most often able to perform sufficiently well to be referred for standardized, nonverbal measures as well. These procedures, accomplished by a trained psychometrist or psychologist, include the performance section of the Wechsler Intelligence Scale for Children—Revised (Wechsler, 1974) and the Leiter International Performance Scale (Arthur, 1952).

The tests included in this section represent but a few of those available for examining the verbal, preschool age child. As you can see, because of the varied formal and informal measures available, these children are relatively easily served. That is, numerous avenues are available for a comprehensive look at their language abilities. Such is not so much the case, however, in attempting to assess the verbal, school age child.

Examining the Verbal, School Age Child

Some children, although somewhat delayed in rate of acquisition, perform sufficiently well in their environments that they are not suspected of having language difficulties until they are unsuccessful in their early, formal education. By the time they are seen for language examination they may be 7 or 8 years of age or perhaps even older. Many times these children are judged by educators as "learning disabled." These children present special diagnostic problems and frequently require the use of our most creative clinical skills. Their language deficits often represent difficulties with the more subtle aspects of our language: advanced syntactic complexity, metalinguistic awareness, and the ability to deal with figurative language.

The child in school has typically achieved the semantic relations discussed previously. Syntactic analysis now assumes greater focus. The Developmental Sentence Scoring (Lee, 1974) or the Language Sampling, Analysis and Training (Tyack and Gottsleben, 1974) procedures are sometimes used to assess these children. However, each of these procedures is somewhat limited in terms of measurements of advanced syntactic complexity. Portions of the Clinical Evaluation of Language Function (Semil and Wiig, 1980) also assess syntactic complexity. This measure also attempts to determine the older child's abilities in areas such as auditory processing, sequencing, and memory. How these abilities relate to overall language remains controversial. Norms are reported by grade level as opposed to age. The Test of Adolescent Language (Hammill et al., 1980) provides a standardized measure of school age children's comprehension and production of syntax and vocabulary. The Fullerton Language Test for Adolescents (Thorum, 1980) provides preliminary norms for its subtests which sample areas ranging from the ability to follow oral commands to the ability to identify homonyms. Each of these tests includes sections that require metalinguistic (e.g., dividing words into syllables) and figurative language (e.g., comprehension of idioms) skills. Pragmatic abilities, however, are not considered.

A spontaneous language sample is probably still the most useful approach to examination of older children, particularly when the clinician seeks to determine syntactic weaknesses. Analysis depends on the clinician's knowledge of advanced syntactic abilities. (The reader is referred to Karmiloff-Smith, 1979.) Although there are relatively few data available on older children's syntactic abilities, one of the most useful guides for analyzing language samples for syntactic structure has been offered by Paul (1981). Language sampling procedures for this age group also vary. Older children interact more conversationally and no longer require toys for focus. Pictures depicting various occurrences and open-ended questions such as "What did you watch on TV last night?" can be used to engage the child in dialogue for the purposes of language sampling.

The previously mentioned checklist of pragmatic attainments (Prutting and Kirchner, in press) provides information at levels through adulthood. The advanced levels include numerous discourse behaviors appropriate for the school age child from both verbal and nonverbal perspectives.

The Piagetian cognitive skills of these children, depending on their ages, are represented in the concrete and formal operations stages. A complete cognitive assessment of these children is best completed by referral to a psychologist skilled in the previously mentioned formal intelligence procedures. In view of their less limited language abilities, these children can also be administered cognitive scales that are not exclusively nonverbal; for example, the Stanford-Binet Intelligence Scale (Terman and Merrill, 1960).

Parent-Child Interaction

In the past decade, numerous studies have been completed to evaluate the influence of the verbal environment on children's language acquisition. There is evidence to suggest that language-disordered children are not always exposed to the rich language environment to which normally developing children are exposed. It is speculated that the nature of the child's language disorder precludes normal interaction with his or her environment. For example, a mother may begin interacting with her child by providing the same input as that provided to a normal child. As the language difficulties emerge, however, the mother may cease to provide as rich an environment for the child. This reduction in quality and quantity of interaction is thought to be due to the reduced responsiveness of the language-disordered child. The influence of the disorder changes the nature of the mother's input.

Emphasis on input has resulted in the inclusion of parents, siblings, and peers in interactional settings with the child during assessment. Such interactions serve a number of purposes. First, the data compiled may be quite a rich source for language sample analysis. We have mentioned earlier that such samples are ideally collected within a variety of settings, and with individuals with whom the child may be most familiar. Second, the data may be used to analyze the input typically received by the child. Such analysis can then be shared with the parent(s). Parents can be helped to understand why their input is such as it is. The analyses can then be used to determine goals for family intervention; that is, specific ways family members' input may be modified to enhance treatment procedures. Some language intervention models make explicit use of parents as intervention agents and parents become an active part of the comprehensive language program provided for the child. Such programs have met with quite favorable success (see, for example, Fey et al., 1978).

INTERPRETING THE DATA

After the clinician has gathered the necessary information about a patient and has scored and analyzed the data, the next step is to closely inspect the results in order to answer the following questions:

1. Does a language problem exist?
2. What is the cognitive status of the child?
3. To what degree, and in what ways, is comprehension difficult for this child?
4. To what degree, and in what ways, is production difficult for this child?
5. Are there speech or hearing variables involved?
6. Do the behaviors of this child indicate audiological, psychological, and/or medical (otolaryngological, neurological) referral?
7. In what type of intervention program should this child be placed (for example: group, individual or both)?
8. Should the parent(s) or other family members be involved in the program?

9. What are the specific goals for language intervention?
10. What procedures will most likely result in achievement of these goals?
11. What is the prognosis for attaining normal language competence?

This last question, of course, will depend on the relationship between the cognitive and linguistic status of the child, organic and environmental factors which may exist, as well as the specific nature and degree of the language disorder.

Once the clinician is satisfied that these issues have been addressed, interpretation to the parent is in order. This topic has been addressed in Chapters 1 and 10. It is important to emphasize that the clinician must approach this task with a great deal of empathy. Webster (1977) has cited four functions which the clinician may need to serve during interactions with family members. These include: 1) providing information; 2) receiving information; 3) clarifying attitudes and feelings regarding the child and his or her disorder; and 4) providing tools for experimenting with behavioral change. Each function requires a great deal of clinical skill, and each may be necessary during the reporting period with the parent(s).

At the beginning of the chapter we introduced you to a hypothetical child, Kent. In the Appendix (this chapter) you will find a tentative plan which might be considered appropriate to his diagnostic evaluation. Such plans reflect decisions you make before seeing a given child and they are colored by your own biases regarding language analysis. Each clinician may vary somewhat in the plans that are devised. Regardless of our viewpoint, we must be prepared to alter these plans if the additional information gained from the parent interview and from observing the child during the first few minutes of the examination suggests that the original impressions of the child were off the mark. It is likely, however, that with sufficient forethought, concern for the child and implementation of solid clinical knowledge and skill, clinicians share the goal of obtaining a comprehensive picture of the child.

ACKNOWLEDGMENTS

We would like to express our gratitude to Joyce Browning Hall and Beverly B. Wulfeck for their reviews and insightful comments regarding the initial outline and first draft of this chapter.

Study Guide

1. Identify and define the four components of the English language.

2. a. What do advocates of the cognition hypothesis say about the relationship between language skill and cognitive attainment?
   b. What do advocates of the correlational hypothesis say about this relationship?

3. Language acquisition is guided or influenced by several significant factors. Identify five factors that guide or influence the acquisition of language.

4. Define and differentiate between language competence and language performance.

5. What is meant by the notion of linguistic constraints?

6. Children with language disorders may be classified under two rather broad categories. What are these categories of classification? Briefly describe some primary difficulties incorporated with each of these two broad categories of classification.

7. Identify three goals or reasons for conducting an evaluation of a child's language abilities.

8. Identify six significant variables that must be addressed in language assessment. Describe why these variables must be addressed.

9. Describe and contrast norm-referenced and criterion-referenced assessment measures.

10. Briefly discuss how the semantic, syntactic, and pragmatic components of language can be evaluated in children with developmental language disorders.

11. Define the following terms

    language
    lexicon
    inflectional system
    elicited imitation
    spontaneous imitation
    delayed imitation
    language disorder

12. Provide examples of two pragmatic skills that a developing child must acquire.

13. Describe the Piagetian stages most likely to be reflected in 1) the very young or prelinguistic child; 2) the verbal, preschool age child; and 3) the verbal, school age child.

14. Discuss the considerations involved in interpreting the data obtained during a diagnostic session with a child suspected of having a language problem.

REFERENCES

Ammons, R. B., and Ammons, H. S. 1948. Full Range Picture Vocabulary Test. Psychological Test Specialists, Missoula, MT.

Arthur, G. 1952. The Arthur Adaptation of the Leiter International Performance Scale. Psychological Service Center Press, Washington, DC.

Ault, R. 1977. Children's Cognitive Development. Oxford University Press, New York.

Bangs, T. E. 1975. Vocabulary Comprehension Scale. Teaching Resources, Boston.

Bates, E., Benigni, L., Bretherton, I., Camaioni, L., and Volterra, V. 1979. The Emergence of Symbols: Cognition and Communication in Infancy. Academic Press, Inc., New York.

Bates, E., Camaioni, L., and Volterra, V. 1975. The acquisition of performatives prior to speech. Merrill-Palmer Q. 21:205–226.

Bloom, L. 1970. Language Development: Form and Function in Emerging Grammars. The M.I.T. Press, Cambridge, MA.

Bloom, L., and Lahey, M. 1978. Language Development and Language Disorders. John Wiley and Sons, New York.

Bloom, L., Lightbown, P., and Hood, L. 1975. Structure and variation in child language. Monogr. Soc. Res. Child Dev. 40:(No. 160).

Boehm, A. 1969. Boehm Test of Basic Concepts. Psychological Corporation, New York.

Brigance, A. 1978. Inventory of Early Development. Curriculum Associated, Inc., North Billerica, MA.

Brown, R. 1973. A First Language: The Early Stages. Harvard University Press, Cambridge, MA.

Bzoch, K., and League, R. 1971. The Receptive Expressive Emergent Language Scale (REEL). Language Education Division, Computer Management Corporation, Gainesville, FL.

Camarata, S., Newhoff, M., and Rugg, B. 1981. Perspective talking in normal and language disordered children. In: Proceedings from the Symposium on Research in Child Language Disorders. The University of Wisconsin-Madison, Madison, WI.

Carrow, E. 1973. Test for Auditory Comprehension of Language. Learning Concepts, Austin, TX.

Carrow, E. 1974. Carrow Elicited Language Inventory. Learning Concepts, Austin, TX.

Chapman, R. 1981. Exploring children's communicative intents. In: J. Miller (ed.), Assessing Language Production in Children. University Park Press, Baltimore.

Colarrusso, R., and Hammill, D. 1972. Motor-Free Visual Perception Test. Academic Therapy Publications, San Rafael, CA.

Creaghead, N., Margulies, C., and Ralph, R. 1980. Evaluation and remediation of pragmatic skills with low functioning children. Mini-seminar presented to the American Speech-Language-Hearing Association, Detroit.

Crystal, D., Fletcher, P., and Garman, M. 1976. The Grammatical Analysis of Language Disability: A Procedure for Assessment and Remediation. Edward Arnold, London.

Doll, E. A. 1965. Vineland Social Maturity Scale. American Guidance Service, Minneapolis, MN.

Dore, J. 1978. Requestive systems in nursery school conversations: Analysis of talk in its social context. In: R. Campbell and P. Smith (eds.), Recent Advances in the Psychology of Language. Plenum Publishing Corp., New York.

Dunn, L. M. 1965, 1980. Peabody Picture Vocabulary Test. American Guidance Service, Circle Pines, MN.

Dunst, C. 1980. A Clinical and Educational Manual for Use with the Uzgiris and Hunt Scales of Psychological Development. University Park Press, Baltimore.

Fey, M., Newhoff, M., and Cole, B. 1978. Language intervention: Effecting changes in mother-child interaction. Paper presented to the American Speech-Language-Hearing Association, San Francisco.

Folger, K., and Leonard, L. B. 1978. Language and sensorimotor development during the early period of referential speech. J. Speech Hear. Res. 21:519–527.

Foster, R., Giddan, J., and Stark, J. 1973. Assessment of Children's Language Comprehension. Learning Concepts, Austin, TX.

Frankenburg, W., Dodds, J., and Fandal, A. 1970. The Revised Denver Developmental Screening Test. B. F. Stolinsky Laboratories, Department of Pediatrics, University of Colorado Medical Center, Denver.

Fraser, C., Bellugi, U., and Brown, R. 1963. Control of grammar in imitation, comprehension and production. J. Verb. Learn. Verb. Behav. 2:121–135.

Frostig, M. 1961. Developmental Test of Visual Perception. Consulting Psychologists Press, Palo Alto, CA.

Gardner, M. 1979. Expressive One-Word Picture Vocabulary Test. Academic Therapy Publications, Novato, CA.

Halliday, M. A. K. 1975. Learning How to Mean: Explorations in the Development of Language. Edward Arnold, London.

Hammill, D., Brown, V., Larsen, S., and Wiederholt, J. 1980. Test of Adolescent Language. PRO-ED, Austin, TX.

Hedrick, D., Prather, E., and Tobin, M. 1975. Sequential Inventory of Communicative Development. University of Washington Press, Seattle, WA.

Karmiloff-Smith, A. 1979. Language development after five. In: P. Fletcher and M. Garman (eds.), Language Acquisition. Cambridge University Press, New York.

Kirk, S., McCarthy, J., and Kirk, W. 1968. The Illinois Test of Psycholinguistic Abilities (Revised Ed.). University of Illinois Press, Urbana, IL.

Lee, L. 1971. Northwestern Syntax Screening Test (NSST). Northwestern University Press, Evanston, IL.

Lee, L. 1974. Development Sentence Analysis. Northwestern University Press, Evanston, IL.

Leonard, L. B. 1979. Language impairment in children. Merrill-Palmer Q. 25:205–232.

Lowe, M., and Costello, A. 1976. The Symbolic Play Test. National Foundation for Educational Research Publishing, London.

Lucas, E. V. 1980. Semantic and Pragmatic Language Disorders. Aspen Systems Corporation, Rockville, MD.

MacDonald, J., and Horstmeier, D. 1978. Environmental Language Inventory. Charles E. Merrill, Columbus, OH.

McShane, J. 1980. Learning to Talk. Cambridge University Press, London.

Mecham, M. 1958, 1971. Verbal Language Development Scale. American Guidance Service, Circle Pines, MN.

Miller, J. F. 1981. Assessing Language Production in Children. University Park Press, Baltimore.

Miller, J. F., and Yoder, D. 1972. The Miller-Yoder Test of Grammatical Comprehension, experimental edition (M-Y Test). The University of Wisconsin-Madison, Madison, WI.

Newcomer, P., and Hammill, D. 1977. Test of Language Development. PRO-ED, Austin, TX.

Nicolich, L. 1977. Beyond sensorimotor intelligence: Assessment of symbolic maturity through analysis of pretend play. Merrill-Palmer Q. 23:89–101.

Paul, R. 1981. Analyzing complex sentence development. In: J. Miller, Assessing Language Production in Children. University Park Press, Baltimore.

Piaget, J. 1963. The Origins of Intelligence in Children. W. W. Norton & Company, Inc., New York.

Prutting, C., and Kirchner, D. 1982. Applied Pragmatics. J. Speech Hear. Disord. In press.

Rees, N. 1975. Imitation and language development: Issues and clinical implications. J. Speech Hear. Disord. 40:339–350.

Schery, T., and Glover, A. 1982. The Initial Communication Processes Scale. McGraw-Hill Book Company, New York.

Semel, E. M., and Wiig, E. 1980. Clinical Evaluation of Language Functions. Charles E. Merrill, Columbus, OH.

Snyder, L. S. 1981. Assessing communicative abilities in the sensorimotor period: Content and context. Topics Lang. Disord. 1:31–46.

Stephens, M. I. 1977. Stephens Oral Language Screening Test. Interim Publishers, Peninsula, OH.

Terman, L., and Merrill, M. 1960. Stanford-Binet Intelligence Scale. Houghton Mifflin Company, Boston.

Thorum, A. 1980. The Fullerton Language Test for Adolescents. Palo Consulting Psychologists Press, Palo Alto, CA.

Tyack, D., and Gottsleben, R. 1974. Language Sampling, Analysis and Training. Consulting Psychologists Press, Palo Alto, CA.

Uzgiris, I., and Hunt, J. 1975. Assessment in Infancy: Ordinal Scales of Psychological Development. University of Illinois Press, Urbana, IL.

Wadsworth, B. 1971. Piaget's Theory of Cognitive Development. Longman, New York.

Webster, E. J. 1977. Counseling with Parents of Handicapped Children: Guidelines for Improving Communication. Grune and Stratton, New York.

Wechsler, D. 1974. Wechsler Intelligence Scale for Children (WISC) (Revised Ed.). Psychological Corporation, New York.

Wolski, W., and Lerea, L. 1962. Michigan Picture Language Inventory (MPLI). University of Michigan, Program of Speech and Hearing Sciences, Ann Arbor, MI.

APPENDIX

Tentative Diagnostic Plan of Kent
(Time Allotted = 3 Hours)

Parent Interview

1. Reconfirm negative birth, medical, and physical development history.
2. Receive parental report of concerns regarding Kent, referral information, home environment, etc.
3. Obtain description of Kent's behavior at home.
4. Obtain complete description of language used by Kent at home, including examples of comprehension and production.
5. Briefly explain assessment protocol, time, etc.

Spontaneous Play and Interaction
(Low Structured Observation)

1. Ten minutes with primary caretaker
   a. to gauge general level of Kent's language functioning in order to insure that the preselected tests and assessment strategies will be appropriate.
   b. to observe caretaker's input, and Kent's responses to such input.
2. Twenty-five minutes with examiner
   a. to obtain sample of Kent's use of semantic, syntactic, pragmatic, and phonological features of language.
   b. to estimate cognitive status through observation of Kent's play behavior.

Norm-Referenced Measures
(High Structured Observation)

1. Test for Auditory Comprehension of Language (Carrow, 1973).
2. Carrow Elicited Language Inventory (Carrow, 1974).

Other

1. Hearing screening.
2. Speech mechanism examination.
3. Revised Denver Developmental Screening Test (Frankenburg, Dodds, and Fandal, 1969).

4

Diagnosis of Speech Sound Disorders in Children

Richard G. Schwartz

Outline

Educational Aims

1. *To describe significant aspects of speech sound behavior in children*
2. *To describe the general course of development of the speech sound system*
3. *To discuss the types and causes of speech sound disorders in children*
4. *To detail the process of diagnosing speech sound disorders in children*

Speakers and listeners share common systems of speech sounds, words and word combinations, conversational rules, linguistic meanings, and general knowledge to communicate orally. Although oral communication may be altered in a number of ways, the most common form of communication disorder in childhood results from errors in speech sound production. In this chapter we will describe speech sound disorders in children. Our discussion begins with a general description of speech sound behavior. Next, we consider the general course of development of speech sound production in children. We also define what speech sound disorders are, make clear what they are not, and specify how frequently they occur. In the remainder of the chapter, we discuss the process of diagnosis of children who produce speech sound errors.

SPEECH SOUND BEHAVIOR

General Considerations

The term *articulation* has traditionally been associated with speech sound behavior. Articulation highlights the role movements of the articulators (lips, tongue, jaw, palate, etc.) play in producing speech sounds. The production of speech sounds cannot be fully understood by only considering the role of articulator movements. Such descriptions reflect an obvious, but by no means the only important aspect of speech sound behavior. In this chapter, we also consider the production of speech sounds within a linguistic and cognitive framework.

Speech sound behavior must be considered within a linguistic framework, in part, because both the production and perception of speech sounds are influenced by the structure of a language. Speech sound behavior must also be studied from general linguistic and cognitive perspectives because both the production and perception of speech sounds play critical roles in determining meaning. Speech sounds may be described in various ways. For example, they may be described in terms of articulatory characteristics, acoustic properties, and linguistic features. Such descriptions enable us to divide speech sounds into groups or classes (e.g., stops, fricatives, nasals, etc.; alveolars, velars, etc.; strident, mellow, grave, acute, etc.; voiced, unvoiced). The manner in which children use and perceive these features appears to depend on the acquisition of a system of more abstract linguistic rules as well as upon the maturation of cognitive, motor, and sensory abilities.

Normal Development

Two general types of speech sound behavior development are of fundamental interest to speech-language pathologists. The first of these is *phonetic development*. Here, speech-language pathologists are concerned with children's acquisition of motor abilities associated with the production of speech sounds and with their acquisition of sensory (e.g., auditory/perceptual) skills needed to perceive speech. Second, speech-language pathologists are interested in *phonological development*. Here, they are concerned with the acquisition of an abstract system of linguistic rules children rely upon to perceive and produce linguistic contrasts (e.g., voicing distinction) and with children's acquisition of linguistic rules used to combine sounds to form words.

We will review the development of speech sound behavior by summarizing five general periods of acquisition.

Period 1: Prelinguistic

The first developmental period begins at birth and ends at approximately 12 months of age or with the appearance of children's first true words. This period can be identified with the label *prelinguistic*. Children gradually progress through five stages of vocalization during this first period:

1. They produce vegetative and reflexive vocalizations (e.g., sucking noises, crying, etc.)
2. They produce voluntary vocalizations (e.g., cooing)
3. They produce vocalizations which include various consonant and vowel combinations and incorporate stress and intonation (e.g., babbling and jargon)
4. They produce long strings of babbling and jargon which are broken up and which "resemble" words in their structure. However, these strings of vocalization are different from true words in terms of the consistency of sound production, meaning, and communicative usage
5. They produce their first true word. (Period 1 ends)

Children in the prelinguistic period are also able to discriminate between some speech sounds. Their discrimination abilities appear limited to distinguishing sounds and syllables devoid of meaning (e.g., /pa/ versus /ba/). For this reason, these abilities reflect phonetic perceptual abilities.

Period 2: Prerepresentational Phonology

The second period begins around 12 months of age and extends to about 18 months of age. I have chosen to identify this period with the label *prerepresentational phonology*. The second period defines the interval over which children typically produce their first 50 words. Children in this period of acquisition are only beginning to develop a cognitive system of mental representation and they generally produce single-word utterances. They vary in the way they produce a word on different occasions (e.g., *dog* [dɔ] [gɔ] [dɔd]). In addition, children in this period of acquisition are apparently selective about the adult words they attempt to say. Different children follow different patterns of word selection. For example, one child may attempt only adult words that take the forms consonant-vowel, (CV) (e.g., *boy*) or consonant-vowel-consonant (CVC) (e.g., *bat*) using labial and alveolar stops or nasals. Another child may follow a different pattern. You should not conclude that the presence of word selectivity indicates that a child does not understand word types which differ from those he or she produces. Rather, you should conclude that the child simply does not produce alternative word forms.

Another characteristic of children in this period of acquisition is that they may produce some words accurately (e.g., *pretty* [prɪti]), yet produce other similar words (e.g., *please* [biz], incorrectly. These instances of correct word productions are referred to as phonological idioms. In some children, the accurate production of some words gradually deteriorates over time (e.g., *pretty* becomes [bɪdi]), so that over time this child's sound production errors become more consistent with those made when other words are spoken. The presence of these behaviors indicates that during Period 2 children do not have a fully established system of linguistic rules or processes into which all new words are incorporated. Children in Period 2 apparently acquire speech largely on a word-by-word basis.

The third period of development extends from about 18 months of age to 3 to 4 years. I have chosen to identify this period with the label *representational phonology*. Children in this period of acquisition produce speech characterized by the presence of many errors which follow consistent patterns or processes. For example, before 3 years of age many children substitute stops for fricatives and/or consistently delete final consonants. Such types of error patterns evident during the production of speech by normally developing children have recently been described in terms of phonological processes or rules. These processes or rules are used to describe children's errors in terms of "simplifications" of adult forms of words. For example, a child's production [dɔ] for *dog* may be termed *final consonant deletion*, whereas production of [tʌn] for *sun* may be termed *stopping*. Students seeking to learn more about these processes or rules are encouraged to read Ingram (1976), Shriberg and Kwiatkowski (1980), and Stampe (1973). More extensive discussion of these processes and rules is provided elsewhere in this chapter.

Period 3: Representational Phonology

Between the ages of 18 months and 3 to 4 years, children begin to acquire mastery over the phonetic inventory of speech sounds of the English language. A large amount of the information we have about the development of speech sound production during childhood has been discussed in terms of the ages at which children master production of speech sounds (Poole, 1934; Prather et al., 1975; Sander, 1972; Templin, 1957; Wellman et al., 1931). The ages at which children achieve production mastery of English consonants is summarized in Table 4.1.

The information provided in Table 4.1 is divided into two parts. In the left hand column the ages at which at least 75 percent of the children tested correctly produced consonants in the initial, medial, and final position of words are listed. The ages at which more than 50 percent of the children

Table 4.1. Normative data for consonant production

	Age of mastery[a]	Age of customary usage[b]
m	3	before 2
n	3	before 2
ŋ	3	2
p	3	before 2
f	3	3
h	3	before 2
w	3	before 2
j	3½	4
b	4	before 2
d	4	2
k	4	2
g	4	2
r	4	3
s	4½	3
ʃ	4½	4
tʃ	4½	4
t	6	2
l	6	3
v	6	4
θ	6	5
ð	7	5
z	7	4
ʒ	7	6
dʒ	7	4

   [a] The age (years) at which 75 percent of the children tested correctly produced the sound in word initial, medial, and final position (Templin, 1957).
   [b] The age at which more than 50 percent of the children tested correctly produced the sound in two of the three word positions (Sander, 1972).

tested correctly produced these consonants in any two of the three word positions are listed in the right column. This information provides a general picture of the development of consonant acquisition and mastery, shows that the process of acquiring consonant sounds is gradual, and indicates that the process is not complete until age 7. Children generally acquire early mastery of nasals, somewhat later mastery of glides and stops, and more delayed mastery over fricatives and affricates. They acquire mastery of vowel sounds by 3 years of age.

These ages of mastery and ages of customary usage provide information only about phonetic (motoric) aspects of production learning. They do not provide information about phonological acquisition (i.e., the learning of linguistic rules and contrasts). They also do not provide information about the types of errors children make. Finally, because mastery data are based on imitated or elicited productions of a small group of words, they may not accurately reflect children's consonant usage or mastery in spontaneous speech. In spite of these limitations, these data are a major source of information concerning phonetic development during this period.

During Period 3, children also begin to recognize that sounds can be used to change meaning and achieve linguistic contrast. The production and perception of linguistic contrasts represents an important aspect of speech sound development.

The fourth period of development extends from approximately 4 to 7 years of age. This period may be identified with the label *phonetic inventory completion*. During this period of acquisition, children master the remainder of the phonetic inventory (see Table 4.1). They also achieve correct production of sounds in multisyllabic words and master some morphophonological rules of English (e.g., the rules governing the use of plural, past tense, and third-person singular endings).

Period 4: Phonetic Inventory Completion

The final period of development extends from approximately 7 to 12 years of age. I have chosen to identify this period with the label *advanced phonology*. In this period, children continue to learn new ways of combining speech sounds to alter meaning. Two factors influence children's learning of phonological rules during Period 5. First, their cognitive development matures to a level that enables children to "understand" formal phonological rules concerned with the derivation of different word forms (e.g., electric/electricity; divine/divinity). Second, they learn to read and write. Learning to read and write may also enhance children's understanding of the relationships between different word forms and their meanings (e.g., difference between noun-verb pairs: 'convict versus con'vict).

Period 5: Advanced Phonology

SPEECH SOUND DISORDERS

Speech sound errors are incorrectly or inappropriately produced speech sounds. Children have speech sound disorders when they produce speech sound errors not typically present in a normally developing peer group. Because it may not always be appropriate to characterize these disorders solely in terms of motor production, I have chosen to use the more general term *speech sound disorders*. Speech sound errors have generally been categorized as sound omissions (e.g., *sun* [sʌ]), sound substitutions (e.g., *sun* [tʌn]), sound additions (e.g., *blue*-[bəlu]), and sound distortions or allophonic errors (e.g., *sun* [ɬʌn]- a "lateral lisp"). Clinicians and researchers alike have found the need to be more specific about how they characterize speech sound errors. For example, substitution errors can be divided into two types: phonemic and allophonic. Phonemic errors are the substitution of sounds of a different phonemic class for intended target sounds. Allophonic errors are the substitution of sounds which do not differ in phonemic class in English (e.g., *ball* [βɔl]: a bilabial fricative instead of a stop). Phonemic and allophonic errors are defined by specifying the actual substitutions that children

Definition

produce or by detailing the patterns of errors (e.g., stops are substituted for fricatives).

Errors can also be classified in terms of context sensitivity. Productions influenced by context are assimilation errors. There are two general types of assimilation: progressive and regressive. In progressive assimilation, a sound which occurs early in the word influences the production of a sound which occurs later in the word (e.g., *back* [bæb]). In regressive assimilation the reverse is true. Namely, a sound which occurs later in the word influences a sound which occurs earlier in the word (e.g., *back* [kæk]). There are other types of assimilation (e.g., prevocalic voicing *top* [dap]; velar assimilation *back* [kæ] or *cup* [kʌk], or labial assimilation *man* [mæm] or *soup* [pup]).

There are also errors which influence the structure of words. Errors of this type include sound deletions or omissions (*dog* [dɔ]), syllable omissions or deletions (*e.g., candy* [kæn]), and reduplications (*ball* [baba] or *water* [wɔwɔ]). Other, less common, types of errors include metathesis (e.g., *pencil* [pɛsnɪl]) in which the order of sounds are reversed, and errors of epenthesis (e.g., *blue* [bəlu]) in which sounds are inserted.

Any or all of these types of errors may be present in the speech of a child with a speech sound disorder. They must, however, be distinguished from developmental errors (i.e., errors that children of that age make in the course of normal development), from sound changes which are often present in the speech of normal adults, and from sound changes which are essential parts of dialect. These distinctions are a critical part of the diagnostic process.

Incidence and Types

The most common communication disorder in childhood results from errors in speech sound production. It has been estimated that speech sound disorders represent in excess of 75 percent of all speech disorders in children (Milisen, 1971). Approximately 10 percent of all children between 6 to 7 years of age are reported to have a relatively severe problem producing speech sounds (Leske, 1981). Thus, children with errors in speech sound production represent the largest group served by speech-language pathologists.

One method used to classify speech sound disorders divides them on an organic versus functional basis. Organically based speech sound disorders are those which result from identifiable physical causes. Functionally based disorders are those which have no identifiable physical basis. This method of classification is very broad and often does not have clear differential implications for treatment. Because physical bases for speech sound disorders cannot be identified in many children with speech sound errors, the majority of children with such disorders are considered to have functionally based problems.

An alternative to the organic/functional method of classification is to categorize speech sound disorders in terms of the level of the speech sound system most prominently affected. Several writers (Winitz, 1969) have drawn a clear distinction between children's learning of motor movements required to achieve acceptable productions of speech sounds (phonetic level) and the learning of more abstract linguistic rules (phonological level). This same distinction has been used (Pollack and Rees, 1972) to differentiate children with deviant or immature phonological systems (phonological speech sound disorders) from children who are unable to plan or execute proper articulatory movements (phonetic speech sound disorders). Consistent with this writer's view that speech sound behavior must be considered in the context of a broadly based cognitive and linguistic system, you will find it important to make the general distinction between *phonetic* and *phonological* disorders.

Phonetic speech sound disorders result from identifiable physical causes (anatomical and physiological disturbances) or from disturbances in motor sequencing or learning. Children with disorders of this type may have auditory/perceptual difficulties (e.g., children with significant hearing impairment) or difficulties actually producing speech sounds. There are a number of identifiable etiologies of phonetic speech sound disorders. Some of the major causes are listed below.

1. Cleft palate and velopharyngeal inadequacy
2. Missing oral-facial structures
3. Hearing impairment
4. Myoneural disturbance
   a. Paralysis or paresis
   b. Motor sequencing and programming problems
   c. Sensory disturbance

Children with phonetic disorders exhibit difficulties in the production of speech sounds which reflect disturbance within the phonetic, rather than the phonological level of the speech sound system. These children share the need for remediation which focuses on the actual production (articulation, motor movement, sequencing) or perception of speech sounds. There are also children in this group whose problem cannot be related to organic or physical factors. For example, some children in this group exhibit isolated or small numbers of sound errors ([ɬ] for [s], lisping). Children with phonetic disorders typically have substitution errors but they do not exhibit significant disturbance in phonological organization or representation.

On the other hand, phonological speech sound disorders result from disturbances in children's organization or representation of linguistic units and rules. In general, children with phonological disorders exhibit errors in speech sound production which can be grouped into patterns (phonological processes) and these patterns differ from those seen in connection with organic (e.g., velopharyngeal inadequacy) disturbance. Children with this type of speech sound disorder may also exhibit more general impairments in language function.

Phonetic and phonological disorders need not be mutually exclusive. For example, children with hearing impairment and cleft palate may have sound errors that are, in part, attributable to their physical deficits and, in part, phonological in nature.

Each of these two broad categories can be divided further. For instance, phonetic disorders may be subdivided into categories based upon the major contributing etiology: hearing impairment, velopharyngeal inadequacy, and so on. The contributing etiology for some children with phonetic disorders is often unknown. For now, such children represent a separate subcategory.

Our current knowledge about children with phonological disorders is limited. Phonological disorders might be subdivided into categories. For example, one might distinguish phonological disorders that are accompanied by a more general language impairment from those that are not. It may also be possible to distinguish phonological disorders on the basis of error types. For example, some older children may have phonological disorders characterized by the production of errors typically made by younger age children, whereas others may have error patterns which are not similar to those made by younger age children.

Speech sound disorders can also be subdivided in terms of severity. Speech-language pathologists often make qualitative estimates of the severity of these disorders. These judgments are often based on such factors as the number of errors, the effect of these errors on speech intelligibility, error consistency, and the frequency of occurrence of sounds on which errors are made. Severity is typically categorized in terms of mild, moderate, and severe disturbance.

EXAMINATION AND DIAGNOSIS: AN OVERVIEW

Screening

One important part of examination of children with potential speech sound disorders is screening. Screening typically requires examination of large numbers of children over brief periods of time. The purpose of screening is to identify those children in need of further testing. Screening procedures require obtaining samples of children's speech by means of directed imitation (e.g., "Say toothbrush"), word elicitation (e.g., "What's this?" or "At night we go to _____."), and/or conversation (e.g., "Tell me what you do in school."). Pictures or objects may also be used to obtain samples. The stimuli used to elicit responses typically sample the more frequently used sounds of English and, for a given child, only those sounds the child would be expected to have acquired would be sampled. There are a number of commercially available screening tests. Some of the more frequently used instruments include: Templin-Darley Screening Test of Articulation (Templin and Darley, 1969), Triota Ten Word Test (Irwin, 1972), Screening Deep Test of Articulation (McDonald, 1968). These provide a convenient, standardized means of conducting screening. Nonstandardized screening tests developed by clinicians can also be used.

An important component of a screening test is the criterion, or *cut-off score*. This score is used to determine whether the child passes or fails. This score is usually stated in terms of total number of errors. The specific types of errors should also be used as criteria. For example, further testing might not be conducted with a 3-year-old girl who consistently substituted [t] for [s], although further testing might be considered for a child of the same age who substituted a lateral fricative ([ɬ] lateral lisp) for [s]. In the first example, further testing might not be conducted because [t] for [s] is a common substitution made by normal developing children of this age. In the second case, further testing might be considered because [ɬ] for [s] does not represent a common substitution and typically would not be expected to change with maturation. Most commercially available screening tests do not take factors such as error type into account. Clinicians should use error type information in their analysis of screening test results.

The cut-off score of a screening instrument should be sufficiently stringent to insure that few children fail who later prove to be within normal limits (*false-positive* identification). The criterion should also not be so lax as to allow many children to pass who later prove to be disordered (*false-negative* identifications). Screening procedures should minimize the likelihood that any truly disordered child passes.

We have emphasized the use of test instruments as the basis for screening. Another important source of screening information comes from the input of adults who have significant contact with children (e.g., parents, other relatives, teachers, physicians, etc.). Any child reported to be difficult to understand by these adults should be evaluated further. Hence, identification of significant difficulty in communication by adults represents a powerful screening technique.

Let us now make some general comments about diagnosis. Here, clinicians are concerned with: **Diagnosis**

1. determining whether a child is, in fact, disordered
2. specifying, in detail, the child's errors in speech sound production
3. determining the type of disorder
4. identifying the factors which cause and/or maintain the problem
5. specifying the severity of the problem
6. formulating a course of therapy
7. offering prognostic statements.

Clinicians need to collect and interpret information gained largely through testing, observing, and interviewing to form a diagnosis.

EXAMINATION PROCEDURES

Examination of children with speech sound disorders requires clinicians to:

1. obtain a comprehensive case history
2. examine the adequacy of the speech and hearing mechanism
3. collect speech samples
4. analyze speech samples
5. test phonological perception
6. examine related abilities (cognition and language).

Obtaining Historical Information

Obtaining comprehensive historical information about the nature, cause, and course of speech sound problems is an essential part of diagnosis. Clinicians often rely upon parents, other relatives, teachers, physicians, the child, and others to obtain such information. Written questionnaires and oral interview techniques can be used for this purpose. The general approaches and specific procedures used to obtain historical information are discussed in Chapters 1, 2, and 10.

As indicated in Chapter 1, historical information about several major areas is obtained when examining people with communication disturbance. The major categories of historical information include:

Conditions related to the onset of the problem
Conditions related to the development of the problem
Previous diagnostic findings
Previous rehabilitative services
General developmental status
Current health status
Educational/vocational status
Emotional/social adjustment
Pertinent family concerns
Other information volunteered by the respondent

For children with speech sound disorders, specific historical information concerning the emergence of and mastery over developmental milestones may be very significant. Identification of factors which may place such children at high risk for speech and language disturbance is also important. It is often useful to determine what sounds informants have heard the child produce and to determine whether the child's errors are consistent or not. Estimation of the child's speech intelligibility may be useful. Identification should be made of circumstances in which the child is more difficult versus easier to understand (e.g., in single words versus sentences; at home versus at the clinic). Information about the child's response to speech disturbance should be gathered. Finally, descriptions of what individuals do when they can not understand the child are often useful.

Other specific types of historical information may be particularly helpful in diagnosis. General information concerning the course and current status of speech sound development may provide information concerning possible etiology. The clinician should be aware of any sudden cessation or deterioration in speech sound development. Description of the child's general responses to auditory stimuli (speech and nonspeech) may serve as preliminary indicators of hearing status. An attempt should definitely be made to identify abnormalities of the speech mechanism or more general physical problems which might directly influence speech sound production and perception.

Examination of the speech and hearing mechanism is an essential part of diagnosis of speech sound disorders in childhood. The primary goals of this form of examination are to identify structural (anatomical) and/or functional (physiological) deviations which might influence or cause disturbances in speech sound production and to determine whether such deviations warrant referral to and examination by other professionals.

Examination of the Speech and Hearing Mechanism

The general approach used in this form of examination has been discussed in Chapter 2. Examination of children with speech sound disorders requires the clinician to specify relationships between oral structure and function and speech sound errors. In particular, attention should be directed to identifying:

1. dental deviations including malocclusion, missing teeth, and presence of dental appliances
2. palatal deviations including repaired and unrepaired cleft palate, genetic signs (submucous cleft palate, lip pits etc.) of clefting, palatal fistulae, asymmetry, and diminished palatal movements
3. tongue deviations including any anatomical differences, asymmetry, and impairments in motion, strength, speed, and tone
4. lip deviations including anatomical differences (e.g., repaired cleft lip) and functional limitations
5. oral facial sensory deficits and other types of facial motor disturbances
6. other potentially significant (e.g., tonsillar enlargement) deviations

Identification of organic factors which may influence speech sound production is typically accomplished by means of visual examination. Specifically, the clinician examines children at rest and as they perform a variety of speech (e.g., diadochokinetic movements) and nonspeech (e.g., pursing the lips) movements. One purpose of this examination is to identify impairments in tone, strength, range, sequence, speed and accuracy of movements. Specific procedures which can be used to conduct such examinations are also outlined by Noll in Chapter 7.

Diagnosis of children with speech sound disorders often requires the clinician to specify relationships between oral structure/function and speech sound errors. Stated differently, clinicians must evaluate the effect of organic deviations on speech sound production. Such judgments are not easy, because the relations among these organic deviations and adequacy of speech sound production are often not direct. For instance, children with malocclusion and/or missing teeth often do not have speech sound errors. Similarly, children with reduced oral diadochokinetic rates may not have speech sound errors. Because the relations among organic deviations and speech sound production are often not direct, beginning clinicians often find it difficult to determine the clinical influence of these deviations. Your confidence in judging the influence of such deviations will improve with further clinical experience.

The hearing function of all children with speech sound disorders must be examined. The procedures to be used in the evaluation of hearing have been outlined in Chapter 2 under Audition and Auditory Perceptual Skills.

Sampling Speech

A central feature of examination and diagnosis is the sampling of a child's speech. Speech sampling for diagnosis differs from that used for screening. Here, sampling is more extensive and should provide an accurate picture of the child's speech use outside of the clinic. Speech samples can be obtained in a variety of ways: using pictorial stimuli, real objects, events, written text, and orally transmitted materials. Sampling may also be completed using elicited imitations of adult words, phrases or sentences, spontaneous utterances, elicited productions (e.g., response to prompts, such as "What's this?"; "You see with your ____"), and oral reading.

Standardized Testing

The most commonly used method of sampling is to elicit productions of single words. This is usually accomplished by administering a commercially available test. The more widely used tests of articulation include: Goldman-Fristoe Test of Articulation (Goldman and Fristoe, 1969), Fisher-Logemann Test of Articulation Competence (Fisher and Logemann, 1971), Deep Test of Articulation (McDonald, 1964), Photo Articulation Test (Pendergast et al., 1969), Templin-Darley Tests of Articulation (Templin and Darley, 1969), and Arizona Articulation Proficiency Scale (Fudala, 1970). The clinician-in-training will want to become familiar with these tests while learning about diagnosis of speech and language disorders.

Most of these tests use pictures to depict and elicit word productions which enable clinicians to determine how well the speaker is able to produce sounds in various word or syllable positions. Some of these tests use imitation and brief sampling of spontaneous speech in addition to elicitation. Some tests require children to read aloud. The advantage of commercially available tests is that they are readily available, are standardized, and in some cases, are accompanied by normative data. In many cases, a score based on the number of errors made by the child can be derived and compared to the scores achieved by normally developing children.

Such tests have some limitations (c.f., Winitz, 1969; Shriberg and Kwaitkowski, 1980). These limitations must be understood if the information gathered from them is to be used appropriately. First, almost all commercially available tests characterize speech sounds in terms of word-initial, -medial and -final positions. One exception is the Fisher-Logemann Test of Articulation (Fisher and Logemann, 1975). Phoneticians have pointed out that such classification of the sound system applies to orthography (written material), but not to speech. It is more appropriate to classify sounds in terms of their syllablic position (e.g., pre-vocalic or syllable initial; post-vocalic or syllable-final, and inter-vocalic or ambisyllabic). With few exceptions (e.g., Comprehensive Articulation Test, Weiss, 1978), most tests also do not sample using items which are weighted to reflect the frequency of occurrence of speech sounds. Thus, an error on a less frequently used sound such as [dʒ] is often equally weighted with an error on a more frequently used sound such as [s]. To keep articulation tests as short as possible and to use test words that can be pictured, sampling achieved by articulation test methods is often limited. In the administration of most commercially available tests, a given sound is sampled in a maximum of three positions and each of these words is elicited only once. This causes two problems. First, because only three contexts are tested, alternative contexts in which a sound may be produced correctly may be overlooked. The Deep Test of Articulation (McDonald, 1964) minimizes this problem by testing each sound in multiple contexts. Second, single elicitation of each word does not enable the clinician to adequately sample production variability.

The choice of test words used in articulation tests may also occasion limitation. For example, in several tests some sounds are elicited in fairly complex words. Although 83 percent of the words children use in spontaneous speech take relatively simple forms of consonant (C) and vowel (V) arrangements (CVC, CV, VC, CVCV, CVCC, CCVC), these forms are represented in 56 to 71 percent of the items of five widely used articulation tests (Shriberg and Kwiatkowski, 1980). Hence, during testing speech sounds are often elicited using words which are more complex than those children typically use. In addition, some tests elicit sounds in words containing bound morphemes (e.g., *witches, cars*), a factor which further complicates the problem of representativeness and structural complexity. Finally, although nouns represent only about 24 percent of the words children use in spontaneous speech (Templin, 1957), a very large percentage of items used in such tests are nouns.

As we have said, most commercially available tests use elicited productions of single words to sample speech sound production accuracy. With the exception of earlier periods of language development, children generally produce speech sounds in words that occur within sentences. Children's productions of speech sounds in single words differ from those produced in sentences. As a general rule, error rate increases as a function of increasing sentence complexity (Schmauch et al., 1978).

The communicative situation typically used during the administration of commercially available tests may also not be representative. For example, it is not common to ask a child to name an object which is pictured and is known to both the adult and the child. Speech and language is used primarily to communicate or to transmit new information, rather than to transmit information that is redundant and already shared between the speaker and listener.

Commercially available tests do provide a convenient, standardized means of obtaining a sample of a child's speech. The results of this form of sampling represents an important tool speech-language pathologists use to determine whether a child is truly disordered, particularly when normative data is available. The results of this type of testing can also be used for other diagnostic purposes in that such results may provide information about error patterns. However, it is important to recognize that a relatively unrepresentative sample of speech may be elicited in this form of testing. Consequently, when such tests are used, they should be supplemented by speech sampling obtained through other means. Above all, the administration of an articulation test should not be equated with diagnosis.

Elicited and Spontaneous Sampling

One form of supplementation to speech sound testing is nonstandardized elicitation. Here, children are requested to produce words or phrases elicited through pictorial, object, event, or written means. In this method, the clinician constructs an examination instrument. This method is nonstandardized only when the clinician fails to select consistent target words or phrases. Clinicians may also individualize targets to sample areas of difficulty identified in screening, spontaneous sampling, and case history taking.

Clinicians can avoid some of the limitations inherent to elicited sampling by carefully selecting stimuli (see Table 4.2 for some examples). One disadvantage of elicitation is that utterances representative of those the child typically uses in spontaneous speech may not be elicited. A child may make errors in spontaneous speech that do not occur in the more constrained situation of elicited sampling. A second disadvantage is the lack of accompanying normative data. In a supplementary role, elicitation can be used to fill gaps. This is accomplished by sampling different contexts, by eliciting additional productions of given words, and by eliciting productions of words, sounds, and syllables not used in other forms of sampling.

Table 4.2.   A source list of words for speech sampling

CVC words				
cup	girl	bug	hole	pen
pat	knife	bird	hit	shirt
mop	bed	bib	bike	door
comb	chair	boat	bead	mouth
bear	man	light	bus	kiss
dish	chip	mouse	hat	rain
phone	bang	walk	juice	boot
dog	more	hop	house	kick
ball	gone	push	nose	mine
bell	book	fall	teeth	cheese
car	moon	give	gum	rock
jack	sock	sit	rip	hug
fish	sun	turn	tear	cook
duck	soap	down	write	coke
lamb	roll	bite	couch	
ring	sit	cough	rug	
doll	cat	hot	fit	

CV and VC words				
toe	boy	tea	eat	ouch
knee	key	hi	go	
no	cow	high	see	
shoe	egg	bye	on	

CCV, CCVC, VCC, CVCC, CCCVC words				
bottle	jump	milk	school	drink
block	clown	hand	throw	stove
spoon	rattle	apple	sneeze	close
fork	horse	broke	bones	
brush	flower	sleep	want	
truck	stick	snow	build	
train	string	cloud	scratch	
box	sky	swing	plane	
table	tree	bread	dress	
plate	clock	glass	drive	
cotton	broom	flag	sink	

Multi-syllabic words				
pillow	daddy	paper	choo-choo	dirty
blanket	brother	pencil	money	TV
trailer	sister	all gone	banana	upstairs
tractor	bunny	heavy	lollipop	open
jumping	rabbit	thank you	candy	
necklace	teddy	soda	cracker	
baby	cookie	puppy	telephone	
mama	water	tiger	tissue	

A second form of supplementation is sampling of conversational or spontaneous speech. Samples of spontaneous speech are often collected in unstructured or free play situations. Clinicians should exert control over sampling obtained in these relatively unstructured situations.

One disadvantage inherent to the sampling of spontaneous speech is the lack of standardization. The lack of standardization may be overcome by choosing a standard core of prompts: various objects, actions, pictures, and verbal stimuli. These prompts or stimuli should be used to sample the range of English speech sounds in a variety of words. Here, a child's speech sound production can be examined using words the child typically produces. The prompts used need not be limited to those which can be pictured. Sounds may be examined in a greater variety of contexts and multiple productions of given words may be examined. Beyond a core of prompts which might be appropriate for all children in a given age range, the clinician may select specific items for individual children. The verbal stimuli clinicians use should facilitate spontaneous speech (Hubbell, 1977). Generally, verbal prompts should be open ended and nondirective, so that minimal constraints are placed on the child's utterances.

There are two situations which may severely limit the utility of spontaneous sampling. The first occurs when there is paucity of spontaneous speech produced. These problems may be minimized by not attempting to collect a complete sample in a single session. Instead, sampling may be attempted over several sessions. The second situation which can influence spontaneous sampling occurs when the child being examined is extremely difficult to understand. Although such a child may readily be identified as disordered, little can be gained from sampling, since the clinician cannot identify what the child is attempting to say. In this situation, the clinician must either forego spontaneous sampling or make alterations in the manner of speech prompting. Stimulus presentation must be highly controlled and presentation of only one or two stimuli at a time can be used to facilitate the determination of the child's target words.

Finally, there is the issue of the length of the sample to be collected. Shriberg and Kwiatkowski (1980) have suggested that a sample of at least 225 words containing approximately 90 different words may provide appropriate sampling. This size sample is reasonable for children who have an average utterance length between one and three words. For children whose average utterance length is larger (four or more words), however, such sampling may yield fewer than 50 utterances. A sample size between 50 to 100 utterances is required for many other types of linguistic analyses (see Chapter 3). Thus, minimum sampling should be 100 utterances and at least 225 words. Although the clinician's role as the interactor in sampling has been emphasized, other individuals (e.g., mother, father, or sibling) may serve in this role.

Imitation and stimulability often also form integral parts of examination and diagnosis. It is often assumed that speech sounds produced as part of imitated responses are more likely to be produced correctly than sounds produced as part of spontaneous speech. This assumption is made because during imitation a perceptual model is presented. This assumption is not always true. For example, the error rates of normal children with vocabularies of 5 to 15 words are comparable in spontaneous versus imitative productions. About the time children acquire their 50th word, they attempt a wider range of words in imitation than in spontaneous production. However, the extent of errors is still comparable. Several studies of young children have shown no differences in the number of errors children make during imitative versus elicited productions of single words (Templin, 1947; Paynter and Bumpas, 1977). On the other hand, investigations of older children show that they make a greater number of errors in elicited naming (Carter and Buck, 1958; Siegel et al., 1963; Smith and Ainsworth, 1967; Snow and Milisen, 1954).

Imitation and Stimulability

Imitative productions are commonly used to examine *stimulability*. Stimulability refers to whether a child can correctly produce an error sound during imitated production or with some phonetic instruction. Take the example "The sun is yellow" which a child produced spontaneously as [dʌ tʌ ɪd lɛlo]. In this example, the child's stimulability for the sound [s] can be examined at a variety of levels. First, the whole sentence could be presented and the child asked to repeat it. Alternatively, the child could be asked to produce only the word *sun* on an imitative basis. The child could also be asked to produce a syllable with [s] in prevocalic position. Stimulability testing typically begins at the sound or syllable level and proceeds to more complex tasks such as words, phrases, and sentences. At any of these levels, stimulability testing may involve the presentation of visual and descriptive cues.

Stimulability has been used to determine whether errors will be corrected without intervention and to formulate prognostic statements. Stimulability data are not always easy to interpret. This is true because stimulability is not always related to children's ability to spontaneously correct errors (Carter and Buck, 1958; Farquhar, 1961; Sommers et al., 1967). Children who are highly stimulable (75 percent correct in imitation of sounds produced incorrectly) appear to be more likely to improve spontaneously. There are, however, children who are stimulable but do not improve without remediation. In some children, spontaneous improvement may be slower than improvement associated with speech remediation. Thus, stimulability data must be interpreted cautiously, particularly when such information is used to make therapy referrals or decisions.

Stimulability data are also used to determine prognosis. Stimulability data, together with mental age and articulation scores are often used to make predictions about the likelihood of successful intervention (Irwin et al.,

1966). Because there are other factors (error type and consistency, etc.) which may also influence success and speed of remediation, stimulability data per se may not provide sufficient information on which reliable prognoses can be made.

Analysis of Speech Samples

The child's speech sound productions must be analyzed after speech has been sampled. Basically, analysis consists of identifying and describing the child's errors. The precise nature of the child's errors often provides important diagnostic information. Consequently, children's productions should be transcribed. Minimally, broad transcription using symbols from the International Phonetic Alphabet should be made of the child's errors. In many cases, narrow phonetic transcription is used (Shriberg and Kent, 1982). The use of narrow transcription should be limited to clearly deviant productions (e.g., labio-dental productions of bilabial sounds, bilabial productions of labio-dental sounds, inappropriate tongue protrusions, etc.). In most cases, accurate transcription of consonants is of primary importance. Transcription of vowels is of secondary importance. Because syllable stress may influence speech sound production, stress should also be transcribed.

Information gained by visual examination provides valuable cues to transcription. Hence, it is important to complete some transcription as testing is conducted. An orthographic (written) gloss of what the child intended to say is exceedingly useful. Sampling sessions should be audiotaped using high quality equipment. Analysis of these recordings serves as supplementation to the transcription process.

After a sample has been transcribed, further analysis is often required. The specific nature and extent of this analysis will depend on the clinician's goals and on the extent of the child's errors. Additional analysis is usually performed to specify six significant aspects of speech sound behavior:

1. production characteristics and constraints
2. selection characteristics and constraints
3. individual errors and error types
4. error patterns
5. variability
6. contrast behavior

Table 4.3 summarizes these forms of analysis.

Before beginning further analysis, the sample should be organized. By now the clinician should have a transcription of the child's utterances, an orthographic gloss, and a description of relevant contextual material (e.g., what was said to or asked of the child, what the child was doing, etc.). There are many possible ways to organize these clinical data. One procedure is to number the child's utterances and write each word the child produced on

Table 4.3. Summary of sample analyses

Analyses	General purpose	Procedure
1. Production characteristics and constraints	Specify a child's phonetic repertoire.	List single consonants, clusters and syllabic structures appearing in a child's productions.
2. Selection characteristics and constraints	Specify the adult forms (e.g., CV, CVC, etc.) and consonants a child tries/does not try to produce.	List forms (e.g., CV, CVC, etc.), single consonants, and clusters (by syllable position) present in the adult words a child attempts.
3. Individual error analysis	Specify individual errors and error types.	List individual and syllabic errors and categorize them in terms of error types.
4. Error pattern analysis	Specify patterns of errors.	Identify and list patterns of errors. Where appropriate use rules or processes to categorize these patterns.
5. Variability	Specify consistency of word production and error patterns.	Identify different productions of given words obtained at various points in the sampling process. Calculate ratios of word variability or optional processes.
6. Sound contrast	Specify contrasts between sounds.	Examine minimal pairs. Identify phone classes for each syllable. Calculate number of phone classes, number of single-member phone classes, and total number of classes. Analyze homonymy.

an orthographic and phonetic basis on individual index cards. If there is some uncertainty about the correct transcription, a pronunciation dictionary can be consulted (e.g., Kenyon and Knott, 1944). Transcription should take into account dialectical variations (Williams and Wolfram, 1977) and general English variations. The cards can then be arranged into categories. For example, cards can be arranged according to the initial sound of the word (e.g., *cheese* goes in a group of words beginning with /tʃ/; *corn* goes with other words beginning with /k/, etc.). It may also be helpful to note whether each production was elicited, imitated, or produced spontaneously and to indicate whether the sound was produced as part of a single-word or multi-word utterance.

**Production
Characteristics and
Constraints**

The basic aim of production analysis is to specify the child's phonetic repertoire. This requires specifying the sounds and syllable structures the child is actually making. In this form of analysis clinicians are not concerned with the accuracy of the child's productions, but rather seek only to identify the repertoire of sounds and syllables a child produces. Simple inspection of the sample can often indicate whether an analysis of vowels is required. Because in most cases vowel analysis is not essential, we will focus on consonant analyses.

Clinicians should initially prepare a table for each syllable position (prevocalic, postvocalic, and intervocalic or ambisyllabic). For each table, sounds may be grouped according to manner and place of articulation. In this way, clinicians can readily identify existing patterns of errors (Schwartz et al., 1980). Consonant clusters should be treated separately. This form of organization enables the clinician to calculate ratios: the number of different words (or syllables) in which given consonants (or syllables) were actually produced in relation to the total number of words sampled.

There may be important aspects of children's speech that are not perceptible to listeners. For instance, Weismer et al. (1981) found that among children who omitted final consonants, some maintained the voicing characteristics of the omitted voiced consonants by increasing vowel duration. These differences were not identified by listener judgments, but were specified by means of acoustic analysis. If dimensions such as vowel duration prove to be clinically significant, adjustments may have to be made to use instrumental forms of examination more routinely.

**Selection
Characteristics and
Constraints**

We noted in a previous section that normally developing children with vocabularies of approximately 50 or fewer words attempt words with certain phonological characteristics, that is, they are selective. This form of selectivity may continue beyond this point in development. Thus, for children with production vocabularies of less than 75 words, analysis of selection characteristics may be extremely informative. For children with more advanced development, this analysis may be unnecessary.

The basic aim of selection analysis is to specify the adult forms (e.g., CV, CVC, etc.) and consonants a child attempts and does not attempt to produce. The procedures for the analysis of selection constraints and characteristics are identical to those used in the analysis of production characteristics and constraints. The same types of ratios used in production analyses (for consonants and syllables) can be calculated in selection analysis.

**Individual Error
Analysis**

The major aim of error analysis is to compare the characteristics of the words attempted (i.e., adult targets) with the child's productions. All correct productions (matches between the child's production and the adult form) and incorrect productions (mismatches) of sounds should be identified. Ratios expressing the number of incorrect productions in comparison with the total number of possible correct productions can be calculated. In calculating these ratios clinicians must distinguish between token ratios (i.e., the number of correct productions of a consonant in the same word in relation to the number of times that word was attempted) and type ratios (i.e., the number of incorrect productions of a given consonant in relation to all different words spoken in which this consonant was present). As in previous analyses, blends or clusters should be treated separately and the syllabic structures of target words can be examined in relation to the syllabic structures present in the child's productions (Ingram, 1981).

Error pattern analysis should be undertaken when numerous errors or a few errors which can be grouped into a pattern(s) are present. Several different approaches have been used to complete this form of analysis. Each of these approaches represents a somewhat different view of phonology and phonological development. One approach is *distinctive feature analysis* proposed by McReynolds and Engmann (1975). Here, clinicians use a distinctive feature system to describe the patterns of segmental speech sound errors. Errors are specified in terms of difference(s) between the linguistic features of intended sound(s) and the child's production of these sounds. The absolute or relative frequency of feature changes for a given sound can also be calculated.

Error Pattern Analysis

One limitation of distinctive feature analysis is that it is exclusively segmental (i.e., speech sound level) in nature. Thus, if a child produces the words *tote* as [toʊt], *top* as [pɑp], yet produces the word *tack* as [kæk], distinctive feature analysis will indicate that the features coronal and anterior are in error. However, this form of analysis will not reveal that the child's production of /t/ was influenced by other consonants in the word. This kind of analysis does not readily permit description of sound and syllable omissions or substitutions of non-English sounds (e.g., bilabial fricatives). There is also considerable debate about the "psychological reality" of distinctive features. There is some evidence to suggest that adults do not group sounds on the basis of distinctive features even when the experimental procedures are designed to facilitate groupings on this basis (Ritterman and Freeman, 1974). Therefore, it may not be reasonable to assume that children would be able to do this readily, even with training. Although McReynolds and Bennett (1972) have found that "training a feature" (e.g., ± continuant) of certain sounds may result in generalization to other error sounds, this does not always occur.

The second form of analysis incorporates the use of *generative linguistic rules* (e.g., Chomsky and Halle, 1968). This form of analysis can be used in conjunction with, or in addition to, distinctive feature analysis. The advantage of using rule-based analysis over feature analysis is that rule-based approaches provide a more formal characterization of error pattern. Generative rules can be written to characterize context-free substitutions for sound classes, features, or individual segments (e.g., fricatives → stops; $\begin{bmatrix} + \text{strident} \\ + \text{continuant} \end{bmatrix} \rightarrow \begin{bmatrix} - \text{strident} \\ - \text{continuant} \end{bmatrix}$; s → t). They also can be written to characterize context-sensitive substitutions with additional notations such as / # _____ (word-initial position), / _____V (prevocalic), / _____# (word-final position), / V _____(post-vocalic), / t V _____(in syllables beginning with /t/, in post vocalic position). Such rules can also be used to indicate context-free or context-sensitive omissions (e.g., t → ø (null or nothing), t → ø / _____#). The information provided by these rules can be examined quantitatively in terms of their relative and absolute frequency of occurrence in relation to features, segments, and sound classes.

A significant problem with rule-based approaches relates to the formality and complexity of the rules. Most clinicians lack the training and experience necessary to write a set of rules for a sample. It is also not clear that this level of formality provides significant clinical information over that provided by less formal approaches. As was the case for distinctive feature analysis, questions can also be raised about the psychological reality of rule-based analysis.

An approach to pattern analysis which has recently received significant attention is called *phonological process analysis*. The application of the term process to normal and disordered development comes primarily from a theory of natural phonology (Stampe, 1973). A process is a mental operation that leads to sound changes. The important part of the definition of a process is that it highlights the merging of normally separate phonological classes (e.g., all fricatives and stops are produced as stops; all CV and CVC words are produced in CV form). The processes are considered "natural" because they reflect natural limitations. The errors to which processes lead are asserted to represent "easier" productions (e.g., it is easier to produce a word without a final consonant than with a final consonant). Our current knowledge concerning what is easy or difficult is still limited. A list of natural processes can be formed, however, using data accrued from slips-of-the-tongue, processes that occur universally across languages, and processes that occur commonly in normally developing children.

A wide range of processes have been suggested (see for example, Shriberg and Kwiatkowski, 1980; Hodson, 1980). Although this wide range of processes presents a somewhat confusing picture, the clinician should remember that the purpose of process analysis is to identify error patterns inherent in the child's productions. The resolution of the issue concerning just how many phonological processes there really are must await future study. For now, it is clear that process analysis provides a useful descriptive tool for examination and remediation planning. A representative list of processes and examples is presented in Table 4.4.

Several published works describing process analyses are available (Hodson, 1980; Ingram, 1981; Shriberg and Kwiatkowski 1980; Weiner,

Table 4.4   Some common phonological processes

Process		Example	
Syllabic processes			
Final consonant deletion[a]		*dog*	[dɔ]
Weak (unstressed) syllable deletion[a]		*candy*	[kæn]
Cluster reduction[a]		*Chris*	[kɪs]
Reduplication		*water*	[wɔwɔ]
Sound change processes			
Assimilation[a]			
Progressive		*duck*	[dʌt]
Regressive		*down*	[naʊn]
Substitution			
Gliding[a]		*rabbit*	[wæbɪt]
Stopping[a]		*see*	[ti]
Fronting[a]		*go*	[doʊ]
		she	[si]
Backing		*thumb*	[sʌm]
Glottal replacement		*bat*	[bæʔ]
Nasalization		*bit*	[mɪt]
Denasalization		*meat*	[bit]

    Although the above production examples for the most part reflect a single process, productions which are the results of multiple processes are common.

[a] Natural processes (Shriberg and Kwiatkowski, 1980).

1979). A general process analysis may be conducted in the following way. Each of the child's productions could be examined to determine the process or processes which describe the errors. Although in many cases a single process may describe a child's production of a given word, often more than one process may be involved (e.g., *truck* [kʌ], consonant cluster simplification, regressive assimilation, final consonant deletion).

Most writers have suggested that analysis should be completed on one production of a given word. Analysis of several, if not all, of a child's productions of a given word can often provide more comprehensive information about the effect and the consistency of the process on the child's speech. Accurate identification of a process is not always simple. For instance, if a child produces the word *cup* as [pʌp], we do not know, on the basis of this production per se, whether the processes of regressive assimilation or fronting are involved. Consequently, the clinician must examine the sample further to determine whether front sounds are substituted for back sounds in cases where such substitutions could not have resulted from assimilation. The clinician must also determine whether there are other instances of substitution of front for back sounds. In some cases, additional words may need to be elicited.

In general, for a sound change to be considered a process, it must influence more than one member of a sound class. Consider a child who simply substitutes /t/ for /s/ and produces other fricatives correctly. Characterizing this behavior as a stopping process adds nothing to our examination information. It is difficult to envision how calling this behavior a process would help in planning remediation. Similarly, identification of processes such as final consonant deletion, consonant cluster simplification, or weak syllable deletion should involve more than a single sound, cluster, or a single word. This would insure that a child does not simply have isolated errors. Other criteria have been suggested (e.g., McReynolds and Elbert, 1981), but given our present state of knowledge and the purpose of such analyses, the criteria just defined should suffice.

Clinicians can also calculate the relative frequency of occurrence of each process. This can be accomplished by constructing a ratio between the number of occurrences in relation to the total number of productions in which that process could occur.

Variability

An important aspect of speech sound behavior is the child's variability in speech sound production. Variability may be related to level of cognitive development, to context and to acquisition processes. Children may produce different errors for the same target. They may produce targets correctly on some occasions and produce them incorrectly on other occasions. Ratios for word production variability may be calculated. For example, if a child produces the word *dog* as [dɔ], [gɔg], and [dɔg] and the word *boat* as [boʊ] and [boʊt], there would be five forms and two types. Similar analyses can be performed to examine the extent of optional or inconsistent processes (Schwartz et al., 1980).

Analysis of Sound Contrast

A final aspect of speech sound behavior that may be examined is the child's system of sound contrast. This type of examination may be particularly important for children who exhibit highly variable behavior and for children with limited consonant repertoires. Contrast behavior can sometimes be examined by identifying minimal pairs (e.g., [pɪn] versus [bɪn]) produced during sampling. Unfortunately, children usually do not produce sufficient minimal pairs during sampling to make such an analysis worthwhile.

There are alternative methods clinicians can use to analyze sound contrast behavior. One method capitalizes on the fact that many children produce given words differently on different occasions. For example, a child may produce the word *see* as [si] and [ti]; the word *sun* as [sʌn], [ʌn], and [tʌn], the word *feet* as [fi]; and the word *play* as [peɪ] and [beɪ]. For this child, sounds [s, ø (null or nothing), and t; p and b] are not used to contrast meaning. Sounds such as these can be grouped into classes called *phone classes*, that is, sounds produced by a child in a given position which do not contrast word meaning. Clinicians can sample production variability to perform analysis of contrast ability. Namely, they can summarize responses in terms of phone classes presented in a child's production system. In the example given earlier in this paragraph, the syllable-initial phone classes in this child's productions were [s~t~ø], [f], [p~b]. Clinicians can also define the total number of phone classes used, calculate the average number of sounds in these phone classes, and determine the proportion of single-member classes.

Another method of examining contrast behavior is to complete an analysis of homonymy (Ingram, 1981). Homonymy occurs when errors in producing one or more words lead to identical productions for different words (e.g., *ball* [bʌ] and *bottle* [bʌ] or *bow* [boʊ] and *boat* [boʊ]). Examining the relative frequency of homonymy may provide information about whether or not contrast is achieved. Information about the extent to which a child may be misunderstood is also gained through analysis of sound contrast.

Phonological Perception

Phonological perception refers to the ability to identify and discriminate linguistically important sound level distinctions among sounds and syllables produced within meaningful linguistic units (e.g., words). Very young infants appear to be able to discriminate among many speech sounds. However, their ability to do this seems limited to phonetic perception. They are able to perceive differences among speech sounds presented as part of non-meaningful syllables. Phonological perception appears to develop later and is associated with the child's achievement of more mature linguistic development.

The relationship between phonological perception and production abilities is still unclear. Research involving older children seems to indicate that perception abilities generally precede production abilities, although for some sounds the reverse may be true (Bernthal and Bankson, 1981). The relationship between perceptual abilities and speech sound disturbance is difficult to ascertain (Winitz, 1969). This difficulty is, in part, related to variations in the test instruments and procedures that have been used to examine children's speech sound discrimination. Three of the more commonly used instruments are the Wepman Auditory Discrimination Test (Wepman, 1958), the Short Test of Sound Discrimination (Templin, 1943), and the Goldman-Fristoe-Woodcock Test of Discrimination (Goldman et al., 1970). In these tests, the stimuli (e.g., use of minimal pairs), the tasks (e.g., same versus different judgments) and the types of responses (e.g., picture identification) combine to make most currently available tests of discrimination clinically problematic (Locke, 1980a). Alternate procedures are available (Locke, 1980b). Locke has suggested using individualized stimuli, yes or no judgments of single-word productions, and has offered some useful procedural alternatives (e.g., ''Is x like A or B?''; ''Which of the following three (stimuli) is different?'').

Some inaccurate perceptions are not clinically relevant. For instance, if a child has difficulty distinguishing between /θ/ and /f/, perceptual training may not be appropriate. This is true because there is a visible distinction between these two sounds which can readily be remediated on a motoric basis (Locke, 1980b). Finally, many children who make production errors have no measureable perceptual difficulty.

Related Developmental Examination: Cognition and Language

There are relationships between cognitive ability and phonological behavior. Thus, examination is often not complete without information about childrens' level of cognitive function. Newhoff and Leonard have provided a summary of procedures clinicians can use to complete cognitive examination in Chapter 3 of this text. Readers should review this material together with additional information offered in Chapter 2.

Examination is often also not complete without data regarding children's general language skills. Determination of whether a child's speech sound disorder is associated with a more general linguistic deficit must be part of the examination process. Again, Newhoff and Leonard (Chapter 3) provide a summary of the procedures clinicians can use to complete language examination.

Linguistic factors have an influence on speech sound behavior. As noted earlier, the syntactic complexity of an utterance, word class (nouns versus verbs) and pragmatic factors (given versus new information) may all influence speech sound behavior. For any given child, the clinician must determine the influence of these factors upon speech sound production. This can be accomplished by comparing word and sound productions in various linguistic contexts. Although the samples collected during original speech sampling may serve as the basis for such analyses, additional sampling may be needed for this purpose. The findings can then be directly applied to the choice and sequence of stimuli, targets, and contexts used in planning remediation.

INTERPRETATION OF DIAGNOSTIC INFORMATION

Identifying Children with Speech Sound Disorders

One step in interpretation of diagnostic information is to determine whether a child actually has a speech sound disorder. This requires interpreting information about normal speech sound behavior. Clinicians rely upon comparative information about the performance of a child in relation to performance data available for groups of normally developing children to make this decision. Normative data accumulated from the responses of relatively large numbers of children at various ages are used for this purpose (e.g., Poole 1934; Prather et al., 1975; Templin 1957; Wellman et al., 1931). These data provide information about the ages at which children acquire speech sounds.

As we have learned, such data may deal with what is termed *speech sound mastery*. The criteria used to determine age of acquisition has varied. For example, Templin (1957) used a criterion of 75 percent of the children tested who correctly produced /s/ in the initial-, medial-, and the final-word position to specify mastery. Poole (1934) used a criterion of 100 percent of the children tested who correctly produced the sound /s/ in all three word positions. Because these are ages of mastery, they represent upper-end values for acquisition. For example, if the norms of Templin, which incorporate a 75 percent criterion of correct production of sounds in all three word-positions are used (see Table 4.1), a 5½-year-old child could be identified as disordered when he or she only articulated /s/ correctly in two positions. Such a child may not be disordered. It is possible that this child's errors were limited to the sound error produced as part of the word in which the third position was tested. It is also possible that this child was about to master this sound. A 4-year-old child who has not yet correctly produced /s/ might not be identified as disordered using Templin norms per se. This is true because age of mastery for this sound is 4½ years.

A second type of norm called *age of customary usage* (Sander, 1972) can also be used to define disorder. Age of customary usage refers to the age at which more than 50 percent of normally developing children examined produced a given sound in at least two word positions (see Table 4.1). Hence, this criterion neither represents mastery nor upper-end performance. For example, using Templin's mastery criterion, /s/ is associated with a mastery age of 4½ years, whereas the age for customary usage is 3 years. Thus, clinicians can obtain a picture of the child's speech sound production status by using both age of customary usage and age of mastery data.

Clinicians clearly rely upon mastery and customary usage information to determine whether a child has a speech sound disorder. In addition, they rely upon clinical interpretation of information gathered about error types and patterns (Ingram, 1976; Shriberg and Kwiatkowski, 1980). For example, types and patterns of errors never or seldom present in normally developing children mark disorder. Types and patterns of errors not typically present in normally developing children of the same age as a child being examined also mark disorder. Determination of disorder also depends upon clinical interpretation of information gathered about error consistency/variability, contrast behavior, and stimulability. Although there are no normative data which take dialectal variations into account, it is important for clinicians to identify such variations and to distinguish them from speech sound errors (Williams and Wolfram, 1977). Finally, identification of significant problems in children's production of speech sounds by teachers and parents can often be relied upon to indicate disorder.

The second concern in interpreting diagnostic information is to describe the nature and types of the child's errors. We have described the procedures used to accomplish this task earlier in this chapter. Production errors must be interpreted to specify the frequency, consistency, and specific patterns

Specifying the Child's Errors

of errors. An attempt should also be made to determine whether linguistic factors influence the child's productions. These interpretations are of great value in formulating a therapy plan.

Identifying Physical Factors Which Cause or Maintain the Problem

After the clinician has determined that a child is disordered and has specified the errors, physical factors which cause or maintain the problem should be identified. Identification of these factors requires interpretation of clinical information gathered as part of the speech and hearing mechanism examination and interviewing. The clinician must interpret this information to determine whether a particular structural problem and/or functional deficit is causing or maintaining speech sound errors. As pointed out earlier, not all structural or functional deficits are clearly related to speech sound disturbance. Consequently, in many cases the clinician will have to make such determinations by relying upon clinical experience and knowledge. The clinician must also determine if a given deficit warrants referral of the child to other professionals.

Determining the Type of Disorder

A fourth concern in diagnosis is determining the type of disorder. Earlier, we indicated that speech sound disorders can be divided into two general types: phonetic disorders and phonological disorders. This division relates to the level of the speech sound system involved.

Several types of clinical evidence can be sought to identify and differentiate phonetic from phonological disorders. For example, identification of known physical causes can be used to identify children with phonetic disorders. In addition, children with phonetic disorders may have isolated speech sound errors and these errors generally neither fall into patterns nor do they meet the criteria for phonological processes.

In contrast, children with phonological disorders generally have errors on several sounds and these errors often fall into patterns that meet the criteria for phonological processes. In addition, children with phonological disorders do not generally have physical deficits which explain their productive sound patterns and they do not have identifiable problems in motor movement or sequencing.

Interpretation of the types and patterns of speech sound errors provide very useful information about disorder type. As a general rule, phonetic disorders are characterized by isolated sound errors, allophonic errors (distortions), sound order errors, or patterns of errors readily attributable to some physical basis. Phonological disorders are generally characterized by pattern(s) of errors which influence all or part of sound classes (e.g., fricatives), and/or word types (e.g., CVC *boat* [boʊ] or CVC *dog* [dɔ]).

Phonological disorders are also diagnosed by determining whether a child has the ability to perceive and produce the error sounds. This determination can sometimes be made by identifying the presence of *phonological idioms* and *puzzle phenomena*. Phonological idioms are words that were produced correctly, or nearly so, when first acquired, although the production of these words gradually deteriorates over time. For example, a parent might tell you that their child accurately referred to his brother as *Chris* [krɪs] when he initially used this word, but more recently his productions of this word were not accurate: *Chris* [kɪ], [sɪs]. This type of behavior, reveals that this child probably has the ability to perceive and produce these error sounds, because at an earlier period, he produced *Chris* accurately. Puzzle phenomena were originally discussed by Smith (1973). This phenomenon is illustrated by the child who clearly produces the word *puddle* inaccurately [pʌgl̩] when this word was intended. During the production of words other than *puddle*, however, this child actually produces the word *puddle* even though another word was intended (i.e., child says [pʌdl̩] for *puzzle*). This behavior reveals that the child has the ability to produce the error sound.

Phonetic and phonological disorders need not be mutually exclusive. Clinical information should be interpreted carefully to determine whether a given child has a phonetic disorder, a phonological disorder, or clinical features compatible with both of these disorder types.

Specifying the Severity of the Disorder

An additional task confronting clinicians engaged in diagnosis is to determine the severity of the disorder. Severity estimates are based primarily upon interpretation of information collected as part of the analysis of the child's speech sound errors. Particular use is made of data gathered about the consistency, the specific kinds and patterns of errors, and the extent of errors. In addition, simply counting the number of sound errors often provides a highly useful, direct measure of severity. Estimation of severity using total error counts should also take into consideration the relative frequency of the occurrence of sounds.

The consistency of error productions must be considered from two perspectives. As a general rule, children who do not consistently produce a given sound or class of sounds incorrectly have less severe problems than those who consistently produce a given sound or class of sounds incorrectly. From the second perspective, children who consistently make the same error on a given sound or class of sounds generally have less severe problems than those who make different errors or are highly variable in their productions of intended sounds.

Finally, some individual types of errors and some patterns of errors may reflect variations in the degree of severity because of their effect on intelligibility and/or because they are more difficult to correct.

Formulating the Course of Therapy

A vital part of diagnosis is interpreting diagnostic findings for the purpose of formulating a course of therapy. Obviously, specification of individual sound errors and error patterns, classification of disorder type(s), identification of causal and maintaining factors, and estimation of severity all contribute to this formulation.

The system of classifying speech sound disorders advocated here is intimately related to speech remediation. In the case of phonetic disorders, remediation strategies are directed toward improving the ability to produce and to perceive specific sounds and phonetic features. Therapy goals are generally stated in terms of motor movement and/or perceptual discrimination objectives. The nature of actual therapy for children with phonetic disorders is largely directed toward some form of motor-oriented production or perception-oriented (identification and discrimination) drill. As a general rule, response generalization to spontaneous speech is more likely to occur when "more natural communication" is used as the base for therapy activity. Although less natural communication activities (e.g., elicited imitation) may need to be used during initial stages of therapy, the clinician should strive to include activities that require more natural communicative responses (e.g., requesting objects or pictures, engaging in conversational speech).

In the case of phonological disorders, remediation strategies and goals are generally directed toward the elimination of error patterns, enlargement of production and selection repertoire through expansion of the lexicon, establishment of contrast behavior, elimination of homonymy, and reduction of variability. In addition, more general language goals (e.g., production of longer and more complex utterances) may often be appropriate. As you recall, phonological disorders reflect disturbances in the cognitive or representational aspects of the speech sound system. Hence, remediation strategies for children with disorders of this type(s) do not generally emphasize motor practice or drill-oriented procedures. Rather, remediation strategies that require more natural communicative responses from the child are emphasized. Emphasis is not placed on the repetition of individual responses. Instead, children are encouraged to produce a rich variety of sounds, of given sound classes and of words. Using selective reinforcement of correct productions, clinicians can increase the likelihood that children will alter patterns. The goal of altering error patterns should be emphasized, whereas the goal of altering production of single sounds should not be stressed.

Therapy should also be directed toward enabling children to recognize the communicative consequences of certain errors and error patterns. Children must learn that changing a sound in a sequence can change meaning. For example, a change in the initial sound of *pen* can result in *den* or *hen*, quite dissimilar referents. At an error pattern level, deletion of final consonants can also result in reduced intelligibility as well as altered meaning. Specific techniques which can be used to assist children in recognizing the consequences of their errors in terms of meaning and intelligibility have been discussed by Weiner (1981). Specifically, Weiner has suggested using activities in which children produce minimally paired (e.g., *boat* versus *bow*) stimuli. A second procedure which might be considered is modeling (see Leonard, 1975, for details).

Specific recommendations concerning the sequence of remediation activities can be made. Four primary criteria which have been used by speech-language pathologists remain appropriate. First, sounds, sound classes, word types, and error patterns which appear earliest should have higher training priority. Second, individual errors and error patterns which have the greatest influence on intelligibility should also have higher training priority. Third, consistency and stimulability criteria can also be used. Finally, individual errors or error patterns which contribute to the perception of "disorder" (e.g., whole syllable omissions) should be considered as a primary criterion for sequencing remediation activities.

Offering Prognostic Statements

The child, parents, teachers, physicians, and clinicians themselves all have an interest in knowing how long it will take and how difficult it will be to remediate a speech sound disorder. We do not have the ability to make categorical prognostic statements. We continue to use information about error types and patterns, etiology, severity, stimulability, and so on to formulate prognostic statements. In general, these statements are based largely on an interpretation of these types of clinical information, general knowledge of speech, cognitive and linguistic development, and the clinician's experience with children having speech sound disorders. Prognostic estimations may be modified as a result of information collected during therapy.

Study Guide

1. Review the significant features of the five major developmental periods of speech sound acquisition.

2. What are some major limitations of the data provided in Table 4.1?

3. How is speech sound behavior in normally developing children related to cognitive factors? To linguistic factors?

4. How may speech sound errors be characterized?

5. How does the system of classifying speech sound disorders proposed in this chapter differ from the traditional method of classification?

6. What are the differences between phonetic and phonological speech sound disorders?

7. List the essential parts of the diagnostic process for children with speech sound disorders.

8. What are some of the limitations of commercially available articulation tests? What are some of the limitations of spontaneous sampling? How might these be remedied?

9. Identify and briefly describe six significant aspects of speech sound behavior which can be analyzed after speech samples have been collected.

10. Describe the major tasks facing clinicians in interpreting diagnostic information.

11. How should the course of therapy for a phonetic disorder differ from the course of therapy for a phonological disorder?

REFERENCES

Bernthal, J., and Bankson, N. 1981. Articulation Disorders. Prentice-Hall, Inc., Englewood Cliffs, NJ.

Carter, E., and Buck, M. 1958. Prognostic testing for functional articulation disorders among children in the first grade. J. Speech Hear. Disord. 23:124–133.

Chomsky, N., and Halle, M. 1968. The Sound Pattern of English. Harper & Row, Publishers, Inc., New York.

Farquhar, M. 1961. Prognostic value of imitative and auditory discrimination tests. J. Speech Hear. Disord. 26:342–347.

Fisher, H., and Logemann, J. 1971. The Fisher-Logemann Test of Articulation Competence. Houghton Mifflin Co., Boston.

Fudala, J. 1970. Arizona Articulation Proficiency Scale: Revised. Western Psychological Services, Los Angeles.

Goldman, R., and Fristoe, M. 1969. Goldman-Fristoe Test of Articulation. American Guidance Service, Inc., Circle Pines, MN.

Goldman, R., Fristoe, M., and Woodcock, R. 1970. The Goldman-Fristoe-Woodcock Test of Auditory Discrimination. American Guidance Service, Inc., Circle Pines, MN.

Hodson, B. 1980. The Assessment of Phonological Processes. Interstate Press, Danville, IL.

Hubbell, R. 1977. On facilitating spontaneous talking in young children. J. Speech Hear. Disord. 42:216–231.

Ingram, D. 1976. Phonological Disability in Children. Edward Arnold, London.

Ingram, D. 1981. Procedures for the Phonological Analysis of Children's Language. University Park Press, Baltimore.

Irwin, J. 1972. The Triota: A computerized screening battery. Acta Symbol. 3:26–38.

Irwin, R., West, J., and Trombetta, M. 1966. Effectiveness of speech therapy for second grade children with misarticulations—Predictive factors. Except. Child. 32:471–479.

Kenyon, J., and Knott, T. 1944. A Pronouncing Dictionary of American English. Mirriam, Springfield, MA.

Leonard, L. 1975. Modeling as a clinical procedure in language training. Lang. Speech Hear. Serv. Schools 6:72–85.

Leske, M. 1981. Prevalence estimates of communicative disorders in the U.S. Asha 23:217–228.

Locke, J. 1980a. The inference of speech perception in the phonologically disordered child. Part I: A rationale, some criteria, the conventional tests. J. Speech Hear. Disord. 45:431–444.

Locke, J. 1980b. The inference of speech perception in the phonologically disordered child. Part II: Some clinically novel procedures. J. Speech Hear. Disord. 45:445–468.

McDonald, E. 1964. A Deep Test of Articulation. Stanwix House, Pittsburgh.

McDonald, E. 1968. Screening Deep Test of Articulation. Stanwix House, Pittsburgh.

McReynolds, L., and Bennett, S. 1972. Distinctive feature generalization in articulation training. J. Speech Hear. Disord. 37:462–470.

McReynolds, L., and Elbert, M. 1981. Criteria for phonological process analysis. J. Speech Hear. Disord. 46:197–204.

McReynolds, L., and Engmann, D. 1975. Distinctive Feature Analysis of Misarticulations. University Park Press, Baltimore.

Milisen, R. 1971. The incidence of speech disorders. In: L. E. Travis (ed.), Handbook of Speech Pathology and Audiology. Appleton-Century-Crofts, New York.

Paynter, W., and Bumpas, T. 1977. Imitative and spontaneous articulatory assessment of three-year-old children. J. Speech. Hear. Disord. 42:119–125.

Pendergast, K., Dickey, S., Selmar, T., and Soder, A. 1969. The Photo Articulation Test, 2nd Ed. Interstate Press, Danville, IL.

Pollack, E., and Rees, N. 1972. Disorders of articulation. Some clinical applications of distinctive feature theory. J. Speech Hear. Disord. 37:451–461.

Poole, I. 1934. Genetic development of articulation of consonant sounds in speech. Elem. English Rev. 11:159–161.

Prather, E., Hedrick, D., and Kern, C. 1975. Articulation development in children aged two to four years. J. Speech Hear. Disord. 40:179–191.

Ritterman, S., and Freeman, N. 1974. Distinctive features relevant and irrelevant stimulus dimensions in speech-sound discrimination learning. J. Speech Hear. Res. 17:417–425.

Sander, E. 1972. When are speech sounds learned? J. Speech Hear. Disord. 37:55–63.

Schmauch, V., Panagos, J., and Klich, R. 1978. Syntax influences in the articulation performance of language-disordered children. J. Commun. Disord. 11:315–323.

Schwartz, R., Leonard, L., Folger, M., and Wilcox, M. 1980. Early phonological behavior in language normal and language disordered children: Evidence for a synergistic view of linguistic disorders. J. Speech Hear. Disord. 45:357–377.

Shriberg, L., and Kent, R. 1982. Clinical Phonetics. John Wiley & Sons, New York.

Shriberg, L., and Kwiatkowski, J. 1980. Natural Process Analysis. John Wiley & Sons, New York.

Siegel, R., Winitz, H., and Conkey, H. 1963. The influence of testing instrument on articulatory responses of children. J. Speech Hear. Disord. 28:67–76.

Smith, N. 1973. The Acquisition of Phonology: A Case Study. Cambridge University Press, Cambridge.

Smith, M., and Ainsworth, S. 1967. The effect of three types of stimulation on articulatory responses of speech defective children. J. Speech Hear. Res. 10:333–338.

Sommers, R., Leiss, R., Delp, M. et al., 1967. Factors related to the effectiveness of articulation therapy for kindergarten, first and second grade children. J. Speech Hear. Res. 10:428–437.

Snow, J., and Milisen, R. 1954. The influence of oral versus pictorial representation upon articulation testing results. J. Speech Hear. Disord. 4(Monogr. Suppl.):29–36.

Stampe, D. 1973. A Dissertation on Natural Phonology. Doctoral dissertation. University of Chicago.

Templin, M. 1943. Study of sound discrimination ability of elementary school children. J. Speech Hear. Disord. 8:127–132.

Templin, M. 1947. Spontaneous vs. imitated verbalization in testing pre-school children. J. Speech Hear Disord. 12:293–300.

Templin, M. 1957. Certain Language Skills in Children. Institute of Child Welfare Monograph Series 26. University of Minnesota, Minneapolis.

Templin, M., and Darley, F. 1969. The Templin-Darley Tests of Articulation. Bureau of Educational Research and Service University of Iowa, Iowa City.

Weiner, F. 1979. Phonological Process Analysis. University Park Press, Baltimore.

Weiner, F. 1981. Treatment of phonological disability using the method of meaningful minimal contrast: Two case studies. J. Speech Hear. Disord. 46:97–103.

Weismer, G., Dinnisen, D., and Elbert, M. 1981. A study of the voicing distinction associated with omitted, word-final stops. J. Speech Hear. Disord. 46:320–328.

Weiss, C. 1978. Weiss Comprehensive Articulation Test. Teaching Resources, Hingham, MA.

Wellman, B., Case, I., Mengert, I., and Bradbury, D. 1931. Speech sounds of young children. University of Iowa Studies in Child Welfare Vol. 5.

Wepman, J. 1958. Wepman Auditory Discrimination Test. Language Research Assoc., Chicago.

Williams, R., and Wolfram, W. 1977. Social Dialects: Differences vs. Disorders. American Speech-Language-Hearing Association, Rockville, MD.

Winitz, H. 1969. Articulatory Acquisition and Behavior. Appleton-Century Crofts, New York.

5

Diagnosis of Phonatory Based Voice Disorders

Bernd Weinberg

Outline

Educational Aims

1. *To describe how human voices are produced*
2. *To identify the roles human voice production plays in the speech act*
3. *To discuss how human voices can become disordered*
4. *To describe how speech-language pathologists evaluate patients with voice disorders*

Human voice production represents an integral part of the speech act. We listen to voices every day. Unfortunately, some people develop problems with their voices. In this chapter, we are concerned with how human voices may become disordered. One task is to describe what the concept of voice disorders means. We also consider the types of voice disorders that exist and provide information about the factors that cause these problems. Finally, our main topic is discussed: a consideration of the procedures speech-language pathologists use to diagnose disordered voice production.

NORMAL ASPECTS OF PHONATION

Phonation refers to the process of producing sound at the level of the larynx. In general terms, pulmonary airflow is channeled through the glottis (opening between the vocal folds) to produce sound, and different basic types of sound result from distinctive patterns of movement of the vocal folds. The two most basic modes of sound production are voicing and whispering, which is the complete absence of voice. Voicing is an important type of phonatory output, because this type of sound provides a primary source of acoustic energy in speech. During voicing the glottis is closed, or nearly so, and subglottal air pressure is directed to the closed or constricted glottis. When a sufficient pressure differential is created across the glottis, the vocal folds are moved to open the glottis. Closing of the glottis is mediated by the elastic forces of the vocal folds and the Bernoulli effect. The cyclical opening and closing of the vocal folds results in the emission of a train of air puffs, which form the recurrent source of acoustic excitation for what we hear as voicing.

Definition of Phonation

A wide variety of sounds are produced during the human laryngeal voicing process. These sounds are marked by a large range of intensity, frequency, and quality characteristics. Thus, essential features of the phonatory process lead to the realization of three primary perceptual attributes of human voices: loudness, pitch, and quality.

Phonation plays several important roles within the speech act. As indicated, one role is to provide a primary source of acoustic energy in speech. This role is, in large part, responsible for the realization of perceived, nonlinguistic differences in vocal pitch, loudness, and quality heard among human voices. Phonation also plays a phonetic role. The presence or absence of voicing or the relative timing of the onset of voicing in relation to articulatory events is a phonetic cue that distinguishes voiced from voiceless consonants. Phonation also plays an articulatory role. For example, the vocal folds are used to form speech sounds known as glottals. In addition, phonation plays a central role in regulating voice fundamental frequency and intensity. It is largely through changes in the physical properties of fundamental frequency

Phonatory Functions

and intensity that linguistically related attributes of speech are realized. Systematic variation in voice fundamental frequency and intensity are used to bring about various degrees or levels of stress and intonation. Thus, phonation plays a linguistic role in mediating the prosodic aspects of speech.

DEFINING VOICE DISORDERS

In this chapter, we discuss disorders of phonation. We are concerned primarily with diagnosis of voice disturbance which results from altered vibratory patterning of the vocal folds during the voiced or voicing mode. We will not discuss changes in human voice which result primarily from nonphonatory factors. Therefore, we will not consider voice disturbances such as excessive nasalization (hypernasality) or diminished nasalization (denasality), which result primarily from altered function of the upper airways or the vocal tract.

We will deal with the dysphonias—disorders of phonation. Any abnormality or deviation in the basic attributes of voice pitch, loudness and quality is considered a dysphonia. A voice disorder exists when the pitch, loudness, and/or quality attributes of a given voice are judged to differ significantly from so-called normal voices of other people of comparable age, sex, and socioeconomic/cultural group.

Rigid, fixed and uniform standards for defining vocal abnormality or deviance do not exist. Despite this well-accepted fact, voice change causes most people to seek the advice of their family physician, a laryngologist or a speech-language pathologist. Clearly, the labeling of a voice as normal/abnormal, deviant/nondeviant, disturbed/not disturbed reflects the background and bias of the individual making the judgment. Patients, parents, friends, physicians, and speech-language pathologists all label, define, and make judgments about vocal adequacy. Fortunately, in most cases clinicians, patients, and family members agree that a voice problem exists, wish to have the problem assessed, and desire treatment for its resolution. The latter observation serves to re-emphasize the fact that labeling of disordered voices is a relative matter which requires problematic production of voice by a speaker and perception of the problem by a listener.

TYPES OF VOICE DISTURBANCE

As indicated earlier, we are concerned with describing the procedures speech-language pathologists use to diagnose voice disorders. Vocal disturbance is present in many different ways and results from a wide variety of causes.

As we have seen, the terms *voiced* or *voicing* are used to mark types of voice production that are quasi-periodic or smooth. As a general rule, normal voicing leads to production of vocal quality that is perceived by the listener as pleasant, smooth, periodic, and tonal. Thus, one primary way voices may manifest deviance is in abnormal vocal quality. Hence, abnormal voicing leads to the production of vocal quality that is perceived by the listener as unpleasant, rough, aperiodic, or atonal. A large number of different voice qualities are heard in clinical practice, and there is no universal agreement about the validity of terms used to describe these qualities. Despite this circumstance, the perception of two major types of vocal quality—roughness/hoarseness and breathiness—provide clear evidence of disturbed phonation.

    As indicated, normal voicing is smooth. Thus, perception of rough or hoarse sounding voice quality reflects deviance. In a similar fashion, normal voicing is perceived as periodic and tonal. Therefore, perception of breathiness and/or roughness in the voice marks a problem, because these qualities signal the presence of aperiodicity, noise, and diminished tonal quality.

Disturbances in Vocal Quality

A second primary way voices may manifest deviance is that they may reflect deviant voice pitch levels and/or pitch patterns. Voice pitch is determined by the fundamental rate or frequency of vocal fold vibration. Pitch deviance may be manifested in voices produced using pitch levels that are conspicuously higher or lower than those used by persons of comparable age, sex, socio-economic, and cultural class. An example of this type of problem is seen in some adolescent males or adult men who consistently use pitch levels appropriate to preadolescent children (persistent mutational falsetto).

    Deviance may also be manifested in disordered pitch patterns. Examples of this type of problem are seen in people who speak with little or no perceptible variation in pitch (monotony), or in persons who use pitch patterns that do not appear to vary appropriately in relation to what is being spoken. Patients unable to clearly realize stress and intonation in speech provide examples of the latter problem. Normal pitch patterning may also be disturbed or marked by the presence of vocal tremor and pitch breaks perceived as rapid, inappropriate, and unintentional fluctuations in pitch.

Disturbances in Voice Pitch Levels or Patterns

A third primary way voices may manifest deviance is that they may reflect deviant voice loudness levels and/or patterns. Deviance of this type is evident in people who speak using vocal or speech intensity levels conspicuously higher or lower than typical for given speaking situations or in people who fail to exhibit variation in intensity or loudness appropriate to the meaning of the spoken utterance.

Disturbances in Voice Loudness Levels or Patterns

Voice Interruptions   Finally, voices may manifest a primary form of deviance when unintentional interruptions or breaks (phonation or voice breaks) occur in voicing during speech.

CAUSES OF VOCAL DISTURBANCE

Abuse and Misuse of the Larynx

We have seen that there are many ways voices may become disordered or reflect disturbance. There are also many causes of vocal disturbance. One major cause of vocal disturbance is abuse or misuse of the larynx. A large number of patients are seen for examination and management of vocal disturbance related to abuse or misuse of the larynx. The abuse may be related to using the larynx excessively or abusing the larynx during speech or during other nonspeech activities—singing, coughing, laughing, crying, throat clearing, and so on. Many authors refer to dysphonias related to abuse or misuse as hyperfunctional disorders or problems. Vocal hyperfunction is associated with a wide variety of vocal symptoms. Patients with vocal disturbance stemming from abuse or misuse have developed inefficient strategies for producing voice and exhibit significant dysphonia. Many patients in this group fail to exhibit clinically observable, laryngeal changes. They merely misuse or abuse their sound producing system and exhibit voice disturbance.

Other patients exhibit clinically observable, laryngeal changes in association with vocal abuse, misuse, and hyperfunction. This observation highlights the view that inefficient use of the larynx may actually lead to organic laryngeal change. The consequences of abuse or misuse may lead to inflammation, vocal fold thickening, vocal nodules, vocal polyps, and contact ulcers. Significant dysphonia often accompanies organic laryngeal changes of these types. Some authors feel that abuse or misuse may not be the sole, primary cause for the laryngeal changes and vocal disturbances just discussed. Rather, they feel there is a catalyst in the etiologic chain for disorders of this type. The catalyst is purported to be emotionally based factors such as stress, incipient anger, repressed agression, and so on (Aronson, 1980). Nevertheless, misuse and abuse continue to be regarded as important etiologic factors responsible for both vocal disturbance and the development of laryngeal change.

Organic Disease, Physical Trauma, and Structural Change

Other major causes for voice disturbance are organic disease, physical trauma or insult, and structural change within the larynx stemming from congenital disorders, glandular disturbance, or tumor formation. Examples of congenital disorders that may produce dysphonia include: laryngomalcia, congenital laryngeal webbing; congenital laryngeal cysts; Cri du Chat syndrome, and so on. Examples of glandular disturbance that may produce dysphonia include: hypothyroidism; hyperthyroidism; acromegaly, and a variety of gonadal and endocrine gland disorders. Examples of tumor formation that may produce dysphonia include: papilloma, intubation granulomas, hemangiomas, and laryngeal cancer. Laryngeal trauma stemming from accidental injury, assault and surgical complications can also produce a wide variety of vocal symptoms. Finally, there are large numbers of laryngeal and systemic diseases, conditions, or illnesses which may produce voice change. For example, various neurological conditions—lower motor neuron syndromes (flaccidity); upper motor neuron syndromes (spasticity); basal ganglion disorders (hypokinetic-Parkinsonism, hyperkinetic-choreas, and dystonias); cerebellar problems (ataxia); brainstem disorders (organic voice tremor)—produce voice change. Voice disturbance is associated with systemic conditions such as arthritis, infectious laryngitis resulting from viral and bacterial infection, allergic responses, colds, and upper respiratory infections. Finally, voice disturbance is associated with the use of a wide variety of drugs and medicines.

A third group of major causes for voice disturbance are psychogenic factors: definable emotional stress and conflict, conversion reactions, psychosexual conflicts, personality disorders, depression, psychoneurosis, and psychoses. Major examples of voice disturbance stemming from psychogenic sources include mutational falsetto and conversion aphonia or dysphonia.

Psychogenic Factors

Finally, some types of voice disturbance stem from undetermined or unknown causes. For example, one major condition—spastic (spasmodic) dysphonia—produces severe voice disturbance and has an undetermined cause.

Undetermined Causes

THE SIGNIFICANCE OF VOCAL DISTURBANCE

We have indicated that most people seek advice when they experience voice change of any type. This response underscores the fact that most people are aware that the voice often provides an indication or symptom of illness. Thus, changes or abnormalities in voice often provide essential signs or symptoms about the status of the speaker's physical and emotional health. One primary clinical concern with patients presenting with vocal change should be to determine whether these changes indicate illness. When possible, the etiology of voice change or disturbance should be found. We have seen that some types of dysphonia result from the presence of serious, life-threatening diseases and conditions (e.g., cancer, papilloma etc.). It is, therefore, important to determine the reason for voice change and to ascertain that voice change is not a sign of threat to the physical or emotional well-

Voice Change May Signal Illness

being of the patient. For these reasons, contemporary speech pathologists are educated from medical as well as rehabilitation perspectives. Evaluation of voice disturbance by speech-language pathologists may contribute information essential to the differential diagnosis of a given patient's overall medical problem.

Voice Change May Interfere with Effective Communication

We have also discussed the roles voice or voicing plays in the speech act. Voice change or abnormal voice symptoms may also be a sign of communication disturbance. In this light, certain types of vocal disturbance may bring about a reduction in speech intelligibility and may cause problems in the efficient transmission and intended meaning of messages. The severity of vocal disturbance may be so great as to interfere significantly with message meaning or understandibility. In other cases, the nature of voice disturbance may give rise to the realization of voice which is aesthetically irritating, if not unacceptable.

Social, Economic, and Personal Influences of Voice Change

Voice disturbance clearly has communicative, social, economic and personal significance. A person's voice is an important source of identification—a signature. Significant or noticeable changes in this signature can alter professional careers and create serious economic hardship. For some people, voice disturbance may be clearly noticeable and significant, although not severe. These forms of voice change are almost always distressing to patients and may create effects of considerable social and economic significance. Altered voice invariably creates a change in family and interpersonal relationships. Voice disturbance may, therefore, interfere with the speaker's social and occupational needs.

DIAGNOSIS OF VOICE DISORDERS

We have considered how human voices may be disturbed and have discussed the factors that cause these problems. We move from there to consider the procedures commonly used to examine and diagnose disordered voice production.

The process of conducting a clinical examination of patients with disordered voice production can be divided into several major parts:

1. Obtain a history of voice disorder.
2. Complete a laryngoscopic and head and neck examination.
3. Examine the functional adequacy of the phonatory apparatus and describe the typical manner of behavior of the respiratory/phonatory apparatus during voice production.
4. Provide a description of patient's voice.

5. Evaluate hearing function.
6. Summarize findings/observations and come to a diagnosis.
7. Recommend treatment options and specify when additional forms of evaluation (need for referral to other specialities) are needed.

History of the Voice Disorder

Typically, the initial step in the clinical evaluation of patients with voice problems is the completion of a thorough history of the voice disorder. Information is gathered to describe the nature of the voice problem, the conditions surrounding its emergence, and the development of the symptoms. As a general rule, the clinician should develop an outline of the information to be obtained. For this purpose, a preinterview questionnaire is often used. A sample questionnaire we use to obtain information from adult patients is provided in Appendix A. When possible, patients complete this form before coming for an examination. We then read the history and use the completed material to pursue areas that merit clarification or verification. Utilization of this history form not only aids significantly in the diagnostic inquiry, but also provides structure and consistency to our management procedures.

Thorough history gathering necessitates obtaining critical types of information. For example, certain types of basic information must be gathered: patient's name, date of birth, address, phone numbers, physician, and so on (see Identifying Information section, Appendix A). In addition, a careful history of the voice problem and conditions or events surrounding its emergence and development must be always obtained. We routinely ask patients to describe their voice problem in their own words. Questions related to the nature of the onset and development of the problem are routinely asked. We believe it is very important to have the patient describe the chief characteristics of the voice problem, the severity of the problem, its cause, and the nature of voice change in relation to various physical and emotional factors (see History of the Problem, Appendix A). Speech-language pathologists must explore family history and information about abuse and use, and environmental and behavioral factors which may influence voice production (see Family and Environmental Information, Appendix A). Finally, a concise, yet reasonably comprehensive health history must be gathered.

Laryngology Examination

A second essential part of the diagnostic process for all patients with voice disorders is the completion of a general examination of the head and neck, including visualization of the larynx. This examination is typically completed by a laryngologist, a physician specializing in the diagnosis and treatment of patients with disorders/diseases of the head and neck. Laryngology examinations are not completed to obtain a prescription for voice therapy or to confirm the presence of a vocal disturbance. The laryngology examination is completed to determine the need for medical treatment, to help identify factors that might limit the ultimate production of normal voice or influence treatment, and to clarify the cause of the vocal disturbance.

Because patients with voice disorders must have a laryngoscopic examination, speech-language pathologists working with individuals having voice problems must develop close professional relationships with consulting otolaryngologists. They will find their professional care of patients enhanced by the development of these close, mutually rewarding ties.

Stone et al. (1978) have developed a Laryngology Consult Form. This form was developed to provide an efficient method for speech-language pathologists to specify the information they need to obtain from laryngologists. We strongly recommend the use of this Consult Form which is reprinted in Table 5.1. Use of this form provides both the physician and speech pathologist with a formal, efficient mechanism for insuring that mutually essential observations are made and recorded on a systematic basis. Our consulting laryngologists use these forms regularly. They merely return completed forms on a given patient to us in lieu of a summary letter and use these forms in their own office charts in lieu of office summaries.

The Laryngology Consultation Form is initiated by the speech-language pathologist who provides a brief statement of the problem, the cause(s) or perpetuating factors, the general treatment plan being considered, and the reasons for the referral (see upper section, Table 5.1). The remainder of the form is completed by the laryngologist. For example, a routine examination by a laryngologist typically includes a systems review of the ears, hearing, nose and sinuses (see items 1 to 3, Table 5.1). In addition, this type of examination includes an assessment of the status of the larynx. Initially, appraisal of the status of laryngeal structures other than the true vocal folds is undertaken. Particular attention is devoted to identifying alterations in the size, shape, and symmetry of non-vocal fold structures and to identifying abnormalities in mucous membrane color or typography (see item 4, Table 5.1).

Visualization of the vocal folds is completed primarily to determine whether vocal fold pathology is present and to specify visually observable abnormalities of vocal fold size and position. Laryngologists use a variety of techniques to visualize the vocal folds. The most widely used indirect method of viewing the vocal folds is mirror laryngoscopy. As the word indirect implies, the interior of the larynx is viewed indirectly by means of a mirror. The physician places a mirror into the mouth and carefully guides the mirror into the oropharynx. A light beam, reflected from a head mirror worn by the doctor, is reflected on the mirror to obtain a view of the interior of the larynx. Using mirror laryngoscopy, the laryngologist can thoroughly examine the interior of the larynx, the pharynx and the base of the tongue. The vocal folds are usually examined as the patient produces sustained vowels, during quiet (tidal) breathing, and during maximal inhalation. Visualization of the vocal folds during these activities provides an opportunity to identify the presence of vocal fold pathology and to specify disturbance in vocal fold size and position (see item 5, Table 5.1). The laryngologist specifically seeks to identify abnormality or difference in vocal fold length and position, mucous membrane color or shape, magnitude or consistency of mucous, and the presence of vocal fold pathology. If vocal fold pathology is present, the laryngologist specifies the nature, appearance, size, and location of the pathology observed.

Examination of the larynx by indirect laryngoscopy is limited by the fact that only visually observable changes can be identified and only gross disturbances can be identified. For example, clinically significant disturbances in the vibratory patterning of the vocal folds during voicing may not be identified during indirect laryngoscopic examination. This is the case because the frequencies of vibration of the vocal folds exceed those capable of being followed by the eye of the examiner. In some patients, complete visualization of the larynx is made difficult or is precluded because a gag reflex is elicited during mirror insertion and placement. Gagging may be eliminated or minimized by spraying a topical anesthetic into the oropharynx. Visualization of the larynx may also be obtained using a fiberoptic laryngoscope. Here, a flexible, fiberoptic bundle is usually inserted into the nose and passed into the pharynx. The fiberoptic bundle carries both a light source and image viewer and the physician views the image through an eyepiece located outside the body.

Comprehensive laryngoscopic examination is not always possible using indirect, mirror laryngoscopy. Laryngologists may also use direct laryngoscopy to obtain full views of the interior of the larynx. In this case, an instrument called a *laryngoscope* is introduced into the mouth and is slowly passed to the level of the vocal folds. The laryngologist carefully inspects structures as the scope is being lowered. Direct laryngoscopy is often used to examine the larynx of infants and young children who have larynges that are difficult to visualize on an indirect basis and may not tolerate indirect examinations. Patients often require general anesthesia during direct laryngoscopy, although in highly cooperative patients topical anesthesia may be sufficient.

The laryngological examination is typically completed by having the physician specify whether conditions influencing altered voice were identified (see item 6, Table 5.1). In addition, the Laryngology Consult Form provides an opportunity for the physician to share information in a free-response format (see Consultant Comments, Table 5.1). Here, the physician can not only embellish upon the results of the laryngoscopic examination, but can express opinions about the patient, recommend treatment approaches, raise questions about the planned intervention suggested by the speech pathologist, and so on. Finally, the laryngologist must provide a medical diagnosis and make some recommendations about future treatment. The need for a medical diagnostic label cannot be underestimated, partic-

Table 5.1. Laryngology Consult Sheet[a]

Refer from _____
Address _____ Phone _____
Refer to _____
Address _____ Phone _____
Client's name _____ Age _____
Address _____ Phone _____

For (indicate specific statement of problem and desired information) _____
Background information (describe voice problem, history, suspected precipitating and perpetuating etiology, and pending intervention or disposition) _____

Consultant's findings (check each item appropriately)

	Normal	Abnormal
1. Ears	( )	( )
2. Hearing	( )	( )
3. Nose and sinuses	( )	( )
4. Larynx (excluding true vocal folds)	( )	( )
Size	( )	( )
Shape	( )	( )
Mucous membrane topography	( )	( )
color	( )	( )
5. Vocal folds		
Length	( )	( )
Thickness	( )	( )
horizontal	( )	( )
vertical	( )	( )
Position	( )	( )
inspiration	( )	( )
phonation	( )	( )
Mucous membrane topography	( )	( )
color	( )	( )
Amount of mucus	( )	( )
Consistency of mucus	( )	( )

6. Conditions influencing altered voice (when indicating "yes" please enter "1" in the space to suggest a precipitating factor and "2" a perpetuating factor)

	Yes	No
Dysplasia	( )	( )
Laryngeal pathology	( )	( )
Malignant	( )	( )
Nonmalignant	( )	( )
Myopathy/neuropathy	( )	( )
Endocrine	( )	( )
Gonadal	( )	( )
Thyroid	( )	( )
Menstrual	( )	( )
Sicca syndrome	( )	( )
Faulty use of the larynx	( )	( )

If vocal fold pathology, indicate on diagrams and checklist (R = right, L = left).

Location		
Anterior commisure	( )	
Anterior third	R	L
Junction of first and middle third	R	L
Middle third	R	L
Junction of middle and last third	R	L
Posterior third	R	L
Posterior commisure	( )	
Superior surface	R	L
Medial surface	R	L
Inferior surface	R	L

Appearance		
Translucent	R	L
Opaque	R	L
White	R	L
Reddened	R	L
Hard, organized	R	L
Soft, unorganized	R	L
Smooth surfaced	R	L
Topographical surface	R	L
Sessile	R	L
Pedunculated	R	L
Pointed	R	L
Rounded	R	L

Size	Lateral dimension		Anterior-posterior dimension	
less than 1 mm	R	L	R	L
1–2 mm	R	L	R	L
2–4 mm	R	L	R	L
more than 4 mm	R	L	R	L

Nature		
Scar	R	L
Polypoid growth	R	L
Nodular growth	R	L
Edema	R	L
Ulceration	R	L
Keratosis	R	L

[a]Adapted from Stone et al. (1978).

162

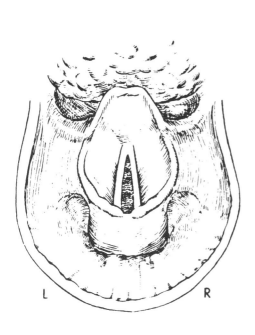

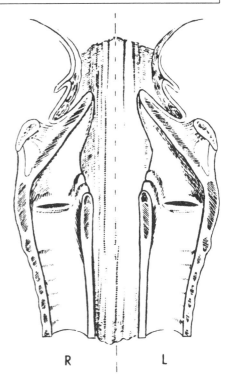

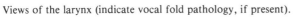

Views of the larynx (indicate vocal fold pathology, if present).

ularly in terms of the legal aspects of clinic practice and the requirements surrounding third party fee reimbursement for service provision. Note should be made of the fact that the laryngologist is not expected to make a recommendation about whether voice therapy is indicated. Although the laryngologist may elect to make such a recommendation, this decision is made by the speech-language pathologist after it has been determined that no factors contraindicating behavioral management have been identified.

Because the results of laryngological examination are often of critical importance, speech-language pathologists in the early stages of their careers should endeavor to view the vocal folds with the consulting laryngologist. Cooperative visualization will enrich the clinician's experiences about the nature and diversity of laryngeal pathology, provide an opportunity for direct communication between the physician and speech-language pathologist about the implications of what has been visualized, may provide the patient with a strong feeling of mutual support and interest, and may enhance the efficiency with which clinical decisions or recommendations are made. Establishment of specialized voice clinics scheduled on a regular or on an as-needed basis provide a fine opportunity for realizing this form of interdisciplinary cooperation.

Examination of Respiratory Function

Contemporary descriptions of normal aspects of human voice production typically embrace aerodynamic-myoelastic principles. Such descriptions highlight the fact that critical aspects of human voice production are mediated chiefly through interactions between respiratory drive and laryngeal adjustment. Thus, examination of respiratory adequacy for voice production represents an essential part of the diagnostic process for many patients with vocal disturbance.

One of the primary functions of the human respiratory system is to supply a sufficient volume of air to the larynx and upper airways during voice production. Hence, one type of respiratory examination involves observing air volume history and movement (kinematic) patterns of the chest wall used during voice production. Normal adults typically expire between 10 to 20 percent of their vital capacity during speech breathing phrases. Thus, normal people expire reasonably small volumes of air (500–1000 cc) during voice production for speech. It is, therefore, highly unlikely that "shortness of breath" or deprivation of lung volume will cause vocal disturbance. Hence, elaborate routine application of pulmonary function studies designed to specify vital capacity or various lung capacities for patients with vocal disturbance are largely unwarranted and unnecessary. Important judgments of volume adequacy often can be made simply through judicious observation of patients.

For example, notation of phrase and sentence length during speech provides important clues about lung volume history. Similarly, timing the duration patients can sustain vowels or counting the number of words or syllables spoken on a single breath can be used to verify volume adequacy. It is important to watch patients as they breathe and speak. For example, normal speakers initiate speech from above resting or tidal breathing levels. Typically, they take about twice as deep a breath to initiate speech as they do during resting breathing and they generally move to higher lung volumes to initiate speech and voice at higher intensity levels. At a clinical level, it is important to verify that patients inhale (about 2 times that of tidal volume) rather than expire before initiating speech or voice. Patients should also produce most of their utterances within the least demanding (mid-volume) portion of their vital capacity range.

Hixon et al. (1973) have shown that normal voice can be produced using a large number of movement patterns of the chest wall. Stated directly there is no single correct way to breathe to produce normal voice or speech. Some speakers are primarily rib cage movers, whereas others rely primarily upon abdominal displacement. Given this situation, routine, instrumental evaluations of the movement patterns of the chest wall during voice production are not warranted or necessary for most patients with voice disturbance. Rather, identification of obvious disturbance (e.g., speaking on inhalation, observable disturbances in control of rib cage or abdomen movement present in association with some major myoneural diseases) can usually be made through judicious observation by the clinician. On the other hand, instrumental analyses of the relations between volume changes and chestwall movement patterns may play a very useful role (i.e., define the origins and/ or factors responsible for speech disturbance) in diagnosis of speech or voice problems seen in patients with neuromotor disturbance.

Finally, it is important to identify patients who have deliberately attempted to alter respiratory activity during voice production or who profess "to know the correct way to breathe." Invariably, such behaviors spell trouble. Most normal-speaking people have no knowledge about how they breathe during voice and speech production. They let the body regulate itself, and in most cases, function will be optimized (Hixon et al., 1973). Use of "known patterns of correct breathing" is likely to spell difficulty, and almost always identifies patients who merit special evaluation, counsel, and perhaps management.

A second primary function of the human respiratory system is to deliver a relatively steady driving pressure to the larynx during voice production. This pressure is called *subglottic* or *subglottal pressure*. During conversational speech, subglottal pressure ranges between 5 and 10 cm H_2O. Hence, a second type of respiratory examination involves determining whether patients are able to supply relatively steady pressures of sufficient magnitude to the larynx.

Direct recording of subglottic pressure during speech necessitates tracheal puncture or placement of a hypodermic needle into the trachea, a procedure clearly not suited for routine clinical use. Netsell and Hixon (1978) have proposed a noninvasive method for clinical estimation of subglottal air pressure. In this method, subglottal pressure is measured during a nonspeech task which requires the client to exhale against an airway resistance that simulates normal phonatory resistance. The airway resistance that simulates normal phonatory resistance is merely a tube with a vent or leak which serves as an analog of glottal resistance. Netsell and Hixon (1978) have stated that "an individual who can generate and sustain 5 cm H_2O for 5 sec, while exhaling against the "leak tube" has sufficient pressure capability to meet most speech requirements." Whether or not the Netsell and Hixon statement is true, this author recommends use of the leak tube or other suitable approaches as simple, noninvasive methods to determine whether patients are able to supply relatively steady pressures of suitable magnitude to the larynx during voice production. An alternative approach to estimation of subglottal pressure generating capabilities of patients is to use peak oral pressure measured during stop consonant production as an estimate of tracheal or subglottic pressure (see Smitheran and Hixon, 1981, for details).

A third factor which deserves attention during examination of patients with vocal disturbance is an estimation of airflow rate through the glottis. Alterations in flow rate through the glottis during the production of vowels may provide important indications of phonatory impairment. During the production of vowels produced in speech or on a sustained basis, airflow rate through the larynx ranges between 100 and 200 cc/sec (0.1 to 0.2 liters/sec). Patients with inefficient valving function of the larynx, characterized in part by the presence of breathiness, often exhibit increased airflow rates, whereas patients exhibiting hyperfunctional laryngeal behavior may exhibit decreased flow rates.

Fortunately, there are a number of ways to obtain noninvasive estimates of airflow rates through the human larynx. Spirometers, pneumotachographs, and simple flow meters can be used to measure flow rates sensed at the patient's mouth. In view of the relative simplicity of obtaining such measures, estimation of glottal flow characteristics should form an essential part of comprehensive voice evaluation.

Finally, there is the issue of measuring glottal resistance. Smitheran and Hixon (1981) have recently commented that the larynx is a valve located between the lower and upper airways. They have indicated that much can be learned about the function of this valve during vowel production by gathering information about the degree of coupling the larynx permits between the larynx and the pharynx. One clinically useful source of information about the degree of coupling is the degree to which the larynx offers opposition to the flow of air through it during vowel production. This opposition is called *laryngeal* or *glottal airway resistance*.

Smitheran and Hixon (1981) have described a noninvasive, method clinicians may use to estimate glottal or laryngeal airway resistance. In this method, subglottal pressure estimates are obtained from measurements of peak oral pressure achieved during stop /p/ production, whereas estimates of glottal flow rate are obtained from measurements of oral flows during the production of vowels /i/ spoken by patients in the form of repetitive /pi/ syllables. This method is clinically easy to implement for clinicians familiar with this type of instrumentation and should also form an essential part of many comprehensive voice examinations.

A fourth essential part of the diagnostic process for all patients with voice disorders is the completion of a detailed perceptual evaluation of the voice. One aim of this phase of the examination process is to describe the characteristics that make a given voice disordered. The clinician should also describe the severity of the dysphonic symptoms, specify conditions or behaviors which elicit or increase the severity of the dysphonic symptoms, and attempt to identify techniques that lessen or eradicate the vocal symptoms.

Description of the Voice

There is no substitute for a thorough perceptual evaluation of voice production by a skilled and experienced clinician. This phase of the diagnostic process is indispensable. Identification of the presence and severity of dysphonic elements forms a critical part of voice diagnosis.

There has been a tendency by many authors to equate perceptual judgments with subjective forms of observation, and to equate observations gathered on non-human, instrumental bases as objective. This form of equation and dichotomy is unfortunate and inappropriate. Most perceptual judgments made about voices by skilled and experienced clinicians have a high degree of face validity and are adequately reliable. Moreover, many perceptual judgments and identifications (e.g., presence of hard glottal attack, high pitch, pitch breaks, aphonia, breathiness, monotone, etc.) can be verified using non-human instrumental methods. When possible, such instrumental verification should be pursued as part of the evaluative process. Although beginning clinicians often tend to undervalue the contributions made by listening to voices, it is worth reiterating that these contributions are indispensable and primary.

There are three primary reasons for completing a thorough perceptual analysis of voice production. First, there is a need to describe the types and severity of dysphonia or voice disturbance. There is also the need to interpret the vocal symptoms in relation to formulating a differential diagnosis. Finally, voice evaluations are completed to ascertain whether a patient should receive voice therapy.

Because a major task for clinicians performing voice evaluations is to describe the types of dysphonia or voice disturbance which might be present, a list of major forms of voice disturbance are tabulated in Appendix B. Clinicians should identify the presence and severity of any of these voice symptoms. To accomplish this task, voice production should be sampled in several contexts:

1. *Voice production in discourse*   Adult patients should read a standard passage (e.g., Rainbow Passage, Fairbanks, 1960, or Grandfather Passage) and engage in conversation. Children not able to read a standard passage should recite a familiar poem, a nursery rhyme, or count, as well as engage in conversation. A reasonably lengthy sample of discourse should be obtained. The clinician should carefully assess voice production as part of the speech act. Initially, efforts should be made to identify the vocal disturbances that are present and to specify the severity of individual elements of dysphonia as well as their collective influence. Use of a checklist such as the one provided in Appendix B may prove helpful in this task.

2. *Vowel prolongations*   All patients should be required to sustain the vowels /i, u, and a/. The patient's task should be to hold voice pitch and loudness constant and to prolong vowels for as long as possible. In this task, the clinician's efforts should be directed principally toward identifying the vocal disturbances that are present and determining that voicing can be sustained for durations sufficient to support adequate phrase length for speech.

3. *Phonational or pitch range*   An estimate should be made of the pitch (fundamental frequency) range of each patient. We use a pitch matching procedure in which patients produce a vowel at pitches elicited by target tones. The primary aims of this task are to identify patients with potential pitch matching problems or those with restricted pitch or phonational ranges. Patients with pitch ranges below one octave clearly exhibit restriction.

4. *Prolonged use of the voice*   Because some forms of vocal disturbance become evident or increase in severity following prolonged use of the speech and vocal mechanism, all patients should be required to count at least from 1 to 100. If vocal disturbance emerges during this counting period or if there is a positive history of vocal problems after exertion or prolonged use of the speech and vocal mechanism, the patient should be required to read for a prolonged period (3 to 5 minutes).

5. *Elicit cough and hard glottal attack*   All patients should be required to cough and to initiate vowels with a hard glottal attack. Impaired ability to elicit a normal cough or elicit vowels with glottal attack suggests problems of vocal fold adduction.

6. *Realization of intonation, stress and voicing distinctions*   Control and regulation of voice pitch (fundamental frequency) and vocal loudness (intensity), together with control over durational aspects of speech, in large part, determine how efficiently a speaker realizes speech prosody. Therefore, routine assessment should be undertaken to determine how well patients are able to achieve intonation and stress contrasts in Amer-

ican English. This is accomplished in a brief test in which patients produce simple sentences in statement-question forms (e.g., ''Bev loves Bob.'' as contrasted with ''Bev loves Bob?''). In a similar fashion, stress contrast realization is assessed by having patients produce sentences in which word and syllable level stress is varied in a systematic fashion. Normal adults are able to realize intonational and stress contrasts in a near-perfect fashion (98–100 percent correct). Thus, patients exhibiting impaired ability to realize stress and/or intonational contrasts may have impaired vocal function reflected in the form of diminished control over voice fundamental frequency and intensity.

In addition, we routinely make certain that patients are able to clearly produce voicing distinctions between cognate pairs (e.g., /p/ versus /b/; /t/ versus /d/; /k/ versus /g/, etc.) of speech sounds in English. The ability to achieve such distinctions is clearly dependent upon control of either the presence or absence of the voicing signal or the relative timing of the onset of voicing in relation to the release of articulatory instructions during stop production (the so-called Voice Onset Time or VOT).

Thus, six tasks are used to elicit voice production in a variety of contexts. A comprehensive description of voice symptoms can be developed from perceptual evaluations of voice production during these six tasks. These tasks were chosen because they enable the clinician to sample a wide variety of types of voice production within a reasonably brief period of evaluation. We routinely obtain tape recordings of patients performing these tasks as part of the evaluative process. It is recommended that these recordings be obtained in a quiet environment (sound proof booth or room) using high quality recording instrumentation. Routine completion of high-quality recordings is important, 1) for medical-legal purposes; 2) for providing speech samples that can be used for additional forms of verification or analysis (e.g., acoustic analysis); and 3) for establishing clinical baseline data. Finally, it is recommended that these recordings be obtained using standardized procedures. For example, we maintain a fixed mouth-to-microphone distance and calibrate the recording system so that instrumental verification and analysis can be completed on both an absolute and a relative basis.

A Brief Note on Optimal Pitch

A fundamental notion embracing much of the literature on appraisal of voice production is the belief that there is an optimal or natural pitch level at which the human vocal apparatus operates with the greatest efficiency. Various clinical techniques have been advocated for locating optimal pitch levels for the speaking voice (Fairbanks, 1960; Pronovost, 1942; Thurman, 1958).

The most prominent approach used to locate optimum pitch level is a technique which requires the patient to hum or sing a scale to determine the level or series of tones at which vocalization is produced most efficiently. Evidence of use of optimal pitch is obtained by having the clinician and/or the patient listen to the humming or singing of scales and identify the tone or series of tones on which an involuntary swell of intensity occurs. This increase in intensity is regarded by proponents of this method as an indicator of increased vocal efficiency and optimum pitch level.

Thurman (1958) has shown that there is serious reason to question the use of the technique just described as a valid indication of specifying optimal pitch. The results of his work failed to provide support for the use of this technique as a method for estimating optimum pitch level. In addition, House (1959) has made the following point:

> When a search for an optimum pitch level is made by intoning vowel sounds at discrete fundamental frequencies throughout a subject's vocal range there probably is a tacit assumption (a) that some sort of optimal physical relationship among the various components of the vocal mechanism will be found, (b) that when this relationship obtains, the laryngeal output will be maximal and will be reflected in a maximum in vocal output at the lips and (c) that the change in over-all level will be perceptible. It might be assumed, furthermore, that vocal effort is constant during the procedures . . .
>
> The description of the clinical procedure leads one to suspect that its proponents intuitively are seeking a condition of optimal "coupling" (in some undefined sense) between the action of the larynx and the supraglottal system. A maximum in laryngeal output, therefore, must originate from activity within the larynx itself and not from some so-called coupling effects. This note attempts to show that maxima in vocal output can be expected when the laryngeal output is constant. Furthermore, it points out that without elaborate controls it would be difficult to detect maxima in laryngeal activity from observations on the vocal output. (pp. 55–56)

Thus, it is now quite clear that clinical forms of appraisal such as those just described are not adequate for locating so-called optimum pitch levels.

This writer believes clinicians should abandon their fervent search for optimum pitch levels during clinical evaluation of patients with voice disorders. Rather, clinicians should search to identify behaviors which lead to inefficient production of voice at any pitch level and seek to establish vocal efficiency at a variety of pitches or fundamental frequencies. Efficiency is achieved by producing voice with as little muscular force as possible. Voice should be produced with no conscious effort on the part of the speaker. In general, voice is produced by relying heavily on background forces (gravity, recoil forces) to power the phonatory apparatus. When active, muscular forcing of the chestwall is used it should be accomplished in a smooth, nonstrenuous fashion, that is, without clinically observable strain or conscious effort. In general, voice production will be optimized by initiating voice at higher lung volumes than by resorting to powering the voice production system at lower lung volumes using strenuous, active, and visually observable chest wall, facial, or neck wall muscle activity.

With respect to pitch level and variability, promotion of efficiency will be realized by having patients produce speech using modal register pitch levels within the low-mid portion of their phonational or pitch ranges, rather than by using the high or low end of these ranges. Highly acceptable speech can be produced using pitch or fundamental frequency variation of less than one-half an octave during connected discourse. Thus, vocal efficiency is achieved by moderating pitch variation, by maintaining pitch levels in the low-mid range and achieving realization of stress, intonation, and emotion using normal, relatively small variation in fundamental frequency and effort or intensity.

Examination of the Speech and Hearing Mechanism

An essential part of the diagnostic process for patients with voice problems is the completion of an examination of the structural and functional integrity of organs used to produce voice and speech. We have already discussed how some forms of this examination can be undertaken in our description of respiratory function testing, in our description of the head and neck examination, and in Chapter 2. We have indicated the need for patients with vocal problems to be examined by a laryngologist and have described what the laryngological examination should accomplish. We have indicated that speech-language pathologists must also conduct their own form of speech mechanism examination and you may wish to review the material in Chapter 2 (see Examination of the Speech Mechanism).

The final phase of mechanism examination includes audiological testing. The form of testing should be commensurate with the needs of the patient. Initially, all patients should receive audiometric screening to determine whether a significant problem might exist. If screening results reveal the need for further testing, a second screening or formal audiometric evaluation should be conducted on subsequent visits (see Chapter 2, Audiological Testing, for further details).

DECISION MAKING

Completion of all phases of the diagnostic process we have discussed provides the clinician with a large amount of information. Thus, the final stage of the evaluation process requires the speech-language pathologist to summarize the information gathered, to interpret this information, to form a diagnosis, and to formulate a management plan.

Referral

In some cases, the information gathered during the evaluative process cannot be brought together to form a definitive differential diagnosis. In these cases, additional information may be needed. The patient may need to be seen by other consultants or specialists (neurologists, endocrinologists, psychiatrists, pediatricians, etc.) to resolve questions. When referral is made to medical specialists, the purpose of the referral should be carefully stated and the types of assistance requested precisely stated. In some cases, speech-language pathologists may wish to refer patients to other speech pathologists either for long-term management or consultation. Management of patients with voice disorders is a complex activity and inexperienced clinicians might enhance both their own skills and the patients progress through referral to and consultation with other colleagues.

Formulating a Diagnosis

In most cases, the information gathered during the evaluative process can be summarized and a diagnosis can be made. For example, the diagnosis of conversion aphonia or dysphonia is made principally on the basis of uncovering a positive history of emotional stress in relation to voice loss or change, identifying normal structure and nonspeech function of larynx during laryngoscopic examination, and eliciting normal ability to fully adduct (close) the vocal folds during such activities as swallowing, coughing, laughing, singing, and/or inspiratory vocalization. Voice disturbances associated with the presence of benign laryngeal lesions such as vocal nodules and contact ulcers are diagnosed principally by identifying these lesions during laryngoscopic examination, uncovering a positive history of specific patterns of abuse or use of the larynx during the interviewing or vocal description phases of the evaluation process, and identifying psychodynamic factors which may contribute further to the development of organic laryngeal and voice change.

In most cases of voice disturbance of organic origin, the specific types of vocal change and their severity are compatable with the findings uncovered in laryngoscopic and medical examination. In cases in which the nature or severity of vocal disturbance is not compatible with medical or laryngoscopic findings, psychogenic factors may also be operating.

Writing Reports and Letters

As we have indicated, in most cases the information gathered during the evaluation process can be brought together and a diagnosis can be made. In these circumstances, a complete report must be written for speech pathology, school, or hospital records. In addition, a letter must be written to conferring physicians summarizing the findings and recommendations (see Chapter 9 for details).

Conferring with Patients

In all cases, the speech-language pathologist should confer with the patient and family. The patient should be informed about the nature of the voice problem, what caused the disorder, and what can be done to improve the voice. Patients should be informed about the prognosis for voice recovery and improvement, the cost, frequency, duration, and nature of therapy recommended or the rationale for not recommending therapy. Finally, patients should be given an opportunity to ask questions and should receive clear, direct answers to these questions.

A BRIEF NOTE ON DIAGNOSIS
FOLLOWING TOTAL LARYNGECTOMY

Cancer of the larynx may necessitate total removal of the larynx. The surgical procedure undertaken in such situations is called total laryngectomy and the individual undergoing such a procedure is referred to as a laryngectomized patient. Total laryngectomy typically necessitates removal of all structures located between the upper tracheal rings and (including) the hyoid bone, forward rotation of the trachea and suturing of the trachea to the base of the neck, and reconstruction of the pharynx and upper esophagus. Total laryngectomy is always followed by an immediate loss of voice, a need to reestablish voice using a nonconventional source, and a need to reestablish speech supported by nonconventional sources of voice excitation, airstream, and articulatory mechanisms.

Major parts of the diagnostic process are already resolved for the speech-language pathologist responsible for laryngectomized patients' speech rehabilitation. For example, the origin of the problem is clear. Namely, voice loss is directly attributable to larynx removal. Second, the severity of the problem is enormous. Patients are unable to communicate satisfactorily to meet their functional needs immediately after surgery without some form of assistance. Third, reliable prognostic indicators which might be used to determine whether a patient will be able to acquire functionally serviceable forms of speech after total laryngectomy are not available. Hence, diagnostic activity for laryngectomized patients is typically devoted to identifying factors which might influence treatment or intervention and formulating a treatment plan.

Identification of factors which might influence treatment can be accomplished through history taking and direct forms of examination (e.g., oral-facial examination, head and neck examination, etc.). Formulation of a treatment plan is relatively straightforward. Restoration of speech and voice for laryngectomized patients is accomplished by teaching patients how to use artificial larynges, teaching them to develop functionally serviceable esophageal speech or developing speech on a surgical-prosthetic basis. A contemporary summary of therapy approaches, goals, and procedures speech-language pathologists use in the treatment of laryngectomized patients is found in Weinberg (1983a,b).

Study Guide

1. What are the major linguistic and nonlinguistic roles phonation plays as part of the speech act?

2. What is a voice disorder? Why are there no rigid, fixed and uniform standards for defining vocal disorders?

3. Identify the major types of voice disturbance.

4. Identify the major causes of voice disturbance.

5. Identify the major parts or steps of the clinical examination used to diagnose patients with voice disorders.

6. Why must all patients with voice disturbance seen by speech-language pathologists undergo laryngoscopic examination which includes visualization of the larynx?

7. Briefly define the following terms or concepts:

phonation	glottis
dysphonia	laryngologist
indirect laryngoscopy	kinematic
resting or tidal breathing	subglottal pressure
glottal resistance	hard glottal attack

REFERENCES

Aronson, A. E. 1980. Clinical Voice Disorders. Brian Decker, New York.

Fairbanks, G. 1960. Voice and Articulation Drillbook. Harper & Row Pubs., Inc., New York.

Hixon, T. J., Goldman, M. D., and Mead, J. 1973. Kinematics of the chest wall during speech production: Volume displacements of the rib cage, abdomen and lung. J. Speech Hear. Res. 16:78–115.

House, A. S. 1959. A note on optimal vocal frequency. J. Speech Hear. Res. 2:55–60.

Netsell, R., and Hixon, T. J. 1978. A noninvasive method for clinically estimating subglottal air pressure. J. Speech Hear. Disord. 43:326–330.

Pronovost, W. 1942. A experimental study of methods for determining natural and habitual pitch. Speech Monogr. 9:111–123.

Smitheran, J. R., and Hixon, T. J. 1981. A clinical method for estimating laryngeal airway resistance during vowel production. J. Speech Hear. Disord. 46:138–146.

Stone, E., Hurlbutt, N., and Coulthard, S. W. 1978. Role of laryngological consultation in the intervention of dysphonia. Lang. Speech Hear. Serv. Schools 9:35–42.

Thurman, W. L. 1958. Frequency-intensity relationships and optimum pitch levels. J. Speech Hear. Res. 1:117–123.

Weinberg, B. 1983a. Voice and speech restoration following total laryngectomy. In: W. Perkins (ed.), Current Therapy of Communication Disorders. Thieme-Stratton, New York.

Weinberg, B. 1983b. Speech assessment and treatment of the laryngectomized patient. In: J. Costello (ed.), Recent Advances in Speech, Hearing and Language. College Hill Press, San Diego, CA.

APPENDICES

A. Pre-Interview Questionnaire for Adults with Voice Disorders

Date _____

I. IDENTIFYING INFORMATION

Name _____ Date of birth _____ Age _____

Address _____

Telephone number (home) _____ (work) _____

Family or personal physician _____

Who referred you to the clinic? _____

Marital status _____ Spouse _____ Age _____

Children: Name _____ Age _____

   Name _____ Age _____

   Name _____ Age _____

Employment history (most recent)

Place	Date	Position
1.		
2.		
3.		
4.		

II. HISTORY OF THE PROBLEM

Describe the existing voice problem. _____

_____

_____

When did you first notice its presence? _____

What were the circumstances? _____

How long has it been present? _____

Do you know why it is present? _____ If so, explain. _____

_____

Have you been seen by an ear, nose, and throat physician?

Yes _____ No _____ Date seen _____

Results/diagnosis _____

Recommendations _____

_____

Estimate severity of the problem: Mild _____ Moderate _____ Severe _____

What other individuals recognize your problem? _____

_____

How would you describe your voice? (check items that apply)

Voice pitch too high _____ Voice pitch too low _____ Voice too loud _____

    Voice too soft _____

Frequent pitch breaks _____ Infrequent pitch breaks _____

Harsh _____ Hoarse _____ Nasal _____ Breathy _____

Montonous _____ Difficulty controlling voice _____

Vocal pitch quavers _____ Vocal intensity quavers _____

Other _____

Do you think your breathing has anything to do with your voice problem? Yes _____ No _____

Have you ever been a mouth breather? _____ If so, when? _____

_____

How has this voice problem affected you? _____

_____

VARIATION OF THE PROBLEM

    List 5 situations in which your voice problem is least troublesome.

1. _____
2. _____
3. _____
4. _____
5. _____

    List 5 situations in which your voice problem is most troublesome.

1. _____
2. _____
3. _____
4. _____
5. _____

What happens to your voice when you get:

    Excited? _____

    Anxious? _____

    Angry? _____

    Depressed? _____

    Other _____

Do you have any pain in your neck, face or ears? Yes _____ No _____

Describe nature of pain. _____

Does your throat hurt during any of these times:

	Yes	No
Morning?	_____	_____
Evening?	_____	_____
After working?	_____	_____
After talking for extended periods of time?	_____	_____

When is your voice better? (check items that apply)

In the morning _____

Midday _____

Evening _____

No change during the day _____

Did you refer yourself to the speech and hearing clinic?   Yes _____   No _____

If no, who referred you? _____

Do you feel the referral to this clinic is appropriate and reasonable one?   Yes _____   No _____

Have you ever received any prior speech, voice, or hearing

Evaluation? _____   Therapy? _____

Agency: _____

Address: _____

Dates: _____

Did prior evaluation or therapy relate to the present problem?

_____

What was the nature of the evaluation and therapy? _____

How effective has prior therapy been in helping you with your problem? _____

_____

Have you, yourself, tried to do anything to help correct your problem? _____   Explain. _____

_____

Was it successful? _____

III. FAMILY AND ENVIRONMENTAL INFORMATION

Family history

Are there other members of the family with voice or speech problems?   Yes _____   No _____

If yes, describe the nature of the problem and relation of person to you in each case. _____

_____

_____

Description of vocal and laryngeal use (daily use and/or abuse):
(check appropriate column)

	Often	Sometimes	Never
1. Talking in a noisy environment			
2. Excessive speaking			
3. Shouting			
4. Screaming			
5. Yelling			
6. Coughing			
7. Clearing throat			
8. Sneezing			
9. Singing			
10. Voice impersonations			
11. Yodeling			
12. Cheering or cheerleading			

Any singing experience? Yes _____ No _____
If yes, please describe. _____
_____

Are you under stress? Yes _____ No _____
If so, check the areas that apply: Marital _____ Professional _____ Other _____
Which of the following adjectives best describes your marital relationship?
Peaceful _____ Stressful _____
Is there a family history of emotional difficulties? _____
Does anyone in the immediate family or among close associates have a similar voice problem? _____
  If so, who? _____
_____

How has your voice problem affected your job status? _____
_____

Is your job basically stressful? _____ Peaceful? _____
How has this voice problem affected your social relationships? _____
_____

IV. HEALTH HISTORY

Describe your present health. _____

Is there a history of:

	Yes	No		Yes	No
Allergies	_____	_____	Numbness	_____	_____
Sinus infection	_____	_____	Paralysis/paresis	_____	_____
Anemia	_____	_____	Incoordination of face or		
Asthma	_____	_____	tongue muscles	_____	_____
Broken nose	_____	_____	Influenza	_____	_____
Bronchitis	_____	_____	Mouth-breathing	_____	_____
Chronic colds	_____	_____	Mumps	_____	_____
Chronic laryngitis	_____	_____	Pneumonia	_____	_____
Chronic rhinitis	_____	_____	Physical defect	_____	_____
Cleft palate	_____	_____	Poliomyelitis	_____	_____
Diabetes	_____	_____	Rheumatic fever	_____	_____
Diphtheria	_____	_____	Scarlet fever	_____	_____
Ear disease	_____	_____	Retarded sexual		
Hearing problem	_____	_____	development	_____	_____
Hearing aid	_____	_____	Syphilis	_____	_____
Emotional difficulty	_____	_____	Typhoid fever	_____	_____
Psychological counseling	_____	_____	Tremor/twitching	_____	_____
Glandular imbalance	_____	_____	Ulcers	_____	_____
Hyperthyroidism	_____	_____	Visual problem	_____	_____
Hypothyroidism	_____	_____	Glasses	_____	_____
Hormone therapy	_____	_____	Whooping cough	_____	_____
Heart trouble	_____	_____	Other _____		
Hypertension	_____	_____	_____		

	Yes	No	
Smoking	_____	_____	How much per day? _____
Drinking	_____	_____	How much per day? _____
Drug use			
(non-medicinal)	_____	_____	

If the answer to any of the above items is "Yes," give the relevant details: _____
_____
_____

List periods of hospitalization or medical treatment:

	Hospital	Date	Reason
1.	_____	_____	_____
2.	_____	_____	_____
3.	_____	_____	_____

List all surgical procedures (related or unrelated to the voice problem). _____

List all prescription and nonprescription medication used over the past year (name the type if you can not remember the generic name, i.e.: aspirin, allergy pills). _____
_____

Have you ever had a trauma to the head or neck?   Yes _____   No _____
Have you ever had a neurological examination? _____   If so, by whom, when, and where? ____
_____

How do you feel this clinic can assist you? _____
_____
_____

List any additional sources of information which may be helpful to us in assisting with your problem. _____
_____

Are there any comments or questions? _____
_____

B. Vocal Attribute Checklist

Vocal pitch
_____ Average pitch level normal
_____ Average pitch level high
_____ Average pitch level low
_____ Pitch variation limited
_____ Monotone
_____ Pitch variation excessive

_____ Pitch breaks present
_____ Vocal tremor present

_____ Falsetto register voice (persistent)
_____ Vocal register problems (inconsistent)
_____ Diplophonia present

Vocal quality
_____ Vocal quality normal
_____ Vocal quality breathy
_____ Vocal quality rough/hoarse
_____ Vocal quality-strain-tense
_____ Aphonia
_____ Other (specify)

Other
_____ Phonation or voice breaks/interruptions present
_____ Shortened maximum phonation duration
_____ Phrase length normal
_____ Phrase length short
_____ Phrase length long
_____ Weak cough
_____ Hard glottal attack

Specify other speech disturbances

Vocal loudness
_____ Average loudness level normal
_____ Average loudness level high
_____ Average loudness level low
_____ Loudness variation limited
_____ Monotone
_____ Loudness variation excessive

Pitch and loudness patterns
_____ Disordered intonational patterns
_____ Disordered stress patterns

Diagnosis of Fluency Disorders

John M. Hutchinson

Outline

Educational Aims

1. *To describe essential features of the speech disorder stuttering*
2. *To define the examination process used to diagnose fluency problems*
3. *To clarify how clinical findings are integrated to form a diagnosis of stuttering.*

In this chapter we consider the process of diagnosis of fluency problems. The information will be presented in three general sections. First, we consider the nature of stuttering. Second, procedures for evaluating speech fluency are discussed. Third, we consider how clinical findings are integrated to form a diagnosis of stuttering.

THE NATURE OF STUTTERING

Historically, there has been considerable disagreement about how stuttering should be defined. Schuell, in her discussions of aphasia, said, "What you do about aphasia depends on what you think aphasia is" (Schuell, 1974, p. 138). That statement could readily be applied to the problem of stuttering. Consequently, many of the definitions of stuttering offered in the literature reflect variations in theoretical positions authors have about the nature of stuttering. For example, in the publication *Stuttering Words* (Speech Foundation of America, 1961), 14 different definitions of stuttering are offered. These definitions range from one by Van Riper who defined stuttering as ". . . a word improperly patterned in time and the speaker's reactions thereto" to another by Sheehan who considered stuttering ". . . a disorder of the social presentation of the self."

Definition and Description

Because he recognized the need for stability and uniformity in the definition of stuttering, Wingate (1964b) formulated a "standard" definition. He based this definition on three criteria: 1) acceptable definitions must identify and emphasize the discriminative features of the disorder; 2) a definition must be amenable to general application; 3) the definition must conform to current understanding about the disorder. Wingate also offered three additional considerations. First, because stuttering is a disorder of speech, he felt that the definition should hinge on speech features, rather than on social or psychological factors. Second, Wingate argued that stuttering should not be defined by enumerating behaviors that are not universally demonstrable among stutterers (e.g., eye blinks, head jerks, etc.). Finally, because the etiology of stuttering is unknown, statements of causality or etiology in the definition are unwarranted. Accordingly, Wingate offered the following definition of stuttering:

> The term stuttering means: a) Disruption in the fluency of verbal expression which is b) characterized by involuntary, audible or silent, repetitions or prolongations in the utterance of short speech elements, namely: sounds, syllables, and words of one syllable. These disruptions c) usually occur frequently or are marked in character and d) are not readily controllable. (p. 488)

In large measure, this definition is acceptable and meets the criteria and considerations just discussed. Three suggested revisions of the definition

will be considered. For example, in later writings, Wingate (1976) emphasized that abnormal interjections (i.e., those judged not to be meditative,
circumstantial, or used for purposes of emphasis) should be identified as
stuttering. This consideration is not immediately apparent in the standard
definition. Second, Wingate expressly excluded repetitive behaviors, in
which the repeated unit is longer than a syllable. For example, a disfluency
of the form "intro . . . intro . . . introduction" would not be labeled stuttering. Wingate's approach to repetitive disfluency may be rather restrictive
in view of the finding that word repetitions are judged as stutterings, particularly when they are frequent (Hegde and Hartman, 1979). Finally, the
recent work of Conture et al., (1977), Freeman and Ushijima (1978), and
others has confirmed the presence of laryngeal aberrations during some moments of stuttering. Perhaps these documented disturbances warrant specification in a definition of stuttering. These additional considerations
prompted the following revision in Wingate's earlier definition:

> Stuttering is a disfluency of verbal expression characterized by: 1) repetitions
> of linguistic units (part-, whole-, or multisyllabic in length); 2) abnormal pro-
> longations (audible or silent) of an articulatory and/or laryngeal posture; and/or
> 3) interjections of extraneous sounds or syllables into the utterance that are
> judged not to be meditative, circumstantial, nor emphatic in nature.

This definition reveals that an individual who does not exhibit repetitions, prolongations, and/or abnormal interjections is not diagnosed as a
stutterer. These three behaviors are considered cardinal features of stuttering.

Accessory Features

People who stutter may exhibit many behaviors not identifiable as cardinal
features. These have often been termed *secondary* or *accessory* behaviors
and include such movements as eye blinking, inappropriate lip protrusions,
head jerking, thigh slapping with the hand, foot tapping, and so on. These
accessory behaviors are usually noted during stuttering. Their prevalence
varies considerably from patient to patient and they may not be present in
some patients. Interestingly, stutterers who do exhibit accessory behaviors
often report that these behaviors occur inconsistently, usually for no apparent reason. Accessory behaviors are often highly disconcerting to listeners. Thus, although they are considered secondary, they are by no means
clinically insignificant and warrant attention in evaluation and remediation.

Other Phenomena

In addition to cardinal and accessory speech behaviors, other behaviors have
been observed in patients who stutter. For example, most confirmed stutterers exhibit *adaptation*, *consistency*, and *adjacency* effects. These effects
are particularly obvious during oral reading. Adaptation occurs when there

is a decrease in the frequency of stuttering over massed (repeated) oral readings of the same passage. Consistency, on the other hand, is the tendency for stuttering to reappear on the same word or words during massed oral readings. Adjacency is a "spreading" phenomenon. Here, during later readings of a passage, instances of stuttering tend to cluster around stuttered words in earlier readings of the material. Historically, speech pathologists have measured the extent of adaptation, consistency, and adjacency as a part of the diagnostic process for stuttering. In recent years, the value of such data has been questioned. This writer agrees with Williams (1978), who noted that there is no evidence that this information predicts improvement in therapy and it does not aid significantly in planning a therapeutic program.

Psychological Features

Although it is universally agreed that communication is vital to effective human interaction and that stutterers experience difficulty communicating, many patients who stutter are remarkably well adjusted. Efforts to pinpoint "typical" psychological problems or unique personality profiles for stutterers as a group have not been productive (see Perkins, 1971; and Sheehan, 1970, for comprehensive reviews of the literature). Several decades ago, Douglas and Quarrington (1952) characterized two general styles of reaction to stuttering. The first style, *interiorization*, dealt with reactions characterized by hiding or masking stuttering, antisocial behaviors, feelings of inferiority, and high levels of anxiety. The second style, *exteriorization*, was reflected by behaviors which minimized efforts to mask stuttering, highlighted good social adjustment and emphasized feelings of acceptance. More recently, Prins and Beaudet (1980) labeled two general defense mechanisms among stutterers: avoidance defense and expressive defense mechanisms. Patients who exhibit avoidance defense mechanisms correspond to Douglas and Quarrington's interiorized style of reaction. Those who exhibit expressive defenses would probably reflect exteriorized reactions. From a diagnostic perspective, it is important to note that Prins and Beaudet found that expressive defenders show more short-element (syllable and speech sound) repetitions and prolongations, whereas avoidance defenders exhibit more long-element (word and phrase) repetitions and interjections.

Incidence and Prevalence

Incidence refers to the number of people who have exhibited a given trait or problem at any time. *Prevalence*, on the other hand, refers to the number of patients who exhibit a given trait or problem at a specific time. The magnitude of prevalence of stuttering is typically lower than the incidence. An excellent review of the incidence and prevalence of stuttering has been provided by Bloodstein (1981). By way of summary, the incidence of stuttering has been estimated to be as high as 10%, whereas the prevalence of stuttering in the United States is estimated to be about 1%.

Etiology

The etiology or cause of stuttering is unknown. Hence, discussions of the etiology of stuttering are largely hypothetical. The etiology of stuttering has been discussed in terms of four general themes: 1) physiological predisposition; 2) learning-based factors; 3) psychoanalytic explanations; and 4) notions of multicausality. In addition, some consideration has been directed to the parents of stutterers, because several etiologic explanations imply that parents play an important role in the etiology and development of this disorder.

Physiological Explanations

A feature of this view is that a general physical condition exists that predisposes the person to stutter. For example, Orton and Travis (1929) suggested that persons who stutter fail to develop hemispheric dominance for controlling speech. Thus, both hemispheres "compete" for speech motor control and the failure to establish hemispheric dominance predisposes the person to stutter. West (1958) suggested that stuttering was an epileptiform disorder and that a moment of stuttering was a type of seizure. In yet another view, Eisenson (1958) considered stuttering the result of sensory and motor perseveration.

These ideas about physiological predisposition to stuttering have been labeled *dysphemic* theories. Most of these dysphemic theories embody the assumption that the physiological predisposition is inherited. Recent evidence, using various contemporary strategies for genetic research, lends support to the credibility of a genetic component to stuttering etiology. In particular, Kidd (1977) and Kidd et al. (1978) have suggested that the relatively high incidence of stuttering in families, together with a sex distribution favoring males, can be relatively well accounted for on the basis of genetic modeling. Hence, although some specific dysphemic agents (e.g., lack of cerebral dominance, seizures, and perseveration) have been largely ruled out as etiologic factors, the possibility of a genetic factor has gained recent support and interest.

Learning-Based Explanations

In its most general sense, *learning* refers to changes in behavior that result from experience (Jones, 1967). One of the earliest and most widely held explanations of the cause of stuttering is Johnson's (1933) "diagnosogenic" theory. In Johnson's view, stuttering is the product of a self-fulfilling prophecy. That is, normal disfluencies that accompany speech development in childhood are labeled *stuttering* by some significant person (usually a parent). Thereafter, the child lives and speaks in an environment characterized by pressure, anxiety, and a familial concern to have the child "rehabilitated." Such an environment is, according to Johnson, conducive to the development of stuttering. Many speech pathologists continue to favor this view today. Others, following the lead of Wingate (1976), regard the normal nonfluencies of childhood and early stutterings as distinctly different classes of behavior.

Another learning-based view of the development of stuttering has been termed the anticipatory struggle hypothesis. Here, the underlying idea ". . . is that stutterers interfere in some manner with the way they are talking because of their belief in the difficulty of speech" (Bloodstein, 1981, p. 43). In other words, expectation of speech difficulty and/or anticipation of disfluency leads to stuttering. Sheehan's notion of an approach-avoidance conflict is one form of this anticipatory-struggle hypothesis. According to Sheehan (1953), stutterers are in a conflict between the desire to speak (which could prompt stuttering) and the desire to remain quiet (which would prevent expression but also prevent stuttering). How the abnormal belief system develops in these anticipatory struggle hypotheses is not well defined. Presumably, this belief system is the product of experience; therefore, it is learned.

Another theory has emerged which may be more directly linked to conventional learning theory explanations of stuttering. This is the two-factor theory of Brutten and Shoemaker (1967). In this view, the stutterer exhibits cardinal features of stuttering (repetitions and prolongations) in response to classically conditioned, negative emotion (Factor One). In an attempt to escape or avoid negative emotion and attendant disfluency, the stutterer engages in secondary or accessory behaviors acquired through instrumental learning (Factor Two).

A final learning-based explanation of stuttering relates to operant conditioning. In this view, most clearly stated by Flanagan et al., (1958), Shames and Egolf (1976), Shames and Sherrick (1963), and it is posited that stuttering behaviors are shaped by their consequences. Accordingly, such theorists state that stuttering obeys the Law of Effect: a behavior that is rewarded will increase in frequency, whereas a behavior that is punished or ignored will decrease in frequency.

Psychoanalytic Explanations

Psychoanalytic explanations of stuttering are less frequently cited than are physiological or learning based theories. From a psychoanalytic viewpoint, stuttering is viewed as neurotic behavior. Explanations are basically tied to either strict Freudian psychoanalytic theory or to neoanalytic interpretations of Freudian theory. Traditional psychoanalytic theory describes stuttering as a symptom complex indicative of fixation at a specific stage of psychosexual development. Bluemel (1935), Coriat (1943), Fenichel (1945), and Glauber (1958) have been the chief proponents of psychoanalytic explanations of stuttering.

Neoanalytic (psychodynamic) interpretations of Freudian theory have been primarily based upon a theory of interpersonal psychology (ego psychology). In this instance, the basic conflict begins with the child's deficient interpersonal relationships with parents. Oral verbal communication is viewed as the essential ingredient to successful interpersonal relationships. Stuttering, therefore, represents the hesitation of the speaker who feels ambivalent and anxious about these interpersonal relationships. Barbara (1965) and Murphy and Fitzsimons (1960) have been the principal advocates of this view of stuttering.

Closely tied to psychodynamic explanations of stuttering is the view that stuttering represents speech phobia (expectancy neurosis). Freund (1966) states that stuttering arises from some specific communicative failure and lacks the symbolic nature of other phobias. Some learning theory based explanations of stuttering characterize the disorder in a similar fashion, therefore it is difficult to make a clear distinction between what can be considered phobic versus learned behavior.

Multicausality   Some theorists argue that stuttering does not develop from a single cause. Rather, they suggest that stuttering may stem from several disparate etiologies (Van Riper, 1982). Unfortunately, these disparate etiologic factors remain unidentified. As a result, this viewpoint is not particularly helpful from either diagnostic or therapeutic perspectives.

Parents of Stutterers   As mentioned previously, theories of stuttering often implicate parents in the onset and development of the disorder. As a result, parents of children who stutter have come under rather extensive experimental scrutiny. Specifically, parents of stuttering children have been evaluated in terms of their adjustment, general attitudes, attitudes toward stuttering, verbal behavior, and standards of fluency. In addition, stutterers' perceptions of parental behavior have been examined (Bloodstein, 1981).

The results of these various evaluations reveal that parents of stutterers are apparently as well adjusted as parents of nonstuttering children. There are some data to suggest that, as a group, they may be somewhat more anxious, critical, or perfectionistic than others (Bloodstein, 1981; Bloom, 1959; Moncur, 1952; Zenner et al., 1978). Using the diagnosogenic concept as a theoretical framework, Kaprisin-Burrelli et al. (1972) analyzed parent-child verbal interactions in stuttering and nonstuttering child-parent groups. The occurrence of positive statements indicating acceptance of the child's feelings or ideas, encouraging verbal output on the part of the child, or encouraging mutual respect between parent and child were compared to negative statements which fostered hostility, distrust, agression, or silence. These investigators discovered that 42% of the statements made by parents of stuttering children were positive, whereas 78% of the statements made by parents of normal children were positive. Further, disfluency decreased when parents were encouraged to use more positive statements. The results of this study highlight the value of examining the nature of parent-child verbal interactions and provide support for the use of parent counseling as part of a therapeutic program.

Although there is some evidence to support the view that parents of stuttering children may be more anxious and may have verbal interactions which differ from those of parents of children who do not stutter, not all investigators and clinicians agree that parents cause or exacerbate childhood disfluency. For example, Shine (1980a) has argued, "There is no conclusive evidence in the literature to support the assumption that parents cause stuttering. Parents may promote stuttering, but they are more likely to be responsible for the remission of stuttering" (p. 340).

One of the most useful descriptions of different ways in which stuttering emerges and develops was offered by Van Riper (1982). After reviewing 44 cases, Van Riper distilled four different "tracks of stuttering." Track I accounted for the behavior in almost half (21) of the stutterers. In this pattern of onset, disfluencies emerged after a period of normal speech. Stuttering onset was gradual, beginning between 30 and 50 months of age. Van Riper noted marked cyclical patterns in both the frequency of disfluency and the severity of symptoms. Periods of remission lasting 1 week or more were observed. Initially, symptoms consisted of effortless repetitions. In time, these repetitions became increasingly more rapid and irregular. In later stages, more prolongations, often associated with tension and tremor were evident. Accessory struggle behaviors such as lip protrusions, jaw jerking, and so on were also evident in later stages of Track I development.

Patterns of Onset

Of the 44 stutterers, 11 were placed in Track 2. Hallmarks of this group were an earlier onset of symptoms and associated delays in speech and language development. The emergence of disfluency coincided with the onset of producing two- and three-word utterances. The disfluency pattern of children in this group was characterized by rapid, irregular repetitions, frequent interjections, numerous revisions, and inappropriate hesitations. Word-finding problems and articulation errors persisted throughout childhood and into maturity. Prolongations and accessory struggle behaviors were uncommon.

Track III onset pattern could be assigned to five of the patients. This pattern of onset could be related to some "traumatic" event in the child's life (e.g., a frightening experience, an abrupt environmental change, etc). After such experiences, initial speech attempts were often "fixations" in which the stutterer could not produce vocalization, ostensibly because of "laryngeal clamping" or glottal occlusion. Struggle behaviors seemed apparent from the beginning, but repetitive forms of disfluency emerged later.

Stutterers with Track IV onset pattern exhibited onset of symptoms much later in childhood, presumably in the primary or middle elementary grades. These youngsters had a history of normal speech for several years before the emergence of disfluency. Their symptoms were marked by very consistent, stereotypical disfluencies, largely of the repetitive type. The pattern of disfluency did not vary significantly over time. Van Riper (1982) viewed this as a deliberate, willful form of stuttering. This form of stuttering may be used, in part, to punish the listener.

Progression of the Disorder

As we have seen, a commonly held view is that stuttering is a unitary disorder which progresses through broadly defined phases or stages of development. Bluemel (1932) became an early proponent of this view by suggesting a "primary" versus "secondary" progression to the disorder. Presumably, primary stuttering refers to relatively effortless, uncomplicated forms of the disorder. Here, children react with minimal awareness or concern to speech repetitions, a central feature of the disorder. Later, secondary stuttering emerges and its progression is marked by tension, struggle, accessory coping behaviors (eye blinks, lip protrusions, head jerks, etc.), and definite emotional reactions to the disorder (anxiety, word and situational avoidances, etc.). Both Bloodstein (1960a,b, 1961) and Van Riper (1954) have attempted to refine the primary-secondary dichotomy by adding additional stages.

As well motivated as these efforts might be, attempts to identify progressive stages of stuttering are fraught with problems. First, there are stutterers who show little or no progression. Some others may improve over time. Second, there is considerable variability in symptomatology, making patient categorization extremely difficult. Third, many clinicians have observed some characteristics of late stages of stuttering in children who may be experiencing normal nonfluency. In short, being aware of the present behavior of the stutterer neither makes clear to the clinician what the behavior has been, nor does it inform the clinician where the patient is headed in the future. Wingate (1976) offers a logical alternative:

> We should abandon the use of words with special and biasing connotations such as "primary," "secondary," "phase," "stage," and the like and instead stay closer to direct and verifiable observation. It would seem most appropriate to speak of stuttering as either "simple" or "complicated" and consider the particular feature of each case individually (p. 67).

Spontaneous Recovery

For a number of years, clinicians have been intrigued by what appear to be a large number of stuttering patients who recover or whose symptoms disappear without appreciable clinical intervention. For example, Andrews and Harris (1964) followed 1000 children from birth to age 16 years. When they concluded their observations, they identified 43 individuals who stuttered. Among this group, most (79%) recovered. Others had what Andrews and Harris called "developmental" stuttering, characterized by early symptom onset (usually between ages 2 and 4) and brief duration of symptoms (less than 1 year). Other individuals were labeled "benign" stutterers. These children generally developed problems after age 4 and experienced difficulty for 1 year.

A second source of information about spontaneous recovery was provided by Cooper (1972). He evaluated 5054 junior and senior high school students and identified 119 students who were stutterers. Sixty-eight students, reported having stuttered at one time, but were now recovered.

Wingate (1964a) identified 50 "recovered stutterers" and examined a variety of factors related to the process of recovery. He noted that although 50 percent of the patients considered themselves "recovered," these people reported recovery in adolescence and noted that their improvement was gradual. In the minds of the respondents, the major factors related to recovery were 1) a change in attitude; and 2) speech practice. The latter was defined as intentionally speaking in different situations and using a variety of techniques (presumably, slow rate, varied prosody, etc.).

The major point of this discussion is to emphasize that spontaneous recovery occurs and that it seems to occur at a relatively high rate. Unfortunately, we have no data other than patient opinions about the factors which mediate recovery. The Stuttering Prediction Instrument (Riley, 1981), to be discussed later, was developed to identify persons likely to recover from childhood disfluencies. Many of the symptoms labeled stuttering in studies of spontaneous recovery may represent symptoms of normal nonfluency (Young, 1975), an issue of importance to be discussed later.

Associated Problems

Speech-language pathologists must remember that people who stutter may have additional problems. Of particular concern are language difficulty, speech sound errors, motor disturbances, and psychological problems. Children who stutter are often identified by parents as delayed in language development (Andrews and Harris, 1964; Morley, 1957). Naturally, such reports have prompted investigators to examine language abilities in children who stutter. For example, Perozzi and Kunze (1969) were among the first to examine stuttering children using language assessment procedures. They evaluated second- and third-grade children who stuttered. Using the Illinois Test of Psycholinguistic Abilities, the Van Alstyne Picture Vocabulary Test, and spontaneous samples of picture description, they noted that, as a group, stutterers were not deficient in language ability.

Perozzi and Kunze speculated that language deficiencies noted by others may be apparent during the preschool years and diminish as the child enters school. Indeed, some support for this notion was provided by Murray and Reed (1977), who examined language skills of seven stuttering (mean age: 5 years) and seven nonstuttering children (mean age: 4;11 years). Dependent variables included scores on the Peabody Picture Vocabulary Test (PPVT), the Zimmerman Pre-School Language Scale, and the Northwest Syntax Screening Test (NSST). The stuttering children exhibited poorer scores for the PPVT, the NSST and the verbal portion of the Zimmerman test. Additional data confirming language problems among pre-schoolers have been offered by Kline and Starkweather (1979) and Westby (1979). Thus, it would appear accurate to view the language difficulties of stutterers as phenomena primarily associated with the preschool years.

Another communication problem frequently associated with stuttering is disturbance in the production of speech sounds. Children who stutter

Table 6.1.   Percentage of stutterers and nonstutterers exhibiting articulation problems

Grade	N	Percentage of stutterers	Percentage of nonstutterers
K–1	25	72.0 (18)	24.0 (6)
2–3	32	18.8 (6)	6.2 (2)
4–5	34	2.9 (1)	2.9 (1)
7–9	24	8.3 (2)	4.2 (1)
Total	115	23.0 (27)	9.0 (10)

From Williams and Silverman (1968).

apparently exhibit more speech sound errors than children who do not stutter (see Table 6.1). Williams and Silverman (1968) surveyed the prevalence of articulation problems in 115 stuttering and 115 nonstuttering children. With the exception of fourth- and fifth-grade children, speech sound errors were much less evident in nonstuttering children.

The reciprocal of this problem can also be examined. For example, children with articulation problems often exhibit more disfluencies than children without these problems, although the disfluencies noted may not constitute bona fide stuttering problems. In this context, Deputy and Hutchinson (1981) reported more interjections, revisions, repetitions, and "articulatory noises" (non-phonemic oral sounds) in 30 children with articulation problems (4;6 years to 6;4 years) in comparison to a control group matched on the basis of age, sex, and IQ.

The major inference to be drawn from these observations is that the speech-language pathologist must consider both articulation and language in the examination of childhood disfluency. Speech pathologists may use some of the examination tools discussed later in this chapter when evaluating children with speech sound errors.

We have learned that when speech-language pathologists diagnose, they usually consider gross and fine motor control (see Chapter 2). Riley and Riley (1980), in a factor analytic study of 76 stutterers, identified a factor characterized by both oral motor and other fine motor problems. Hence, clinicians should be prepared to engage stutterers in tasks that measure oral and general fine motor coordination during the diagnostic process.

Earlier, it was mentioned that stutterers react to stuttering in one of several ways. Speech-language pathologists should be alerted to psychological problems, especially problems judged to be disproportionate to the communicative difficulty being experienced by the patient. There is some evidence to suggest that some people who stutter exhibit increased levels of autonomic reactivity (i.e., physiological disturbances in response to stress), lower levels of aspiration, increased levels of suggestibility, and increased levels of behavioral rigidity. A small number of stutterers may be psychologically maladjusted to the degree that psychological or psychiatric consultation is warranted. The role of the speech-language pathologist in these instances is discussed in Chapter 10.

EXAMINATION

The majority of our discussion will deal with examination of disfluency. It would not be prudent to conclude that examination of disfluency per se should be equated with diagnosis of stuttering. Conture (1982) has said:

> Speech-language pathologists need to consider the context of the stutterer's life in order to see the individual who stutters as a person, as a functioning individual interacting on a number of levels with a number of people, and as a person, like you and me, unique and without duplicate. (p. 4)

Thus, speech-language pathologists have a responsibility to get to "know" their clients. They do not only examine disfluency, but they also consider the physical, environmental, and emotional factors that may contribute to stuttering.

As speech pathologists examine patients who stutter, four basic objectives should be kept in mind:

1. The clinician must secure sufficient background information regarding the history of the disorder.
2. A complete description of the overt behaviors and patients' reactions to these behaviors should be obtained.
3. A decision should be made about the need for therapy. If possible, the nature of the therapy should be specified.
4. The speech pathologist needs to identify whether associated problems (communicative or otherwise) are present and ascertain the degree to which they relate to the disfluency problem itself.

In this chapter, we discuss only that historical information to be gathered that is directly related to disfluency and not that which may be common to general examination of patients with communication problems (see Chapter 2 for these details). This discussion is not intended to minimize the importance of obtaining information about prenatal problems and birth history, developmental progress, general medical status, socio-economic position, educational history, socialization patterns, and so on. Indeed, information about these factors may impact significantly on disfluency problems, and such information warrants careful attention.

Obtaining Case History Information— The Interview

Specific interviewing skills are addressed in depth in Chapter 10 and will not be considered in depth here. Two considerations directly related to interviewing parents of disfluent children or adults who stutter merit attention here. First, clinicians should avoid subjecting the parents or patients to unduly probing personal questions. As a general rule, every question should be clinically relevant; questions should not be asked to fulfill the personal interests or needs of the clinician. Second, parents and patients may enter the interview situation with feelings of guilt and anxiety. It is not helpful to add to the degree of guilt or anxiety. The adoption of an open, empathetic, nonjudgmental attitude by the clinician will serve to minimize these negative feelings, thereby establishing a more favorable communicative relationship.

It is recommended that both parents be involved in the initial interview when a child is being examined. Significant discrepancies between the reports of parents concerning their perceptions of the problem, their relationships to their children and their opinions regarding what should be done to solve the problem are often relevant in clinical practice. If intervention is needed, the parents should be unified in their views. Clinicians may need to spend time resolving potentially injurious discrepancies uncovered during the interview process.

Given these preliminary considerations, the clinician should obtain historical information pertaining to the following basic areas:

1. the presenting problem
2. history of the disorder
3. reactions to the problem
4. precipitating factors
5. nature of the disfluency

A listing of possible questions that could be asked of parents or adult stutterers is provided in Appendix A.

Direct Examination of Disfluency

Direct examination of disfluency involves analyzing actual, overt behaviors which form integral parts of the act of speaking. Clearly, a primary task is to secure an adequate speech sample. Disfluency is known to vary as a function of speech task (Deputy and Hutchinson, 1981; Stocker and Usprich, 1976; Van Riper, 1982). Therefore, speech samples should be obtained while the client is engaged in several different speech tasks.

With children, three speaking tasks can be used: conversation, picture description, and paraphrase. Conversation and picture description are self-explanatory. Paraphrase necessitates the retelling of a story. An oral reading task should also be used if the child can read. At least a 300-word sample should be secured. Definitive interpretation of the significance of variation in disfluency as a function of speech task cannot be made. However, such information may assist the clinician in constructing task hierarchies in therapy. For example, if a child were very disfluent during picture description and became progressively more fluent in conversation and paraphrase, paraphrase could be used as the initial task in therapy. Indeed, Shine (1980b) has offered precisely this approach in the development of a program entitled, Systematic Fluency Training for Young Children. The samples obtained should be tape recorded for systematic analyses. Videotape recordings are also often very useful for this purpose.

It is recommended that clinicians obtain a monologue sample of at least 300 words from adult patients. This sample can be obtained by having the patient talk about his or her job, hobbies, favorite pastimes, education, and so on. In addition, a 300-word sample of oral reading should be obtained and a similar amount of conversation should be elicited. Picture description is typically unnecessary with adult patients.

At least four types of analyses should be completed after the speech samples have been collected. Historically, the most common form of analysis is to calculate total frequency of stuttering. Overall frequency counts do not provide a complete description of stuttering behavior; therefore clinicians often find it helpful to obtain frequency counts of specific types of stuttering. Counts of specific types of stuttering are called *topographical analyses*. Here, clinicians tally the frequency of syllable repetitions, prolongations, interjections, and so on. Third, determination of the severity of stuttering is warranted. A fourth analysis is designed to define linguistic attributes or correlates of disfluency.

Total Stuttering Frequency

One of the major contributors to any clinical impression of stuttering is the total frequency of stuttering behavior (Van Riper, 1982). Total stuttering frequency provides one of the best measures of disfluency, situational variation, and task variability, and it provides a useful measure of change accompanying therapy. Total stuttering frequency should be expressed as a percentage of the total number of syllables spoken. Clinicians have often expressed total stuttering frequency as a percentage of the words spoken. Unfortunately, words may be quite variable in terms of syllabic number. Hence, the syllabic base provides a more useful referent.

Topographical Analysis

As we have seen, sole dependence on total stuttering frequency for description of the stuttering may serve to mask variations in component behaviors. Identification of variations in component behaviors is important for at least two reasons. First, there is evidence to support the view that particular forms or types of stuttering respond better to certain treatment strategies. Hence, choice of therapy may partially depend on the topographical profile of the stutterer. Second, certain clinical approaches may extinguish or minimize some forms of stuttering, yet not alter or aggravate others. Periodic and frequent topographical analysis during the course of therapy often serves to uncover these differential influences.

Several approaches to topographical analysis have been suggested. A widely used system was proposed by Johnson (see Johnson et al., 1963) and later revised by Williams et al. (1978). In this system, the clinician tabulates

frequency data for: 1) interjections; 2) part-word repetitions; 3) word repetitions; 4) phrase repetitions; 5) revisions; 6) incomplete phrases; 7) broken
words; 8) prolonged sounds; 9) dysrhythmic phonation in words; and 10)
tension pauses. This system is not recommended for three main reasons.
First, as suggested earlier, the use of "the word" as a base for repetition
counts is problematic. For example, "I I I I went to the show" would be
regarded as the same form of disfluency as "He came down with tuberculosis
tuberculosis tuberculosis." Second, some forms of disfluency are not mutually exclusive. For example, a broken word may be a prolongation in the
middle of the word. Third, some categories are poorly defined. For example,
Williams et al. (1978) have noted that a dysrhythmic phonation

> . . . may be attributable to prolongation of a phoneme, an accent or timing which
> is notably unusual, an improper stress, a break, or any other speaking-behavior
> infelicity not compatible with fluent speech and not included in any other cat-
> egory. (p. 265)

Clearly, dysrhythmic phonation is a "wastebasket" category. What is a
"break?" What is a "speaking-behavior infelicity?"

A system of topographical analysis which alleviates many of the problems encountered in the systems of Johnson et al. and Williams et al. was
suggested by Wingate (1976). Wingate employs a base called an *elemental
disfluency*. Elemental disfluencies occur on linguistic units equal to or
smaller than the syllable. Thus, in Wingate's formulation, descriptions in
fluency which extend beyond a syllable are not judged to be principal components of stuttering. Rather, they are viewed as accessory verbal features.
Wingate's protocol is summarized in Table 6.2 and the categories are self
explanatory. In using Wingate's approach, speech-language pathologists can
tabulate speech-related movements and ancillary body movements as the
patient speaks, while frequency counts of the cardinal characteristics and
verbal features of stuttering are obtained from tape recordings.

Severity Estimation   There are at least three reasons to estimate severity. First, estimates of
severity constitute a powerful and convenient way of summarizing the
patient's behavior. Second, measures of severity can be used to evaluate the
effectiveness of therapy. Finally, severity data may assist in choosing therapeutic approaches and procedures. For example, a child whose stuttering
is characterized by few disfluencies of only fleeting duration may not be a
good candidate for therapies which involve extensive modification of actual
stuttering simply because the behavior occurs too infrequently to activate
the techniques.

Two general approaches are used to obtain severity estimate. The first
involves having a clinician make an overall estimate of severity ("very severe," "severe," "moderate," "mild," "very mild," or normal). This approach is characterized by questionable interjudge reliability. A second ap-

Table 6.2.   System of topographical analysis of stuttering
behaviors suggested by Wingate

Cardinal features
1. Audible elemental repetitions
2. Silent elemental repetitions
3. Audible prolongations
4. Silent prolongations
   (Interjections that are elemental should be included
   in the above categories)

Accessory features
1. Speech-related movements
   a. Compressed lips
   b. Lingual posturing
   c. Mouth held open
   d. Holding breath
2. Ancillary body movements
   a. Blinking eyes
   b. Dilating nostrils
   c. Raising eyebrows
   d. Grimacing
3. Verbal features
   a. Repetition of syllable strings
   b. Interjections (longer than one syllable)

Adapted from Wingate (1976) p. 49.

proach uses a rating tool. One tool is the Stuttering Severity Instrument
(SSI), which requires obtaining a sample of reading and a speech monologue
(Riley, 1980). If children are nonreaders, they are shown a series of pictures
that depict a story. The clinician then evaluates the verbal responses in terms
of total frequency of disfluencies, the duration of the longest disfluencies,
and the degree to which physical concomitants are present (e.g., distracting
sounds, facial grimaces, etc.). Scores for these three variables are then combined to provide an overall severity score which may be converted to a
severity rating and percentile placement. Although the interjudge reliability
of scores obtained using the SSI with children fall in the fair to good range,
the instrument has not yet been fully tested with adults, nor has it been
adequately validated. Our experience suggests that the instrument under-
estimates severity, particularly with adults having more severe forms of the
disorder.

Clinicians should note that the types of severity estimation discussed
focus exclusively upon observable speech events associated with stuttering.
The actual severity of stuttering problems is not solely defined by the severity of speech disfluency. Overall severity of this disorder is undoubtedly
related to a variety of emotional and environmental factors.

It is useful to determine the impact linguistic variables have on the frequency   *Linguistic Attributes*
of stuttering. There is considerable evidence to suggest that disfluency does   *of Disfluency*

not occur on a random basis. For example, Williams et al. (1968) noted that stuttering occurs more frequently on content words that on function words. Wall et al. (1981) observed higher rates of stuttering at clause boundaries and at the beginning of sentences. Therefore, the clinician might consider the parameters of word type, syntactic location, topic controls (e.g., topic initiation, topic maintenance), speech act (representatives, directives, etc.), in their analysis of speech performance. These types of linguistic information may be used to suggest helpful communication strategies between parent and child, or to plan therapeutic approaches in a clinical setting.

Examination of Attitudes

Earlier in the chapter, it is suggested that stutterers approach communication with various interpersonal styles. These styles reflect stutterers' attitudes about the speech problem in relation to the general process of communication. It is important to examine these attitudes. At least three reasons to examine attitudes may be offered.

First, examination of attitudes can be very important in determining a stutterer's motivation for therapy. If the stutterer exhibits little or no negative emotion with respect to the disorder and feels socially effective, interest in an intensive program of speech therapy may be minimal. Conversely, if the stutterer has a high degree of intolerance for the problem and feels socially disadvantaged, motivation to engage in therapy may be high.

Second, the patient's attitudes may partially dictate the therapeutic approach. By way of example, if a stutterer is extremely fearful of social contact and dislikes displaying stuttering publicly, therapy which relies heavily upon "outside" assignments early in treatment may be quite inappropriate. On the other hand, patients who are more open and gregarious often can benefit from such a clinical approach.

Finally, examination of attitudes about speech and stuttering may reveal important issues that merit attention later in therapy. Stutterers may exhibit undesirable, irrational, or unrealistic emotional responses to their problems. Occasionally, patients express a sense of being victimized. Here, stuttering is perceived as something which cannot be changed or controlled. It is not uncommon for a stutterer to feel inferior, unaccepted, and unloved, despite the potential for establishing strong and healthy personal relationships. Other stutterers often report that without their speech problems, the "sky would be the limit." In short, there would be little or nothing that they could not achieve or accomplish. Obviously, attitudes such as these can be destructive, not only to the patient's emotional health, but to the progress of therapy as well. Failure to deal with these attitudes could result in unsuccessful treatment.

For the most part, examination of attitudes is made on an informal basis. The clinician discusses and counsels. It is unrealistic to expect full disclosure of a given patient's attitudes toward stuttering in an initial interview. Accordingly, the therapist should remain attentive to patients' evaluations of their speech, their environment, and their communicative relationships.

Several paper-and-pencil inventories are available that can assist in the examination of attitudes. It would be appropriate to have patients complete several of these inventories, at least one during the initial evaluation and others early in therapy if treatment is recommended. Three attitudinal inventories that can be used are the Stuttering Severity scale (Lanyon, 1967), the Scale of Communication Attitudes (Erickson, 1969), and the Stuttering Problem Profile (Silverman, 1980).

The Stuttering Severity (SS) scale is a rather comprehensive inventory (Lanyon, 1967). In this inventory, the stutterer must respond "true" or "false" to 64 statements. Some of the statements relate to speech behavior (e.g., "Sometimes my jaws seem to lock together when I talk."), some are related to avoidance patterns (e.g., "I tend to avoid introducing myself."), and still others concern attitudes (e.g., "I hate to stutter."). In the original research on the SS scale, differences in the responses to these 64 items discriminated between 50 stutterers and 50 nonstutterers as well as among mild, moderate, and severe forms of stuttering (Lanyon et al., 1978). Lanyon et al. have shown that SS scale results provide information about two rather different but related dimensions of stuttering: behavioral and attitudinal (sensitivity, social anxiety, and avoidance) dimensions.

The Scale of Communication Attitudes (S-Scale) deals more directly with the stutterer's ". . . feelings about his speech and his attitudes toward interpersonal communication in general" (Erickson, 1969; p. 711). This scale has 39 true-false items (e.g., "I would like to introduce a speaker at a meeting," "I am a good mixer," "I often feel nervous when talking," or "I feel pretty confident about my speaking").

An important investigation of the S-Scale was completed by Andrews and Cutler (1974). They reasoned that attitude change should accompany improvement in stuttering, particularly as the stutterer returns to normal activities after formal treatment. Hence, Andrews and Cutler sought to determine whether responses to the S-Scale items would reveal such attitudinal adjustments. Accordingly, they administered the 39-item S-Scale to 25 stutters at three points in time: before therapy; when fluency was achieved in the clinic; and after transfer had been made to everyday situations. They discovered that 15 items were not suitable for repeated administration, resulting in a 24-item inventory (S24). This shorter form, along with the longer version, were given to an additional 12 stutterers at the same stages in therapy. Andrews and Cutler found that the S24 was more reliable and valid than the 39-item S-Scale and that attitudes toward speech became normal only after patients experienced fluency in everyday situations. The S24 scale seems to represent a useful clinical instrument of particular value in planning therapy and assessing clinical progress.

The Stuttering Problem Profile (SPP) offers rather different insights to patients' perceptions about stuttering (Silverman, 1980). The SPP is not a test, per se. Rather, the SPP consists of 86 statements made by stutterers after therapy (e.g., "I now rarely anticipate stuttering," "I am relatively relaxed in speaking situations," or "I talk as much as most people"). The patient's task is to circle those statements ". . . you would like to be able to make at the termination of therapy that you don't feel you could make now" (Silverman, 1980; p. 122). The major purpose of the SPP is to identify goals for therapy. In addition, Silverman feels that the SPP can be used to individualize therapy, to facilitate communication between client and clinician regarding expectations, to aid in motivation, and to help in determining when therapy might be terminated.

To this author's knowledge, there is no published instrument that provides a measure of attitudes of young children who stutter. Information about attitudes of children who stutter is obtained largely by means of informal probes during conversation with the child. In this regard, the reader is referred to the discussion about talking with children in Chapter 10.

Speech Modification

The ability to modify stuttering patterns is a critical aspect of speech behavior which must be dealt with in the examination of persons who stutter. There are several reasons for completing this type of examination. First, attempts at stuttering modification or fluency enhancement permit the clinician to observe the degree of flexibility (or rigidity) a patient exhibits with respect to altering stuttering behaviors. Second, this form of examination provides the clinician with important information about the comparative effects of various speech modification techniques. Third, experimentation with speech modification methods can serve to promote discussion between the patient and clinician about those approaches to speech modification with which the patient feels most comfortable. This last point is of particular clinical importance, because clinicians need to compare the patient's long-term fluency potential with the speech modification approaches that appear to have immediate utility. Some speech modification approaches are designed to enhance (reinforce) fluency to the exclusion of stuttering. Other approaches are designed to modify stuttering in such a way that the tension patterns associated with moments of stuttering are reduced so that speech "moves forward" with a minimum of effort. Contemporary speech modification approaches used with stutterers are summarized in Table 6.3. Fluency enhancing conditions such as unison speaking or reading, shadowing, or the use of direct suggestion to the patient to "talk better" are not listed in this table. Operant behavior modification approaches which depend upon the clinician's use of specific types of reinforcement (positive and negative) are also not listed. The techniques listed in Table 6.3 represent approaches to modifying disfluent speech.

Table 6.3. **Summary of contemporary speech modification techniques for stutterers**

Technique	Description
Prolonged speech	Either through modeling or DAF,[a] the clinician seeks to prolong the duration of sounds, usually with a slow, well-controlled transition between sounds and syllables.
Gentle onset/airflow	The stutterer is directed to initiate vocalization with a stable egressive airflow and gentle onset of phonation. Biofeedback assistance is available with some commercial programs.
Rhythmic pacing	Usually pacing involves synchronization of words or syllables with the beat of a metronome. Over time, most programs increase the rate of beating and utterance length per beat.
Reduced speech rate	The stutterer maintains a reduced rate, usually beginning with single word productions and advancing to longer, more complex utterances. Normal phrase boundaries and prosodic features are maintained.
Reciprocal inhibition	Use of deep relaxation training and construction of a hierarchy of feared speech situations form the basis of this therapy.
Masking	The stutterer speaks in the presence of high intensity masking noise. Usually, this involves wearing a portable, voice-initiating masking unit.
EMG biofeedback	The patient, by monitoring muscle action potentials, attempts to reduce tension in various sites (e.g., jaw, lips, larynx).
Reduced articulatory effort	The stutterer minimizes articulatory tension by bringing the specific articulatory patterns of ongoing speech into conscious attention.
Response contingent management	The stutterer is either punished verbally or physically for disfluency. Alternatively, tangible or verbal reward may be offered for periods of fluency. Time-out from speaking has also been used as a response contingency for stuttering.

[a] DAF, delayed auditory feedback.

The patient's ability to utilize and be emotionally comfortable with a variety of these speech modification approaches is an important part of differential diagnosis, particularly with respect to therapeutic planning.

No matter what longer term therapeutic approach(es) is recommended and initiated, early clinical contact should be regarded as trial therapy. Trial therapy should be carefully evaluated before a long-term commitment is made to the patient. In this respect, Conture (1982) has suggested:

> Before we begin a protracted therapy regime, we inform our clients that we plan to initiate what I call *trial therapy*. With adults this trial usually lasts from three to six weeks. We inform the client . . . that a judgment will be made . . . regarding the continuation of therapy. (p. 114)

Let us now illustrate how some of the techniques presented in Table 6.3 might be used in clinical practice. If a stutterer exhibited a high percentage of repetitive forms of disfluency, pacing or slowed speech rate might be used on a trial basis (Hutchinson and Norris, 1977). This is not to suggest that other techniques are not effective in modifying repetitive disfluencies. Rate control and pacing have been shown to be helpful. On the other hand, if a patient exhibited a large number of prolongations associated with laryngeal tension and hyperadduction, techniques that stress gentle onset of voicing and airflow may represent logical choices. These strategies are often used to modify tension and struggle that is often present during voice onset. In contrast, there is evidence to suggest that laryngeal features of stuttering may not respond well to pacing (Hutchinson and Norris, 1977) or masking (Dewar et al., 1979). If the clinician has electromyographic instrumentation, electrode placement in the laryngeal region could be used as a biofeedback device to monitor laryngeal tension and attempts could be made to reduce it (Guitar, 1975). A stutterer exhibiting numerous prolongations apparently without significant laryngeal components might respond quite well to either prolonged speech, reduced articulatory effort, and/or gentle onset/airflow approaches. This would seem to be particularly true when labial and mandibular tremors are present (Hutchinson and Navarre, 1977; Hutchinson and Watkin, 1976). Whereas the use of punishment has a rather spotty record of success, time-out has been shown to be useful with a wide variety of clients (Adams and Popelka, 1971; Costello, 1975; Haroldson et al., 1968). Use of response-contingent reward for fluency has been rather promising in children who stutter (Manning et al., 1976; Shaw and Shrum, 1972).

If, during the interview, the clinician identifies significant situational anxiety related to speech, reciprocal inhibition may represent an appropriate therapeutic approach. Reciprocal inhibition is a particularly useful form of therapy for mild stutterers with high levels of situation anxiety. Unfortunately, reciprocal inhibition may not lend itself well to trial therapy, simply because it may take many sessions before significant improvement is noted. Clinicians might consider using the deep relaxation component of reciprocal inhibition therapy during evaluation and very early in the trial therapy program.

These suggestions for trial therapy may not be universally effective. That is, a stuttering patient who exhibits repetitive forms of disfluency may not respond to pacing as suggested earlier, but might respond well to masking or to slowed speech. When clinicians prepare to engage in trial therapy several alternative forms of fluency enhancement should be considered.

Other Examination Considerations

As suggested earlier, examination of disfluency per se should not be equated with diagnosis of stuttering. There are other significant dimensions of behavior that warrant consideration. For example, communicative problems other than disfluency are common among children who stutter. Consequently, clinicians should be prepared to examine communicative function in a broad context. In particular, examination of the form (semantics), structure (syntax), and contextual use (pragmatics) of language is important (see Chapter 3 for details). Information obtained about linguistic features of speech production may have a direct bearing on disfluency itself. Children should be examined in terms of their speech sound production ability. Speech sound errors can add to the communication problem by reducing intelligibility, increasing parental concern, and causing further frustration to the child. In some patients, language and speech sound problems may be more significant than the disfluency problem. In these patients, the language and speech sound problems may warrant greater therapeutic attention. It is this author's opinion that therapy directed toward speech sound production and language will not lead to an increase in disfluency when care is taken to minimize and control stress within the therapy program. Other aspects which merit routine examination include hearing, voice production, and adequacy of the speech mechanism. Procedures for accomplishing such examinations are provided elsewhere in this book (see Chapters 2, 5, and 8).

Speech-language pathologists should also consider parent-child interactions. As mentioned earlier, parents may offer a large number of "negative" statements when talking with their children. When this behavior is observed, the content of such statements should be carefully specified. During subsequent parental counseling, these negative statements can be identified and efforts must be made to reduce their number.

We have also learned that adult stutterers frequently exhibit anxiety. Anxiety may be situational and/or trait related. In either instance, useful information about the nature of the patient's anxiety can be gathered by interviewing. In the case of speech situation anxiety, a hierarchy of feared situations can be constructed by asking the patient to rank order the difficulty of those situations experienced in daily living. These might be presented in terms of areas relevant to the patient, for example, home life, school, work, social situations, demand situations, and so on. It is often possible to construct such a hierarchy both within and among these broad areas. The extent to which the presence of trait anxiety can be probed by means of interview will depend upon the interviewing skill and experience of the clinician. This topic is discussed in Chapter 10.

Information about specific situational (speech) anxiety can also be gathered from the Speech Situation Checklist (Brutten and Shoemaker, 1974). This instrument gives little information about trait anxiety. *Trait anxiety* refers to general responses to situations that may or may not demand speaking. The Fear Survey Schedule (Wolpe and Lang, 1969) is a paper-and-pencil inventory used to gather information about generalized anxiety. This schedule consists of 108 items which may be associated with fear or unpleasant feelings. Patients respond to these items by rating the severity of their anxiety using a five-point scale. In addition to the Fear Survey Schedule, two other paper-and-pencil instruments suggested by Wolpe (1973) may be used to gather information about anxiety. The first is the Willoughby Schedule. High scores on the Willoughby Schedule suggest "neurotic" reactivity in the form of interpersonal difficulty and emotional sensitivity. The second instrument is the Bernreuter Self-Sufficiency Inventory. This instrument consists of 60 questions dealing with self sufficiency and requires only yes-no responses. In this context, it should be noted that reciprocal inhibition therapy is often ineffective for patients with high levels of trait anxiety. Identification of very high scores on any of these three tests may indicate that referral to a counselor, clinical psychologist, or psychiatrist is warranted.

ANALYSIS OF THE FINDINGS: DIAGNOSIS

When the examination process nears completion, the speech pathologist has accumulated a considerable amount of information and must now integrate the findings to answer three basic questions:

1. Is stuttering the problem?
2. If it is, what should be done about it?
3. If something is done, what is the prognosis for improvement?

Is Stuttering the Problem?

Determining the existence of stuttering in young children can be very difficult. There are no definite guidelines that permit clear differentiation between early stuttering and the normal nonfluencies that often accompany speech maturation. Nearly all clinical approaches speech pathologists use to make the diagnosis of stuttering in young children are based upon a "danger sign" principle. Here, clinicians search for certain symptoms and ascertain the frequency with which these danger signs occur. If a child exhibits these signs, the diagnosis of stuttering can be made with greater confidence.

Ainsworth and Fraser-Gruss (1981) have offered a hierarchy of danger signs. These signs, arranged from least to most serious, include the presence of:

1. multiple repetitions
2. schwa conversions (/gə, gə, gə, gem/ as opposed to /ge ge ge gem/)
3. prolongations
4. tremors
5. rises in pitch and loudness during the moment of stuttering
6. struggle and tension
7. moments of fear (fleeting facial expressions suggestive of anxiety)
8. avoidance of sounds, words, and situations

This particular system, although popular, has two major weaknesses. First, not all of these danger signs have been validated. Second, some of the signs are neither easily quantified nor reliably detected (e.g., moment of fear).

Because of these two problems, this author has developed an alternative approach based upon the danger sign principle. In this approach, the clinician obtains a 300-word sample of conversational discourse. Picture description and paraphrase should not be used to obtain the sample, because paraphrase and picture description responses may provide speech samples which are not representative of those used in everyday communication. Based upon an analysis of this speech sample and parent interview data, the clinician searches for certain mandatory signs. The confidence in forming a diagnosis of stuttering is increased through positive identification of additional confirmatory signs.

Mandatory Signs

In the approach developed by this writer, a child must exhibit one or more of four mandatory signs to be diagnosed as a stutterer. The more signs the clinician observes, the more firm (or less tentative) the diagnosis. One danger sign is the presence of elemental repetitions. Namely, a positive danger sign is elicited if a child exhibits more than 10 elemental repetitions per 100 words of discourse (Johnson et al., 1959). Normal children exhibit about 2 elemental repetitions for every 100 words of discourse. A second danger sign is the presence of audible or silent prolongations. Any child exhibiting audible or silent prolongation at a rate exceeding 2 prolongations per 100 words of discourse exhibits an indication toward stuttering (Johnson et al., 1959). There is a large pool of evidence supporting the view that laryngeal dysfunction is a part of stuttering. Hence, identification of repetitions or prolongations produced with apparent glottal occlusion, glottal flaring (breathy productions), or vocal fry represent a third danger sign. A small number of experts have suggested that schwa conversion or vowel neutralization is suggestive of incipient stuttering, (Adams, 1977, 1980; Ainsworth and Fraser-Gruss, 1981; Curlee, 1980). Thus, if the vowels produced within elemental repetitions involve schwa conversions or are neutralized, a fourth danger sign has been uncovered.

Confirmatory Signs

At least six additional signs may be used to confirm the diagnosis of stuttering:

1. presence of accessory features (speech-related, ancillary body, and verbal accessory features)
2. awareness of and ability to describe the problem
3. avoidance of words, sounds, or situations
4. expressions of frustration related to speech efforts
5. lowered self-esteem
6. ability to construct a clear hierarchy of feared-speech situations

It must be recognized that some, if not all, of these confirmatory signs can be found in some people who do not stutter. Some stutterers exhibit few or none of these confirmatory signs.

Even after a clinician has tabulated the mandatory and confirmatory signs for a child, the clinician may still be in a quandary about whether or not a diagnosis of stuttering should be made. Clinicians should be very cautious about applying the label *stuttering*. This caution is not meant to imply that clinicians should be reluctant to proceed with intervention. In fact, the first line of treatment might be parent counseling combined with frequent re-evaluation of the child. Often counseling combined with re-evaluation of changes that occur without direct treatment resolve disfluency problems in children. If disruptions in speech fluency persist or worsen, direct intervention may be warranted.

One published instrument has been developed (Stuttering Prediction Instrument, Riley, 1981) to predict "chronicity" of disfluency. Using this instrument, the clinician can obtain scores in four areas: 1) reactions to stuttering (both by parent and child); 2) part-word repetitions; 3) prolongations; and 4) total frequency of stuttering. A total score is then derived and presumably a decision concerning chronicity is possible. Although this tool has promise, further analysis of the reliability of scores resulting from the use of this instrument and additional longitudinal data are needed before the Stuttering Prediction Instrument can be considered a valid tool for differentiating stutterers from those who are normally disfluent. Clinicians are also encouraged to read the work of Adams (1977, 1980), Curlee (1980), and Zwitman (1978) for additional approaches to the problem of differentiating between normal disfluency and stuttering.

Diagnoses in Older Children and Adults

The diagnosis of stuttering is not particularly difficult in older children and adults. Usually, people have had a long history of disfluency and the diagnosis has been made long ago. In Conture's (1982) view, such stutterers exhibit elemental repetitions and prolongations that are predictable parts of their speech. Moreover, these disfluencies have been persistent over relatively long periods of time and are consistent with certain sounds, words, and/or situations.

With older children and adults, the clinician is concerned primarily with describing existing speech behaviors, identifying emotional, social, and environmental factors that contribute to the stuttering problem, and clarifying the patient's potential to modify speech patterns during the diagnostic process. The making of judgments about whether a patient's disorder is stuttering is seldom necessary except in situations in which speech behavior might be confused with fluency problems associated with certain neurological conditions.

It is beyond our scope in this chapter to consider, in detail, forms of therapy that may be used with children and adults who stutter. The issue of diagnosis cannot be discussed, however, without some comment about directions for clinical management. One meaningful way of considering decisions regarding therapy is to subdivide disfluent patients into three general groups: 1) young nonstuttering children; 2) young stuttering children; and 3) older stuttering children and adults.

What Should Be Done?

As suggested earlier, when clinicians encounter a child for whom the diagnosis of stuttering cannot be made reliably, the principal focus of therapy is on the parents. There are certain standard kinds of information imparted in most parent counseling programs. For example, parents are usually advised about how they should react to disfluencies. Information concerning the development of speech and language and about the possible etiology of stuttering is often also presented. Parents may be taught to improve listening and interpersonal skills. Finally, general guidelines for behavioral management, particularly with respect to discipline, can be helpful (Zwitman, 1978).

Considerable information is often gathered during the examination process that might be used in counseling. For example, during the interview the parents might identify certain people who are reacting inappropriately to the child's disfluency and a discussion should take place about how the parents can resolve this problem. As another example, parents might express considerable frustration over the cyclical disappearance and reappearance of disfluency. The clinician should plan to set aside a portion of counseling time to discuss this problem in order to relieve the anxiety and frustration parents express over the variability in disfluency. In the process of examining young children, rather serious problems in parent-parent or parent-child interactions may be uncovered. Resolution of some of these problems may extend beyond the clinician's expertise. In such cases, appropriate referrals should be made to counselors or psychologists who specialize in marriage and family therapy.

When a young child is diagnosed as a stutterer, both the parents and the child should be directly involved in therapy. With parents of stuttering children, all that has previously been said regarding counseling is appropriate. In addition, parents become part of the actual therapy team, helping the clinician implement behavior changes required within a particular treatment strategy. It is particularly important to determine parents' ability and willingness to assume this responsibility as part of the diagnostic process.

Several important factors must be considered before initiating therapy for children. Initially, some attention should be given to the tracks described by Van Riper. Efforts should be made to determine which track most closely defines the behaviors of a given child. Children exhibiting Track I characteristics are usually candidates for any of the standard procedures for intervention appropriately adapted to children. On the other hand, children with Track II characteristics may require some language remediation in conjunction with stuttering therapy. Rate control therapies also seem appropriate for such children. Children with Track III characteristics who experience considerable speech-related anxiety would profit from reciprocal inhibition and, perhaps, rather extensive counseling. Children with Track IV characteristics might require psychological services as an adjunct to the speech therapy. To some degree, these track-specific therapy suggestions are speculative. Careful attention to the topography of disfluency and to the response to trial therapy are often critical in the selection of an appropriate clinical strategy. Finally, severity of disfluency and patient attitude may be the key determinants of the form of therapy to be recommended. Attitude per se may be the critical factor used to determine whether or not therapy services are offered.

By the time a stutterer reaches the adolescent or adult years, the track of development may be somewhat more difficult to discern. However, case history information is often sufficiently revealing to permit track identification. As with childhood stutterers, topography of stuttering, response to trial therapy, severity of the problem, and attitude must all be considered in deciding whether therapy is appropriate and, if so, what form it should take. As the stutterer matures, parents play an increasingly less significant role. More responsibility is shifted to the patient. In addition to individual therapy, adolescent and adult clients often benefit from group therapy experiences. Group therapy can be especially helpful for clients who interiorize their feelings and have little social support. Attitudinal data can be very important to the making of decisions about the value of group therapy for a particular stutterer.

What Is the Prognosis?

We agree with Van Riper (1973) that the clinician is obligated to provide some statement about prognosis for improvement at the conclusion of an evaluation. There are very few strong predictors of successful therapeutic outcome. Three important factors must interact in just the right way for therapy to succeed. First, clinician variables must be considered. Clinicians cannot establish strong therapeutic relationships with all patients, a factor that can influence therapeutic progress. Further, not all clinicians have expertise or feel comfortable working with the variety of available clinical programs used for patients who stutter. Clinicians need to broaden their expertise whenever possible to enable a wider range of services to be provided. Second, there are the variables related to therapy; for example, time and frequency of therapy, therapy constraints, reinforcement schedules, types of reinforcement, forms of fluency shaping, and so on, that may determine therapy outcome. Third, patient variables must be considered. Such factors as motivation, therapy history, social network, family environment, personality, and so on, bear significantly on prognosis. Many of these factors can be evaluated in the diagnostic process, but it would be naive to assume that all can. Therefore, statements of prognosis must be formulated with caution and care.

A number of factors have been identified that relate to prognosis: the stutterer's developmental track, the topography of disfluency, severity of the problem, response to trial therapy, and so on. We simply do not know precisely how these factors interact on a prognostic level. For example, some patients with severe forms of stuttering are not always the most difficult to remediate. We have been very successful with some Track III stutterers who Van Riper implies would be most resistant to treatment. Some patients who respond very well to trial therapy, ultimately fail to respond well during long-term treatment.

Perhaps the variables of client motivation and environmental support are the two most powerful predictors of therapeutic outcome. There is little question that stuttering therapy works (see Andrews et al., 1980). However, nearly all authorities agree that regardless of how capable the clinician is or how powerful the therapy might be, prognosis for improvement is diminished when patients are not strongly motivated to help themselves, and when there is not a supporting attitude among parents, spouses, and significant others.

Study Guide

1. a. How does Wingate (1964) define stuttering?
   b. How does the author of this chapter define stuttering?

2. Describe the major themes used to explain the etiology of stuttering.

3. Identify the major characteristics of the four tracks or patterns of onset of stuttering described by Van Riper (1971).

4. Speech-language pathologists should have four basic objectives in mind as they undertake diagnostic evaluations of patients who stutter. What are these objectives?

5. a. How are total frequency counts of stuttering occurrences obtained?
   b. Why is it important to obtain total frequency counts of stuttering occurrences?

6. a. What is meant by topographical analysis?
   b. Why is it important to complete topographical analysis?
   c. What are the essential features of the system of topographical analysis suggested by Wingate (1976)?

7. Why is it important for the clinician to assess attitudes as part of diagnostic evaluation of patients with fluency problems?

8. Briefly describe techniques speech-language pathologists can use to modify speech behavior in patients who stutter.

9. When the assessment process nears completion, speech-language pathologists must integrate their findings to answer three basic questions. What are these questions?

10. a. What are the four mandatory signs the writer of this chapter uses in the diagnosis of stuttering?
    b. What are six confirmatory signs that may be used to confirm the diagnoses of stuttering?

11. Define the following terms or concepts:

    adaptation   anticipatory struggle hypothesis
    consistency   secondary stuttering
    incidence   primary stuttering
    prevalence   spontaneous recovery
    diagnosogenic   elemental disfluency

REFERENCES

Adams, M. 1977. A clinical strategy for differentiating the normally nonfluent child and the incipient stutterer. J. Fluency Disord. 2:141–148.

Adams, M. 1980. The young stutterer: Diagnosis, treatment, and assessment of prognosis. In: J. L. Northern (ed.), Seminars in Speech, Language and Hearing (Vol. 1). Brian C. Decker, New York.

Adams, M. R., and Popelka, G. 1981. The influence of "time-out" on stutterers and their disfluency. Behav. Ther. 2:334–339.

Ainsworth, S., and Fraser-Gruss, J. 1981. If Your Child Stutters: A Guide for Parents (Revised) Speech Foundation of America, Memphis.

Andrews, G., and Cutler, J. 1974. Stuttering therapy: The relation between changes in symptom level and attitudes. J. Speech Hear. Disord. 39:312–319.

Andrews, G., and Harris, M. 1964. The Syndrome of Stuttering (Clinics in Developmental Medicine, No. 17). Spastics Society Medical Education and Information Unit, London.

Andrews, G., Guitar, B., and Howie, P. 1980. Meta-analysis of the effects of stuttering treatment. J. Speech Hear. Disord. 45:287–307.

Barbara, D. 1965. New Directions in Stuttering: Theory and Practice. Charles C Thomas, Springfield, IL.

Bloodstein, O. 1960a. The development of stuttering: I. Changes in nine basic features. J. Speech Hear. Disord. 25:219–237.

Bloodstein, O. 1960b. The development of stuttering: II. Developmental phases. J. Speech Hear. Disord. 25:366–376.

Bloodstein, O. 1961. The development of stuttering: III. Theoretical and clinical implications. J. Speech Hear. Disord. 26:67–82.

Bloodstein, O. 1981. A Handbook on Stuttering, 3rd Ed. National Easter Seal Society, Chicago.

Bloom, J. 1959. Child training and stuttering. Speech Monogr. 26:132–133(abstract).

Bluemel, C. 1932. Primary and secondary stammering. Q. J. Speech 18:187–200.

Bluemel, C. 1935. Stammering and Allied Disorders. Macmillan Publishing Co., New York.

Brutten, G. 1975. Stuttering: Topography, assessment, and behavior-change strategies. In: J. Eisenson (ed.), Stuttering: A Second Symposium. Harper & Row, New York.

Brutten, E., and Shoemaker, D. 1967. The Modification of Stuttering. Prentice-Hall, Inc., Englewood Cliffs, NJ.

Brutten, E., and Shoemaker, D. 1974. Speech Situation Checklist. Unpublished manuscript. Southern Illinois University, Carbondale.

Conture, E. 1982. Stuttering. Prentice-Hall, Inc., Englewood Cliffs, NJ.

Conture, E., McCall, G., and Brewer, D. 1977. Laryngeal behavior during stuttering. J. Speech Hear. Res. 20:661–668.

Cooper, E. 1972. Recovery from stuttering in a junior and senior high school population. J. Speech Hear. Res. 15:632–638.

Coriat, I. 1943. The psychoanalytic conception of stammering. Nerv. Child. 2:167–171.

Costello, J. 1975. The establishment of fluency with time-out procedures: Three case studies. J. Speech Hear. Disord. 40:216–231.

Curlee, R. 1980. A case selection strategy for young disfluent children. In: J. L. Northern (ed.), Seminars in Speech, Language, and Hearing (Vol. 1). Brian C. Decker, New York.

Deputy, P., and Hutchinson, J. 1981. Hesitations in the speech of children with misarticulations. Asha 23:748–749(abstract).

Dewar, A., Dewar, A. D., Austin, W. T. S., and Brach, H. M. 1979. The long term use of an automatically triggered auditory feedback masking device in the treatment of stuttering. Br. J. Disord. Commun. 14:219–229.

Douglas, E., and Quarrington, B. 1952. The differentiation of interiorized and exteriorized secondary stuttering. J. Speech Hear. Disord. 17:377–385.

Eisenson, J. 1958. A perseverative theory of stuttering. In: J. Eisenson (ed.), Stuttering: A Symposium. Harper & Row, New York.

Erickson, R. 1969. Assessing communication attitudes among stutterers. J. Speech Hear. Res. 12:711–724.

Fenichel, D. 1945. The Psychoanalytic Theory of Neurosis. Norton, New York.

Flanagan, B., Goldiamond, I., and Azrin, N. 1958. Operant stuttering: The control of stuttering behavior through response-contingent consequences. J. Exp. Anal. Behav. 1:173–177.

Freeman, F., and Ushijima, T. 1978. Laryngeal muscle activity during stuttering. J. Speech Hear. Res. 21:538–562.

Freund, H. 1966. Psychopathology and the Problems of Stuttering. Charles C Thomas, Springfield, IL.

Glauber, I. 1958. The psychoanalysis of stuttering. In: J. Eisenson (ed.), Stuttering: A Symposium. Harper & Row, New York.

Guitar, B. 1975. Reduction of stuttering frequency using analog electromyographic feedback. J. Speech Hear. Res. 18:672–685.

Haroldson, S. K., Martin, R. R., and Starr, C. D. 1968. Time-out as a punishment for stuttering. J. Speech Hear. Res. 11:560–566.

Hegde, M., and Hartman, D. 1979. Factors affecting judgments of fluency: II. Word repetitions. J. Fluency Disord. 4:13–22.

Hutchinson, J., and Navarre, B. 1977. The effect of metronome pacing on selected aerodynamic patterns of stuttered speech: Some preliminary observations and interpretations. J. Fluency Disord. 2:189–204.

Hutchinson, J., and Norris, G. 1977. The differential effect of three auditory stimuli on the frequency of stuttering behaviors. J. Fluency Disord. 2:283–293.

Hutchinson, J., and Watkin, K. 1976. Jaw mechanics during release of the stuttering moment: Some initial observations and interpretations. J. Commun. Disord. 9:269–279.

Johnson, W. 1933. An interpretation of stuttering. Q. J. Speech 19:70–76.

Johnson, W., and associates 1959. The Onset of Stuttering. University of Minnesota Press, Minneapolis.

Johnson, W., Darley, F., and Spriestersbach, D. 1963. Diagnostic Methods in Speech Pathology. Harper & Row, New York.

Jones, J. 1967. Hearing. Harcourt Brace, and World, Inc., New York.

Kaprisin-Burrelli, A., Egolf, D., and Shames, G. 1972. A comparison of parental verbal behavior with stuttering and nonstuttering children. J. Commun. Disord. 5:335–346.

Kidd, K. 1977. A Genetic perspective on stuttering. J. Fluency Disord. 2:259–269.

Kidd, K., Kidd, J., and Records, M. 1978. The possible causes of the sex ratio in stuttering and its implications. J. Fluency Disord. 3:13–23.

Kline, M., and Starkweather, C. 1979. Receptive and expressive language performance in young children. Asha 21:797(abstract).

Lanyon, R. 1967. The measurement of stuttering therapy. J. Speech Hear. Res. 10:836–843.

Lanyon, R., Goldsworthy, R., and Lanyon, B. 1978. Dimensions of stuttering and relationship to psychopathology. J. Fluency Disord. 3:103–113.

Manning, W. H., Trutna, P. A., and Shaw, C. K. 1976. Verbal versus tangible reward for children who stutter. J. Speech Hearing Disord. 41:52–62.

Moncur, J. 1952. Parental domination in stuttering. J. Speech Hear. Disord. 17:155–165.

Morley, M. 1957. The Development and Disorders of Speech in Childhood. Livingstone, Edinburgh.

Murphy, A., and Fitzsimons, R. 1960. Stuttering and Personality Dynamics. Ronald Press, New York.

Murray, H., and Reed, C. 1977. Language abilities of pre-school stuttering children. J. Fluency Disord. 2:171–176.

Orton, S., and Travis, L. 1929. Studies in stuttering: IV. Studies of action currents in stutterers. Arch. Neurol. Psych. 21:61–68.

Perkins, W. 1971. Speech Pathology: An Applied Behavioral Science. C. V. Mosby Co., St. Louis.

Perozzi, J., and Kunze, L. 1969. Language abilities of stuttering children. Folia Phoniatrica 21:386–392.

Prins, D., and Beaudet, R. 1980. Defense preference and stutterer's speech disfluencies: Implications for the nature of the disorder. J. Speech Hear. Res. 23:757–768.

Riley, G. 1980. Stuttering Severity Instrument for Children and Adults. C. C. Publications, Tigard, OR.

Riley, G. 1981. Stuttering Prediction Instrument for Young Children. C. C. Publications, Tigard, OR.

Riley, G., and Riley, J. 1980. Motoric and linguistic variables among children who stutter: A factor analysis. J. Speech Hear. Disord. 45:504–514.

Schuell, H. 1974. The treatment of aphasia. In: L. F. Sies (ed.), Aphasia Theory and Therapy. University Park Press, Baltimore.

Shames, G., and Egolf, D. 1976. Operant Conditioning and the Management of Stuttering. Prentice-Hall, Inc., Englewood Cliffs, NJ.

Shames, G., and Sherrick, C. 1963. A discussion of nonfluency and stuttering as operant behavior. J. Speech Hear. Disord. 28:3–18.

Shaw, C. K., and Shrum, W. F. 1972. The effects of response-contingent reward on the connected speech of children who stutter. J. Speech Hear. Disord. 37:75–88.

Sheehan, J. 1953. Theory and treatment of stuttering as an approach-avoidance conflict. J. Psychol. 36:27–49.

Sheehan, J. 1970. Stuttering: Research and Therapy. Harper & Row, New York.

Shine, R. 1980a. Direct management of the beginning stutterer. In: J. L. Northern (ed.), Seminars in Speech, Language, and Hearing (Vol. 1). Brian C. Decker, New York.

Shine, R. 1980b. Systematic Fluency Training for Young Children. C. C. Publications, Inc., Tigard, OR.

Silverman, F. 1980. The stuttering problem profile: A task that assists both client and clinician in defining therapy goals. J. Speech Hear. Disord. 45:119–123.

Speech Foundation of America. 1961. Stuttering Words. Speech Foundation of America, Memphis.

Stocker, B., and Usprich, C. 1976. Stuttering in young children and the level of demand. J. Childhood Commun. Disord. 1:116–131.

Van Riper, C. 1954. Speech Correction: Principles and Methods 3rd ed. Prentice-Hall, Inc., Englewood Cliffs, NJ.

Van Riper, C. 1973. The Treatment of Stuttering. Prentice-Hall, Inc., Englewood Cliffs, NJ.

Van Riper, C. 1982. The Nature of Stuttering. 2nd Ed. Prentice-Hall, Inc., Englewood Cliffs, NJ.

Wall, M., Starkweather, C., and Cairns, H. 1981. Syntactic influences on stuttering in young child stutterers. J. Fluency Disord. 6:283–298.

West, R. 1958. An agnostic's speculations about stuttering. In: J. Eisenson (ed.), Stuttering: A Symposium. Harper & Row, New York.

Westby, C. 1979. Language performance in stuttering and nonstuttering children. J. Commun. Disord. 12:133–145.

Williams, D. E. 1978. The problem of stuttering. In: F. L. Darley, and D. D. Spriestersbach (eds.), Diagnostic Methods in Speech Pathology. 2nd Ed. Harper & Row, New York.

Williams, D. E., and Silverman, F. 1968. Note concerning articulation of school-age stutterers. Percept Motor Skills 27:713–714.

Williams, D. E., Darley, F., and Spriestersbach, D. 1978. Appraisal of rate and fluency. In: F. L. Darley, and D. D. Spriestersbach (eds.), Diagnostic Methods in Speech Pathology 2nd Ed. Harper & Row, New York.

Williams, D. E., Silverman, F., and Kools, J. 1968. Disfluency behavior of elementary-school stutterers and nonstutterers: The adaptation effect. J. Speech Hear. Res. 11:622–630.

Wingate, M. 1964a. Recovery from stuttering. J. Speech Hear. Disord. 29:312–321.

Wingate, M. 1964b. A standard definition of stuttering. J. Speech Hear. Disord. 29:484–488.

Wingate, M. 1976. Stuttering: Theory and Treatment. Irvington, New York.

Wolpe, J. 1973. The Practice of Behavior Therapy. Pergamon Press, New York.

Wolpe, J., and Lang, P. 1969. Fear Survey Schedule. Educational and Industrial Testing Service, San Diego, CA.

Young, M. 1975. Onset, prevalence, and recovery from stuttering. J. Speech Hear. Disord. 40:49–58.

Zenner, A., Ritterman, S., Bowen, S., and Gronhovd, K. 1978. Measurement and comparison of anxiety levels of parents of stuttering, articulatory defective, and normal-speaking children. J. Fluency Disord. 3:273–283.

Zwitman, D. 1978. The Disfluent Child. University Park Press, Baltimore.

APPENDIX

Sets of Possible Questions for the Intake Interview with Either a Parent of a Disfluent Child or an Adult Stutterer

Parent interview	Interview of an adult

Presenting problem

Parent interview	Interview of an adult
1. Could you describe your child's speech problem in your own words?	1. Could you please describe, to the best of your ability, the speech problem you have?
2. What prompted you to contact this clinic?	2. What prompted you to contact this clinic?
3. Have you been aware of any speech difficulties in your child? If so, please describe. (For use when child has been detected in screening.)	

History of the disorder

Parent interview	Interview of an adult
1. When was the disfluency problem first noticed and by whom?	1. Can you recall when the stuttering problem was first detected and by whom?
2. Were there any special circumstances that related to the onset?	2. Do you recall or were you told of any special circumstances that surrounded the onset of stuttering?

3. Did you or anyone do anything about it initially?	3. Can you review the history of the disorder with reference to changes in behavior?
	   a. Periods of remission
	   b. Periods of extreme severity
	   c. Changes in symptoms
	   d. In general, better, worse, about the same

4. Since the problem was first noticed, have there been any changes?
   a. Periods of remission
   b. Periods of extreme severity
   c. Changes in symptoms
   d. In general, better, worse, about the same
	4. Do you think there is anything in your medical history that is related to the problem?

5. Do you think there is anything in your child's medical history that might be related to the problem?	5. Do you feel that there is anything in your psychological history that is related to the problem? Have you ever seen a counselor, psychologist, or psychiatrist? If so, can you tell me the nature of the problem?
6. Do you think there is anything in your child's psychological or social history that might be related to the problem?	6. Does anyone in your family stutter or does any family member have a related speech problem?
7. Could you describe any family history of stuttering? Is there any family history of other speech problems?	7. Please review the different times when you have had therapy.

218

Parent interview	Interview of an adult
8. Has your child received any speech therapy? If so, could you describe when he received therapy and what was done?	8. Can you tell me what you did in therapy each of those times?
	9. What did you like about these therapies, if anything? What did you dislike, if anything?
	10. Did any of the therapies work to improve your speech?

Reaction to the problem

Parent interview	Interview of an adult
1. Do you think your child is aware of his speech problem? If so, is this a subtle awareness or a very clear awareness?	1. Can you tell me a bit about your feelings toward your stuttering?
2. How does your child react to his speech problem?	2. Why do you think it has happened or what do you think caused it?
3. Has he ever labeled or described his problem? How?	3. In general, how have others reacted to the problem:
	a. Parents
	b. Brothers and sisters
	c. Spouse
	d. Children
	e. Employers/employees
	f. Close friends
	g. Teachers/professors
	h. Others
4. Do you think he avoids any situations because of his speech?	4. How do you react to these various reactions? For example, how do you react to _____? (irritation, pity, amusement, etc.)
5. How have others reacted to the problem?	5. Do you find yourself avoiding any situations or people because of your stuttering? If so, please describe.
a. Mother	
b. Father	
c. Brothers and sisters	
d. Grandparents	
e. Friends	
f. Teachers	
g. Others	
6. Have any of these reactions altered the person's relationship to your child? If so, how?	6. Do you feel your stuttering has affected your social life? If so, how?
7. How concerned are you about the problem?	7. Has your stuttering hampered your educational and/or occupational progress? If so, how?
8. How have you handled the disfluencies at the moment they occur?	8. How significant a problem is it?
	9. If therapy were indicated, how much time or energy would you be willing to devote to it?

Parent interview	Interview of an adult

Precipitating factors

1. I will identify some situations. To the best of your ability, you describe the impact of these situations on your child's fluency?
   a. Relaxed, but not tired
   b. Playing with friends
   c. Playing with brothers and sisters, parents
   d. Playing with one friend as opposed to a group
   e. Talking with parents, but not excited, casual
   f. Explaining something
   g. Excited but happy (Christmas, birthday, etc.)
   h. Angry
   i. Concerned about others (hurt sibling, sick pet, etc.)
   j. Tired
   k. Talking in front of a group of adults
   l. Talking to parents when they are upset, but not at child
   m. Confessions
   n. Talking to parents when angry at the child
   o. Impatient listeners
   p. People who give negative reaction to the child's speech
   q. Interrupted
   r. Afraid
   s. Competing
   t. Upset
   u. Strangers
   v. Teachers
   w. Grandparents
   x. Recitations
   y. Others
2. Are there any particular words upon which your child has difficulty?
3. Are there any particular sounds upon which your child has problems?

1. Can you identify any situations where you could anticipate normal speech?

2. Can you pick out any situations when you expect notable difficulty in speaking.
3. Do you think anxiety or tension is in any way related to your stuttering? (It is recommended that the *Southern Illinois Speech Checklist* be administered and the information obtained should be integrated with answers to this question.)

Parent interview	Interview of an adult
4. Can you predict when the child is apt to have more disfluency.	4. Do you consider yourself generally anxious, tense, or "high strung"?
5. Do you think the child can predict when s/he will have difficulty speaking.	5. Are there any particular words upon which you have trouble?
6. Are there any agents or conditions that prompt fluency (singing, choral recitation, etc.)	6. Are there any sounds that give you particular difficulty?
	7. Can you generally predict when the stuttering will happen or does it come "out of the blue"?
	8. Are there any particular emotions that are associated with improved speech? Poorer speech?
	9. Are there any agents or conditions that prompt fluency (singing, choral recitation, etc.)?

Nature of the disfluency

1. Can you describe the exact type of speech problem? (Here, it may be necessary to mimic various forms of repetition, prolongation and interjection.)	1. Would you consider the stutterings I have seen up to this point fairly typical?
2. Does your child seem to struggle when he speaks or are his disfluencies relatively effortless?	2. What other symptoms or kinds of stuttering have you experienced, if any? Do you do those now?
3. Have you ever seen any secondary behaviors not directly related to the speech? (Here, it will often be necessary to mention examples: lip protrusions, eye blinking, head jerking, pinching self, foot tapping, etc.)	3. What does it feel like physically when you're in a stuttering episode?
4. Have you noticed any unusual changes in the pitch and loudness of the voice when s/he is having trouble?	4. Do you have any particular places in your body that feel tight or tense when you stutter?
5. Are there any particular sites of tension in the body when he is having trouble?	5. Does anything else happen to you physically when you stutter (sweating, flushing, butterflies, heart pounding, etc.)?
6. Have you noticed any tremors in the lips, jaw or neck?	6. Do you have any devices or tricks you use to control stuttering?

7

Diagnosis of Speech and Language Disorders Associated with Acquired Neuropathologies: General Considerations and Aphasia

J. Douglas Noll

Outline

In Chapters 7 and 8 we describe speech and language problems in patients with certain disorders of the nervous system. These chapters should be read together, because they were prepared to complement one another. Our primary task will be to review the process of speech and language diagnosis for patients exhibiting three major forms of communication disturbance: aphasia, apraxia of speech, and dysarthria. In Chapter 7 we consider how speech and language functions are organized. The next discussion concerns how mental confusion and generalized intellectual impairment are reflected in disordered communication. We conclude Chapter 7 by considering the problem of aphasia, a condition of impaired expression and comprehension of language due to some specific form of brain damage. Here, we learn about the forms of linguistic impairment patients with aphasia may exhibit, the systems professional workers use to classify aphasic patients, and approaches workers use to examine patients with aphasia.

In Chapter 8 we consider the problem of apraxia of speech, an articulatory disturbance resulting from impaired motor programming for speech. We will also consider dysarthria, a disturbance resulting from damage to the nervous system causing impaired neuromuscular control of the structures (larynx, tongue, lips, etc.) used in speech.

A NEUROLOGICAL MODEL OF ORAL COMMUNICATION

Before describing these major forms of neurologically based communication problems, we will discuss how normal speech and language functions are organized. Obviously, talking requires a relatively intact central and peripheral nervous system. Active movements of the body, no matter how simple or primitive, occur only as a result of direct muscle stimulation and contraction. Muscle tissue contracts in response to bioelectric stimulation of the muscle fibers from selected nerve impulses. The muscle movements involved in walking, sitting, eating, and talking are initiated and controlled by nerve impulses which originate in the brain. In the case of speech, the complex neural stimulation of the speech mechanism must be controlled to produce precise, rapid articulatory movements. Let us explore some of the neurological relationships between the brain and speech-language abilities.

Levels of Activity

In studying the neurological bases of speech and language, it is helpful to consider oral communication in terms of ordered levels. In order to talk, the speaker goes through a sequential series of steps. There are at least four distinct steps, or levels of activity. First, we generate the concepts or thoughts about what we wish to say. We call this process ideation. Second, these thought processes are put into a specific symbolic system using the linguistic rules of the speaker's language. At this level the words we will use to convey the intended message are selected. The third step involves the conversion or translation of these linguistic units into neuromotor commands that initiate the orderly and sequential innervation of the motor nerves. The neural innervation results in the fourth level of activity, the actual execution of movements of the speech mechanism essential to the production of speech output.

A schematic representation of the four levels of activity associated with oral communication is illustrated in Figure 7.1. This representational model has been described by Hutchinson and Beasley (1976) and Schow et al. (1978). In Figure 7.1 there are arrows between levels, and these arrows point in one direction. The arrows are to be read, "leads to." Thus, Level I leads to Level II, which in turn leads to Level III, which in turn leads to Level IV, which results in the actual utterance. In order to say something, then, one moves temporally from Levels I to II to III to IV. Before we can symbolically encode a message (Level II), we must first go through a process of conceptualization (Level I). The translation of motor program units (Level III) is derived from the encoded message (Level II), which in turn triggers the nerve impulses causing the speech mechanism to move (Level IV). Intuitively, the levels are arranged in a hierarchical order from central to peripheral, or higher to lower.

The notion of sequential arrangement of neurological events associated with oral communication is not particularly new. For example, Hughlings Jackson in 1878 proposed that the nervous system acts as a series of hierarchically controled levels, and that lower levels are dependent upon control from higher levels, not unlike what has been described here. Porch (1981) described these four levels of communication in the following way:

> Once the decision is made to generate a response and the output modality is selected the process of *conceptualization* takes place. Storage banks containing the response repertoire are scanned; then the components for the concept are selected and *encoded* into a sequence of response units typical of the selected modality and appropriate for conveying the concept. Next, during the process of *formulation*, the response units carrying the [encoded] concept are formulated into a series of neural patterns which excite the final stage of output, expression. *Expression* of the idea takes place when the formulated neural patterns cause the contraction and relaxation of the expressors, the muscles involved in the operation of that modality. (p. 26)

Speech versus Language

When we try to characterize the processes involved in oral communication, we often try to distinguish between speech and language. Although both speech and language are involved with oral verbal communication, each refers to separate aspects of that process. Perkins (1977) defines language as the internal, symbolic formulation of ideas according to semantic and grammatical rules, and speech as the observable expression and production

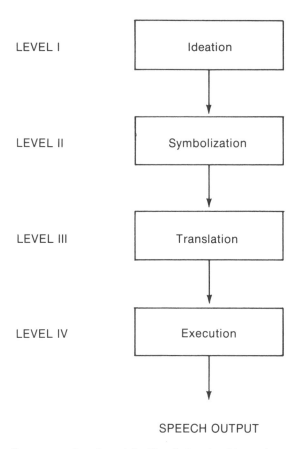

LEVEL I — Ideation

LEVEL II — Symbolization

LEVEL III — Translation

LEVEL IV — Execution

SPEECH OUTPUT

Figure 7.1. Representational model of levels involved in oral communication.

of language. This definition of language is consistent with the one given in Chapter 3: "... language is a code whereby ideas about the world are represented through a conventional system of arbitrary signals for communication" (Bloom and Lahey, 1978, p. 4). We learned in Chapter 3 that this language code is made up of four components: phonology, semantics, syntax, and pragmatics. Whitaker (1976) defines speech in terms of the processes related to direct articulatory movements. Thus, language is the more inclusive, abstract function; speech is more tangible and peripheral. How do speech and language viewed in this way fit into the outline of the four levels of oral communication: *ideation, symbolization, translation,* and *execution*? Clearly, language is a function represented by Level II, symbolization. Speech is the function represented by Level IV, execution. But what about Levels I and III? Is "ideation" a language process? Is "translation" a function of language or of speech as we have defined these terms?

For many years, philosophers and psychologists have argued about whether cognition is a verbal activity. Do we use some kind of "inner language" to create our thoughts? Is thinking a form of implicit or subvocal "speech"? In the previous paragraph, Perkins defined language in terms of the formulation of ideas. If ideation ("formulation of ideas") is a part of the process of cognition, then presumably thought would be mediated through language. Others would argue that mental functioning and language usage are separate and independent. The controversy continues, and the issue probably cannot be resolved to everyone's satisfaction.

What about Level III, translation? If symbolization is a language function and execution is a speech function, what is involved in the motor neural programming of the encoded message? Is this language or speech? This writer considers Level III to be primarily a speech function. We frequently examine patients who, because of certain types of brain damage, only have impaired motor programming for speech and retain their language competence. Darley et al., (1975) report that such patients have difficulty with articulation skills, but do not have major difficulty with comprehension, formulation, and expression of language.

The implication of all this is that programming neural events for speech, as represented by Level III, should be regarded as an operation separate from symbolization, as represented by Level II. This does not mean that motor programming is independent of language formulation. Indeed, none of the four levels in the model is completely independent. They interact in a very complex way. However, each level seems to make a unique and recognizable contribution to the total process of oral communication.

Neuropathologies of Speech and Language

Figure 7.1 can also be used to provide a systematic way of considering neurologically based speech and language disorders. If the four levels of oral communication are valid, there should be a differential effect on the speech output depending upon which of the four functions is disrupted. Neurological damage which results in impaired intellectual, ideational, and mental functions (Level I) should cause a type of communication disorder which differs from one in which the damage brings about impaired symbolic functions (Level II). Likewise, neurological damage influencing motor programming for speech (Level III) should have distinctive speech effects, and these effects should contrast with dysfunction of Levels I, II, and IV. We should be able to analyze characteristics of a patient's speech and make a reasonable interpretation about which of the four functions shown in Figure 7.1 is impaired.

The diagnostician acts something like a detective. Based upon information obtained from the patient's clinical history and from analysis of characteristics of the patient's impaired speech and language usage, clinicians attempt to discover whether the problem is one of intellectualization, symbolization, programming, or motor execution. This discovery is possible only if the function represented by each of the four levels exerts a particular and identifiable influence in the ultimate speech output.

Probably most, if not all, disorders of oral communication caused by neurological damage can be placed under one of the following four headings:

mental-verbal dysfunction
aphasia
apraxia of speech
dysarthria

These four broad diagnostic categories correspond to the four levels of oral communication described. This is represented in Figure 7.2.

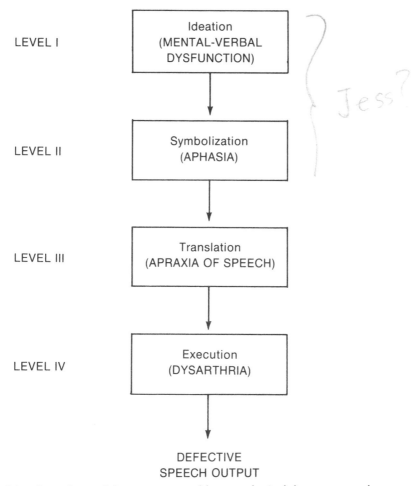

Figure 7.2. *Disorders of speech-language caused by neurological damage at each of the four levels of oral communication.*

Patients with mental-verbal dysfunction exhibit generalized intellectual impairment, psychosis, or confusion. Their speech output is quite restricted or is irrelevant. On the other hand, patients with aphasia have a disturbance of symbolization. They are responsive, alert, and have intact cognitive functions. However, their specific use of language is disrupted. Generally, receptive as well as expressive language functions are impaired. That is, aphasic patients have some difficulty comprehending or understanding what is said to them, and they have problems talking. On the other hand, the patient with apraxia of speech has intact verbal or language skills, but cannot sequence or recall speech motor movements. Apraxia of speech is a translation problem which results in articulatory disturbance. Finally, dysarthria is a neurologically based disorder which results from direct damage to the actual motor pathways which innervate specific musculature of the speech mechanism (larynx, tongue, lips, soft palate, etc.) Thus, dysarthria is an execution problem.

A word of caution—patients seldom exhibit isolated disruption of just one of the functions described in Figure 7.1. Patients typically demonstrate problems in several speech and language functions and they do so simultaneously. Any of the four neurogenically based communication problems can coexist in any or all combinations. When there is damage to the brain, more than one system is often affected, simply because of the nature of neurological lesions. However, the different functions may not be impaired with equal severity. One purpose of differential diagnosis is to determine the patient's primary deficit. Which one of the four levels of oral communication is most seriously affected? The patient may not have normal abilities for the other three levels, but to what degree of severity are they also impaired? Are these other impaired processes of little consequence relative to the major communicative deficit?

MENTAL-VERBAL DYSFUNCTION

As we have seen, Level I has been designated ideation. More processes are incorporated within this level than simply one's use of verbal intelligence. All mental or conceptual functions are important in any thought process. Emotional patterns, state of awareness, psychosensory responses, and so on, are as much a part of ideation as is verbal intellectual performance. There are two acquired conditions reflecting disturbed ideation which result in disordered oral communication: mental confusion and generalized intellectual impairment. Wertz (1978) has provided a complete description of these conditions and the associated speech and language characteristics. Much of the material in this section is drawn from that particular reference.

The hallmark of patients with mental confusion is their disrupted contact with reality. They have difficulty comprehending or fully recognizing their immediate environment. Memory also tends to be faulty. As a result, their speech and language behavior is peculiar. They are often disoriented about time and place. That is, they are unaware of or are in error about their understanding of where they are at the moment. They also reflect this problem by giving erroneous information about places they have lived in the past. They firmly believe that what they are telling you is true. When the author was at the Mayo Clinic he saw a patient with mental confusion caused by encephalitis. The patient lived in Illinois. He neither had homes in any other state, nor had he ever lived in any place other than Illinois. Note the following conversation:

Language of Confusion

Examiner: Tell me, where are you from?
Patient: Whatcha may call it.
Examiner: Where do you live?
Patient: Well, you can almost spit across into Woodcrest there.
Examiner: What state is that in?
Patient: This state.
Examiner: What state is that? What state do you live in?
Patient: Do I live in? I'm resting in any state.
Examiner: Do you live in New York?
Patient: No, I live in Pennsylvania.
Examiner: Do you live in Pennsylvania, or is your home in Illinois?
Patient: I have a home in Illinois, and I also have a home in Florida.
Examiner: Where do you live?
Patient: My home right now is strictly in Los Angeles.
Examiner: Los Angeles? Which state is Los Angeles in?
Patient: I don't know which one you mean.
Examiner: Let's talk about your home in Illinois. What town do you live in there?
Patient: It's not in a town.
Examiner: Well, near what town do you live.
Patient: Los Angeles.
Examiner: This (hospital chart) says that you live in (name of city), Illinois. Is that right?
Patient: No. Not now.
Examiner: Let me ask you about this very moment. Where are you right now?
Patient: Right now, from what I read long, long time ago, I'd be right in the middle of a world.
Examiner: What town is this we're in?
Patient: This should be out in—I can't keep track.
Examiner: We're in Rochester, Minnesota. Can you remember that?
Patient: Oh, yes, I know that. I'm trying to think of—no one's trying to think of a particular name. Because Rochester gave him the same adieus.

Examiner: I wanted you to tell me where we are right now.
Patient: You're south of Westmont, and you're south again of the other ones.
Examiner: No. We're in Rochester, Minnesota. Can you remember that?
Patient: Oh, yeah, that part.
Examiner: Where are we?
Patient: Rochester, Minnesota.

Another patient interviewed at Mayo Clinic was asked where he was at that moment. He stated that he was standing guard duty at Great Lakes Naval Training Station. These patients tend to give information in a very matter of fact fashion without any apparent recognition of the incongruity of their statements. One would think the patient ought to realize he obviously was not outside on guard duty on the naval base just then.

Another feature often observed in the language of confused patients is confabulation. Confabulation is the detailed fabrication of imaginary experiences. Patients who confabulate are not consciously lying, because they are convinced that their experiences are genuine. They seldom show any attempt to self-correct their responses. The interview with the confused patient mentioned earlier was held in an ordinary examining room. Part way through the session, the patient suddenly looked around the room and said, "I was wondering where the fireplace was; I was just wondering where it went to." The examiner answered, "We don't have a fireplace in here." In a very matter-of-fact fashion, the patient said, "I brought it in." He was quite certain that he brought a fireplace with him, and was perplexed by its absence.

Wertz (1978) describes a patient who had never met Helen Keller, and yet when asked who she was, replied as follows:

Patient: Helen Keller? I know her well. She would come to give a talk and I would carry her slides.
Clinician: Who was she?
Patient: She? She was a lady who was supposed to be good, but I really didn't think so myself.
Clinician: Did she have any problems?
Patient: Problems? Oh yes! She had problems, all kinds of problems. But I was too busy carrying slides.
Clinician: What kinds of problems did she have?
Patient: You name it, and she had it. But she never had any difficulty with her slides. I carried those as you might remember.
Clinician: Did she have problems with her eyes or ears?
Patient: Oh my yes! She had problems with her eyes, with her ears, with her nose, with her mouth, with her chin. Lots of problems

It usually is not productive to help patients realize that they are confabulating, even though they may describe a sequence of events that are completely illogical. These patients "know they are right."

Confused patients talk in a way which is irrelevant, bizarre, and often does not make much sense. This becomes most apparent in rather open-ended language situations (Wertz, 1978). For example, confused patients' responses "wander" when giving biographical information, describing situational pictures, explaining a television show, and so on. There is little opportunity for these patients to exhibit irrelevancy when they are simply instructed to name objects and pictures or to point and gesture.

Once again, we return to the post-encephalitic patient from Mayo Clinic. The examiner handed a door key to this patient and asked, "What do you do with a key?" The patient promptly said:

> Well, there's things you can do with 'em. First of all you want to get 'em like that. You use it to open the door to get out of the house, and you use the door when you open the door to get the peep out of the bottles outside to dry your rim. And then you gotta take this in. Open another faucet so the water will come out the bottom—be clean and clear—so that the thing can get a good one. You bring it in, throw it on the bim, and it runs on the bim. You wash it off. You take a couple of little rye bims for yourself to get that stuff out of your face, and get yourself warmed on. Wash yourself off—your hands. You have to get off the dirt through your legs and whatever else. You get some apeace to wash your face off and your hands and stuff to wash the stuff off. You gotta go from there—you gotta get it through your rib with the compalants that you don't get no stuff out of it.

There are several things to notice about this response. It was spoken at a fairly normal rate, was delivered fluently and spoken with few, if any, hesitations. At the beginning, the patient was performing reasonably well in that he indicated a key is used to "open the door to get out of the house." However, notice that he quickly drifted away from the topic and his responses became quite inappropriate to the task at hand. It appears that his responses triggered successive associations which led him further from the stimulus. What do bottles, faucets, washing hands and face, and so forth have to do with a door key? This is an example of irrelevant and bizarre language usage which results or is associated with lack of clarity in thinking processes.

This patient also used quite a lot of jargon, such as, *rye bims, compalants, apeace. Jargon,* in this context, refers to "gibberish" or made-up words. Jargon is produced by patients with different kinds of neurogenically based communicative problems, even those with adequate intellectual abilities. Patients with aphasia and apraxia of speech may also produce jargon on occasion. As a consequence, the presence of jargon does not differentiate one group of impaired speech and language patients from another. Furthermore, all these patients may produce a similar form of jargon.

**Generalized
Intellectual
Impairment**

Some patients lose some of their intellectual capacities due to brain damage. These patients are simply not as alert or as intellectually capable as they were before their illness. Another name we sometimes give to this condition is *dementia*.

The ability to understand abstract concepts requires some degree of cognitive or intellectual ability. In order to abstract, one must be able to generalize or reason. On the other hand, concrete functions are generally more simple, immediate, and refer to the here and now. Thus, demented patients are inclined toward more concrete attitudes. This inclination is reflected in general behavior as well as in the use of language. The vocabulary and language usage of demented patients tends to be more restricted. There is limitation in the variety or spontaneity of speech output, as noted for example in an over-reliance on stereotypic responses. Horenstein (1971) reports that such patients speak less often and simply say less when they do talk. Their verbal responses tend to be perseverative and concrete. Espir and Rose (1970), however, report that vocabulary ability may be retained until late in the course of dementia. The features of oral communication produced by demented patients may reflect disorientation, irrelevance, poor recall and retention, abnormal affect, reduced spontaneity, and so on. They have difficulty concentrating and attending to the tasks. Memory loss may also be quite apparent.

There are a variety of examination procedures which can be used with the patient suspected of having intellectual deterioration. The patient might be asked to define some words or to explain the meaning of some common proverbs. By carefully evaluating the qualitative nature of the patient's responses, you might be able to make some judgments about the patient's ability to use verbal abstracting skills. Another approach is to ask the patient some general information questions. Consider the following interview with a patient having mild intellectual deficits:

Examiner: When do we celebrate Christmas?
Patient: (long pause) Twenty-fifth, isn't it?
Examiner: What is the capital of the United States?
Patient: I can't think. (long pause) I can't remember.
Examiner: Who is the President of the United States?
Patient: Nixon; is it Nixon? (That was correct)
Examiner: Who was before him?
Patient: Johnson. (Correct)
Examiner: And before him?
Patient: I don't know.
Examiner: Do you recall who discovered America?
Patient: Columbus.
Examiner: Do you remember the date?
Patient: No.
Examiner: How many states are there in the United States?

Patient: Thirty-six, is it?
Examiner: Who was the first president of the United States?
Patient: Abraham Lincoln.
Examiner: Who was President during the Civil War?
Patient: Jefferson?

This patient demonstrates several characteristics common to demented patients. They tend to be very unsure of their answers. This is reflected in the number of times they answer questions with a rising inflection. These patients also tend to express an inability to perform, frequently resorting to "I don't know" in handling questions (Wertz, 1978). Halpern (1972) described patients with generalized intellectual impairment by indicating that they have an "across the board" depression of mental faculties, personality changes, emotional lability, dull and bland behavior, and some memory loss.

Confusion and general intellectual impairment have been placed under the single diagnostic heading of mental-verbal dysfunction. Although these two conditions were defined and discussed separately, in fact there are probably more similarities than differences between them. Both confusion and dementia involve a disturbance of higher level cognitive or conceptual processes. In other words, patients with confusion and dementia demonstrate a breakdown of the ideational functions represented by Level I in the model we have discussed. Actually, it is very difficult to differentiate between these two types of patients based upon their use of speech and language. Confused and demented patients often exhibit comparable symptoms. For instance, because demented patients are not very alert or capable of adaptive responses, they tend to be less cognizant of their environment, which is one of the features of confusion. Wertz (1978) has pointed out that some patients may appear to be confused as a direct result of generalized intellectual impairment. Both types of patients have memory deficits, difficulty concentrating, and decreased ability to attend to stimuli or tasks at hand. Also, they tend to deny and/or fail to exhibit significant awareness of their deficits.

Dementia and Confusion: A Unidimensional Process

There are other reasons to combine confusion and dementia under one diagnostic category. There is some evidence to suggest that confused and demented patients have similar types of brain damage (Halpern et al., 1973). These patients show rather diffuse, generalized, or nonlocalized damage, often influencing both cerebral hemispheres. On the other hand, patients with aphasia, apraxia of speech, and dysarthria are more inclined to have more focal or localized lesions, which are quite specific and identifiable to a particular part of the brain. In a subsequent section of this chapter and in chapter 8, we discuss the probable lesion sites for these latter problems.

Another way in which confusion and generalized intellectual impairment correspond is in the general principles of management. A heavy reliance is placed on social interaction for these patients. Many of these patients respond to a program called *reality orientation* (Folsom, 1968; Phillips, 1973; Wells, 1969). In this approach, patients are continually reminded throughout the day of basic information, for example, their names, what day it is, the next meal, and so on. An orientation board listing such essential and meaningful information is kept near the patient at all times. The entire program staff personnel participate in encouraging the patients to achieve habitual recall. Also as a part of this approach, a rigid, simple daily schedule is established with a set routine. Simplifying the environment for the confused and demented patients will help them to make their life more predictable and manageable.

The speech-language pathologist probably does not have a primary role in therapy with the demented or confused patient. The approach described in the previous paragraph is certainly not the traditional therapy program one associates with speech-language pathology. Wertz (1978) points out that there is a generally held opinion that these patients do not profit from speech and language therapy. To counteract this view, however, he gives a number of suggestions of things to be done by the speech-language pathologist. We have more obvious and direct functions in the management of aphasic patients, patients with apraxia of speech, and patients with dysarthria.

It is often difficult and perhaps unnecessary for the speech-language pathologist to attempt to differentiate language of confusion from language of generalized intellectual impairment. As a general rule, the clinician needs only the broader diagnostic label: mental-verbal dysfunction. The basic question which the diagnostician must try to answer is whether the patient has a specific speech-language problem or a more basic, pervasive, cognitive, conceptual problem. If the patient appears to have intact intellectual abilities, but impaired use of speech and language, one would suspect aphasia, apraxia of speech, or dysarthria. If, on the other hand, the patient is not alert, seems disoriented, is out of contact with reality, or has obvious deterioration of intellectual capacities, the clinician would consider mental-verbal dysfunction.

APHASIA

Aphasia is a disturbance of formulation, expression, and comprehension of language symbols. Aphasia results from fairly localized brain damage, usually in the cerebral cortex surrounding the Sylvian fissure of the left hemisphere. As such, aphasia represents a disruption of the language functions involved in Level II, symbolization. The problem is likely to influence symbolic processes in any or all of the verbal modalities: speaking, writing, reading, numerical skills, telling time, and so on.

There are several different receptive and expressive linguistic impairments which might be observed among aphasic patients. In the examination of the patient's use of language, the diagnostician will want to determine the extent to which these impairments are present.

Forms of Linguistic Impairment

Aphasic patients with disturbances in the comprehension of spoken language hear the speaker but have difficulty understanding what is being said. The problem tends to become worse as utterance length or complexity is increased. Patients also tend to have more difficulty when there are competing signals or when there is a rapid change in the nature of content of the message. Patients' ability to comprehend may depend upon the general familiarity of the words used, the length and informational content of the spoken message, grammatical complexity, and the intellectual demands of the message.

Impaired Auditory Verbal Comprehension

Many aphasic patients have reduced auditory retention span. Keenan (1975) has indicated that the patient cannot listen effectively to spoken instructions which are long or complex. Patients may be able to process single words or short sentences much more accurately than phrases or longer sentences. Halpern et al. (1973) reported that impaired auditory verbal retention span is a fundamental component in aphasia.

Anomia refers to word-finding difficulty. The patient is unable to evoke, retrieve, or recall a particular word. The problem is most evident in the case of nouns, but this may be because nouns constitute a large proportion of a speaker's word use. The presence of anomia reflects a reduction in available vocabulary. Some patients, unable to evoke an elusive word, substitute another word, phrase, gesture, or use circumlocutions (i.e., they talk around or about the specific word).

Anomia

The usual method for testing word-finding problems is confrontation naming. In this task, the patient is simply instructed to name a series of pictures or objects. Holland (1980) incorporates a functional communication approach by having patients role-play a series of real-life situations.

Eisenson (1973) defines paraphasia as "any error of commission modifying the individual word (sound and morpheme substitution) or of word substitution in the spoken or written production of a speaker or writer" (pp. 14–15). Eisenson is referring to the two types of paraphasias frequently mentioned in the clinical literature on aphasia: literal paraphasia and verbal paraphasia. Paraphasia constitutes the major behavioral consequence of word retrieval difficulties.

Paraphasias

Literal paraphasia is often called phonemic paraphasia. In this type of paraphasia, the patient produces inconsistent errors of some sounds of words. The use of the term literal is derived from the notion of alphabetic letters, which in earlier literature meant the speech sounds ("phonemic").

Here, a patient might say "lipe" for "life", or "lan" for "man." According to Goodglass and Kaplan (1972), certain phonemic features such as the vowels and number of syllables of the target words are preserved in the utterances spoken by patients with literal paraphasia. If, however, the errors are grossly distorted, jargon or neologisms might result. In this case, the words are unintelligible to the listener.

Verbal or semantic paraphasias are errors in which a real word is inadvertently substituted for the intended one. Usually the errors are "in class." That is, the speaker substitutes a word of somewhat related semantic meaning to the target word (for example, "knife" for "fork" or "paper" for "pencil"). These errors are not intentional, conscious, or deliberate word substitutions for those which the patient cannot recall. Rather, the errors are linguistic consequences of word retrieval failure by the patient.

Agrammatism and Paragrammatism

Some aphasic patients demonstrate an impairment in the use of grammar. *Grammar*, or *syntax*, refers to the structure and order of words in an utterance according to the established rules of the language. Many clinicians differentiate between two forms of impaired grammar: agrammatism and paragrammatism.

Patients with agrammatism tend to omit some of the "little words" during attempts at connected speech. These are the so-called function words, such as prepositions, articles, pronouns, and conjunctions. These words serve as grammatical markers which provide the actual syntactic structure to sentences. Patients with agrammatism produce what some people call "telegraphic speech" because their responses resemble a telegram. Only the main or key words are used. A different type of grammatical impairment is noted in patients with paragrammatism. Patients with paragrammatism use a variety of syntactic forms in connected speech, but they occasionally make inappropriate use of pronouns, inflectional endings of verbs, conditional clauses, or prepositional phrases.

Two aphasic patients who exhibit errors of syntax in their speech are included in the film entitled, *Verbal Impairment Associated With Brain Damage*, by Martha Taylor Sarno (United States Public Health Service, 1966). The conversation with one of the patients is as follows:

Examiner: Tell me, what did you do last weekend?
Patient: I—some washing—a dress.
Examiner: Did you do anything else?
Patient: Some reading—a paper.

In response to the question, "Where did you go yesterday?", the other patient said:

"Well, in the morning yesterday, I droving to the office, but then later my friends picking me up. We ate together lunch."

The first patient is demonstrating agrammatism, whereas the second patient exhibits paragrammatism.

Many brain-damaged patients exhibit perseveration. They continue a par-   *Perseveration*
ticular response long after it is appropriate. For example, in a confrontation naming task, the examiner might present a picture which the patient names. On subsequent pictures the patient still answers with the name of the first picture. The patient is having difficulty shifting the response.

Perseveration can sometimes be observed in instances of literal para-phasia in which phonetic error patterns recur. Eisenson (1973) gives the example of an aphasic patient who, when asked to say the sentence "Per-sistence is essential to success," said "Mesastense is instans to sesatins." Note the repetitive nature of the error sounds, such as the /st/ and /ns/ clusters.

Eisenson (1973) makes the cogent observation that perseveration tends to increase when any of the following conditions exist: 1) the aphasic patient is confronted with difficult, new contexts; 2) the patient is experiencing fatigue; 3) situations change rapidly; and 4) the patient is in a state of anxiety and feels the need to say something, despite his inability at the moment to say what is required. Eisenson goes on to say that perseveration may in-dicate the demands being made by the clinician are excessive. In this case, the patient is unable to respond appropriately, and the unconscious repetition of a previous act is a natural consequence. The clinician should alter the pace or change the activity to reduce perseveration.

Aphasic patients differ with regard to the fluency of their connected, spon-   *Impaired Verbal*
taneous speech. Traditionally, patients have been identified as being either   *Fluency*
fluent or nonfluent. Benson (1979) gives one of the more complete and cur-rent descriptions of these two forms of aphasic language use. The nonfluent patient with aphasia produces decreased verbal output, usually fewer than 10 words per minute with obvious effort. Facial grimacing and articulatory struggle are likely to be visible. The nonfluent patient produces very short word groupings. Actually, most responses are disjointed, single-word ut-terances. An interesting feature of nonfluent speech is altered prosody. Fluent aphasia is the opposite of nonfluent aphasia. The quantity of verbal output is essentially normal. There is little apparent effort during talking. Fluent speech is characterized by facile articulation and a reasonable rate of speech. Phrase length is usually adequate and melodic pattern is normal. The patient may exhibit occasional pauses when a specific word cannot be recalled on demand. When this happens, the patient may substitute a de-scriptive phrase or may resort to circumlocution. The fluent aphasic patient also frequently uses general, nondescript words like "thing," "stuff," "it." As a consequence, such patients produce spoken messages that tend to flow

quite smoothly. Nonetheless, there is a deficiency of meaningful content words. Little actual information is conveyed, resulting in what some clinicians call "empty speech."

Classification of Aphasic Patients

Patients with aphasia may be divided into several different groups, types, or syndromes. One way patients can be grouped is according to overall severity of the impairment, that is, mild, moderate, severe. Clinicians and researchers have also developed classifications of aphasia based upon the nature of the verbal impairment.

There are several reasons why a speech-language pathologist would want to classify aphasia based upon the nature of verbal impairment. Classification provides a systematic, structured way of looking for both similarities and differences in patterns of language usage by aphasic patients. Classification also provides a common frame of reference that speech-language pathologists can use to interact with professional colleagues. A final matter for discussion is the approach used in speech-language therapy. Of course, we treat each aphasic patient as an individual case. However, as Benson (1979) correctly points out, "Recent advances in language therapy techniques suggest that some varieties (syndromes) of aphasia respond best to certain techniques and future advances may well demonstrate even greater specificity between the variety of aphasia and the most favorable treatment technique" (p. 138).

An Aphasia Classification System

Brown (1972), Schuell (1965), and Sies (1974) have provided detailed historical reviews of the development of various classification systems used by people interested in aphasia. The system which is most current and probably used by most individuals incorporates all or some of the following categories of aphasia:

Broca's Aphasia
Wernicke's Aphasia
Conduction Aphasia
Transcortical Motor Aphasia
Transcortical Sensory Aphasia
Transcortical Mixed Aphasia
Anomic Aphasia
Global Aphasia

Each of the eight major types of aphasia mentioned above can be differentiated in terms of the kinds of verbal impairments discussed earlier in this chapter. As a matter of fact, reasonably good classification of patients can be accomplished using only three verbal processes: speech fluency, auditory verbal comprehension, and ability of the patient to repeat words and sentences presented by the examiner.

Figure 7.3 was devised by Gerald Canter (1979) at Northwestern University. In this figure, Canter shows how each of the eight types of aphasia can be identified using the three verbal processes just discussed. The "plus" symbol (+) is used to indicate that the specific function is intact or at least fairly good. The "minus" symbol (−) is used to indicate that a specific function is relatively impaired. In interpreting Figure 7.3, one must understand that a plus does not necessarily indicate that the specific function is normal, and a minus does not necessarily indicate that a function is completely defective. These are relative matters.

We now discuss some of the types of aphasia in terms of the material provided in Figure 7.3. As we can see, patients with conduction aphasia have most difficulty repeating words and sentences spoken to them, although they have adequate auditory verbal comprehension skills. The speech output of patients with conduction aphasia is also fairly fluent. On the other hand, patients with Broca's aphasia have nonfluent speech and some problems in repetition, but they understand the speech of others. Patients with Wernicke's aphasia have difficulty comprehending spoken language and repeating utterances, yet their speech is reasonably fluent.

Global aphasia and anomic aphasia require special mention. The former is represented by minuses in all three functions; the latter by pluses. The patient with global aphasia has severe impairment, exhibiting depressed performance in all verbal skills. Global aphasic deficits cut across all language

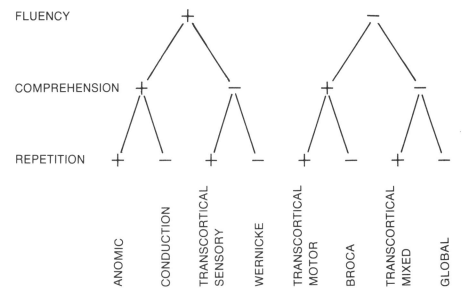

Figure 7.3. Diagnostic flow chart of major types of aphasia. (Reprinted with permission from G. J. Canter, 1979)

modalities. Patients with this form of disturbance show no particular strength in any verbal function. Patients with anomic aphasia, on the other hand have minimal difficulty with speech-language functions. Their major problem is isolated word-finding difficulty. Otherwise, their speech is fluent and grammatically well formed. Auditory comprehension is generally quite good. Their speech often lacks substantive words. In conversational speech, they may resort to circumlocutions. Goodglass and Kaplan (1972) give the example in which, instead of the statement "I had an operation on my head," the anomic patient might say "I had one of them up there," or "I had a thing done up where your hair is." The patient with anomic aphasia might be able to name most objects quite promptly, but the naming deficit becomes evident when the patient is asked for less familiar names or is asked to name parts of objects ("teeth" of a comb, "band" of a watch, "eraser" on a pencil). Because their problems are generally not severe, many of these patients function fairly well in most communicative situations, because they develop strategies for coping with the occurrence of isolated word-finding problems.

In order to evaluate the ability of a patient to repeat, the examiner gives a series of words, phrases, or sentences to the patient, and observes whether the patient can reproduce the words exactly as presented. There may be word substitutions, omissions, additions, or reversals; syntactic errors; paraphasias; and so on. One might expect the degree of difficulty in repetition to directly reflect the amount of impairment in auditory verbal comprehension. The patient with minimal problems in auditory verbal comprehension might be expected to have minimal difficulty repeating something said by the examiner. Similarly, you might expect the patient with marked difficulty in auditory comprehension to also have marked difficulty in repetition. In clinical practice, these two functions do not necessarily go hand-in-hand. Some patients with good auditory comprehension skills are unable to repeat an utterance to the examiner. Conversely, some patients with significant problems in auditory verbal comprehension surprisingly are able to repeat or "parrot" an utterance spoken to them.

One should clearly identify the types of aphasias characterized in Figure 7.3 by a discrepancy between the ability to repeat and the ability to comprehend on an auditory basis. These discrepancies or types of aphasia are marked by a plus (+) for comprehension and a minus (−) for repetition, or vice versa. In conduction and Broca's aphasia, the ability to repeat is poorer than auditory verbal comprehension. On the other hand, in transcortical sensory and transcortical motor aphasia, the situation is reversed. Namely, the ability to repeat is better than the ability to comprehend. Thus, relative strength or liability in one of these functions does not imply what ability will be in the other. Later, we will describe why this discrepancy can occur in aphasia. The book by Goodglass and Kaplan entitled *The Assessment of*

Aphasia and Related Disorders (1972), provides a more lengthy and complete description of the system of classification we have been discussing.

So far, we have described major types of aphasia based upon behavioral aspects of patients' speech and language deficits. Types of aphasia can also be identified in terms of areas of damage within the brain. After all, the most logical explanation as to why there are different types of aphasia is that damage to different parts of the brain results in different effects on patients' verbal abilities. The speech-language pathologist provides important clinical information about the aphasic patient's language problems, whereas the physician's findings are used to determine the nature, extent, and site of the pathology. Both sets of information contribute to the diagnosis of the disorder. Relations between anatomical and clinical findings helps us understand the neural mechanisms underlying the aphasias.

Site of Lesion

We begin this discussion by describing a theory of the relationship between brain and language proposed by Geschwind (1970) and embellished by Brookshire (1978) and Canter (1979). We must emphasize that the theory which follows is highly speculative and overly simplistic. Unquestionably, brain function is more complex than the theory would suggest. Theory description does help us think about how speech and language functions could be processed in the brain, and as Brookshire (1978) says, based upon our knowledge of the aphasias, "the brain seems to behave as if these events occur" (p. 26).

In most individuals, the left hemisphere is the dominant half of the brain for verbal processes, specifically speech and language. A lateral view of the cerebral cortex of the left hemisphere is shown in Figure 7.4. Some of the major landmarks are identified. The cortical areas most important for speech and language abilities are located in the frontal, parietal, and temporal lobes surrounding the Sylvian fissure. We will describe each of these areas and identify what function each area seems to have.

Another name for Heschl's gyrus is the *primary auditory cortex*. This gyrus is located in the superior-posterior surface of the temporal lobe, an area active during the perception and recognition of auditory stimuli. Activity in this area is also important to our ability to discriminate sounds, even nonverbal sounds, like differentiating a finger snap from a car horn. Wernicke's area is positioned slightly below Heschl's gyrus, in the mid-temporal lobe. Auditory verbal comprehension and the retrieval of words and grammatical rules depends upon adequate functioning of this area of the brain. Symbolization requires adequate form and function of Wernicke's area.

Broca's area is located in the posterior-inferior region of the frontal lobe. This area of the brain is located just in front of the primary motor cortex or the pre-central gyrus. Broca's area is assumed to be involved in

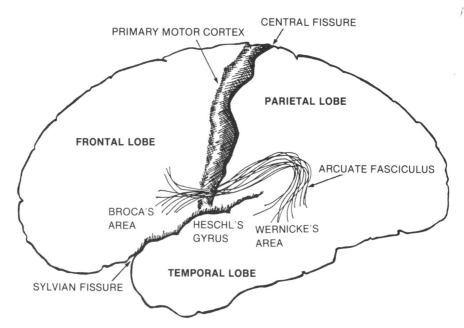

Figure 7.4.   Lateral view of cerebral cortex of left hemisphere.

the programming, timing, directing, and coordinating of activity of speech musculature.

Association fibers refers to those nerve axons which interconnect different areas of the cortex. The term *fasciculus* is also used to refer to association fibers, and there are names for each of the major fasciculi in the brain. The arcuate fasciculus is one set of association fibers. These fibers sweep through the cerebrum to interconnect Wernicke's area with Broca's area. These interconnections permit transmission between the area of the brain important for audition and the area of the brain important for speech production. As Brookshire (1978) stated, ''The arcuate fasciculus is thought to be the major pathway by which the acoustic-phonemic 'patterns' of words are transmitted forward to Broca's area for motor encoding'' (p. 25).

The theory of Brookshire (1978), Canter (1979), and Geschwind (1970) proposes how each of these areas contributes to various speech and language processes. For example, in order to comprehend a spoken message, the primary auditory cortex (Heschl's gyrus) makes some elementary analyses of the acoustic signal. This information is then ''sent'' to the auditory association area (Wernicke's area) where ''meaning is extracted'' from the verbal message, which is really a process of decoding.

What happens when we simply want to speak a sentence spontaneously? In some complex way, Wernicke's area is involved in the selection of appropriate words, neurally coded according to learned semantic and grammatical rules of the language. This encoded sentence is then "sent" to Broca's area via the arcuate fasciculus, where it is translated into a sequence of neural commands. That information, in turn, is relayed to the appropriate parts of the primary motor cortex where nerve impulses are then sent along the various motor pathways to the anatomical structures needed for speech production.

The theory implies that the entire circuit is involved when a person repeats something he or she has heard. Heschl's gyrus is active when one perceives and discriminates spoken messages. Wernicke's area is active when one interprets and recodes messages, which are then sent to Broca's area. At this point, messages are converted into neural codes of movement commands, and sent to the primary motor cortex for actual execution.

We can now consider the probable location of brain lesions associated with the major types of aphasia. Broca's aphasia most likely occurs from lesions to Broca's area or to the fiber tracts which innervate this area. Patients with Broca's aphasia have difficulty planning and coordinating the sequence of movements necessary for fluent, smooth speech production. As a consequence, they typically exhibit effortful and awkward articulation, short utterances, and some transpositions of phonemes. Vocabulary and grammatical forms tend to be restricted because of the relative paucity of expressive language usage. In patients with Broca's aphasia, Wernicke's area is usually not affected. Therefore, auditory verbal comprehension may be unimpaired. Patients with Broca's aphasia are able to hear themselves and realize that they are having difficulty producing speech. They can monitor speech on an auditory basis and generally are able to recognize their errors. They will usually struggle to self-correct speech errors as they are speaking. This pattern adds to the nonfluent, disrupting character of their speech output.

Wernicke's aphasia generally seems to result from damage to the auditory association area in the left temporal lobe, that is, Wernicke's area. As a consequence of this type of lesion, patients with Wernicke's aphasia usually will have impaired auditory verbal comprehension, and therefore some difficulty in repetition tasks. Their speech tends to be quite fluent, however, and is characterized by reasonably good grammatical form. They generally show considerable language output, but the content of this output is quite defective. Language output tends to be disorganized, rambling, devoid of substantives and action words, and lacking in specific meaning. Brookshire (1978) gives this example of a sentence spoken by a Wernicke's aphasic patient: "I went down to the thing and did it, but it wasn't there, so I came around." Patients with Wernicke's aphasia almost always have a marked word-finding problem, and reading ability is usually impaired as well. Their writing tends to parallel the content of their speech.

Probably because of their impaired auditory comprehension, patients with Wernicke's aphasia have defective auditory monitoring of their speech output. They appear to be unaware of their speech errors. There is little evidence of self-correction or of any real effort to alter what they are saying.

Conduction aphasia results from a disruption of the arcuate fasciculus. Remember that this is the network of association fibers which transmits encoded messages from Wernicke's area to Broca's area. Thus, in conduction aphasia, two areas of the brain are disconnected. Patients with conduction aphasia exhibit adequate auditory verbal comprehension because the primary auditory area and the auditory association area are intact. Likewise, the speech output is reasonably fluent because Broca's area is undisturbed. Because the connection between the auditory areas and the area for planning and execution of motor speech is interrupted, however, these patients have difficulty repeating what they hear. This illustrates how ability to repeat an utterance can be impaired while auditory comprehension is intact. Brookshire (1978) has suggested that reading aloud will also be impaired because that function probably also requires transmission from Wernicke's area to Broca's area. But, interestingly enough, silent reading or reading comprehension is generally good.

We have tried to emphasize the importance of the region surrounding the Sylvian Fissure of the dominant hemisphere as being important for speech and language functions. Normal speech and language requires very complex interactions between this portion of the brain and the rest of the brain for knowledge, intentions, perceptions, and other cognitive processes. That is, for normal speech and language skills, Wernicke's area, Broca's area and the arcuate fasciculus do not function independently from the rest of the brain. Geschwind et al. (1968) explain that this is exactly what happens in the transcortical aphasias. The region surrounding the Sylvian fissure, represented by the Wernicke-Broca area complex, is isolated from the rest of the brain by a band of damaged brain tissue. Thus, Wernicke's area, Broca's area, and the pathways between them can continue to perform their functions. In this circumstance, there is little intervention of control or abstract intellectual processing. Therefore, patients with transcortical aphasia can repeat what is said to them, although they seemingly attach very little meaning to their responses. As a matter of fact, patients with transcortical aphasia sometimes demonstrate automatic, apparently involuntary repetition of almost everything, a condition referred to as *echolalia*. In other words, they show the enigmatic feature of impaired auditory verbal comprehension in the face of relatively strong ability to repeat an utterance spoken by the examiner.

There are several specific types of transcortical aphasia. For example, transcortical motor aphasia occurs from an anterior cerebral lesion, in the region surrounding Broca's area. Except for the ability to repeat, these patients resemble patients with Broca's aphasia. On the other hand, transcortical sensory aphasia arises from posterior lesions outside of Wernicke's area, probably behind the arcuate fasciculus. Such patients present the empty, fluent speech similar to that produced by Wernicke's aphasic patients, except for their uncanny ability to repeat what is said to them. Finally, transcortical mixed patients probably have fairly extensive anterior as well as posterior lesions, although the Wernicke's-Broca's complex is preserved. Thus, they exhibit severe impairment, similar to global aphasia, but are able to perform some repetition tasks.

Speech and Language Examination of the Aphasic Patient

The speech-language pathologist needs to make a thorough examination of patients' verbal skills. This is needed to determine the type of aphasia and to provide a basis for formulating an appropriate program of therapy. There are several commercially available tests of aphasia which can be used to examine patients' verbal skills. The most common tests are: Examining for Aphasia (Eisenson, 1954), Minnesota Test for Differential Diagnosis of Aphasia (Schuell, 1965), Porch Index of Communicative Ability (Porch, 1981), Boston Diagnostic Aphasia Examination (Goodglass and Kaplan, 1972), Sklar Aphasia Scale (Sklar, 1973), Aphasia Language Performance Scales (ALPS) (Keenan and Brassell, 1975), and Communicative Abilities in Daily Living (Holland, 1980). In each of these tests, a series of tasks are presented to sample patients' verbal behaviors. Most of the tests provide items which sample patients' abilities in oral output, written output, auditory input, and visual input. Oral and written output are examined by analyzing both quantitative and qualitative aspects of speech production and writing completed in response to test items. *Auditory input* refers to the ability to comprehend spoken language, while *visual input* specifies reading skills.

The actual organization of different tests of aphasia vary. These tests are typically divided into four major sections: oral and written output and auditory and visual input. Different terminology is often used to refer to these four processes. For example, Keenan and Brassell (1975) simply use the descriptive headings of talking, writing, listening, and reading. Sklar (1973), on the other hand, refers to the four sections of his test as oral encoding, graphic encoding, auditory decoding, and visual decoding. Encoding is the process of generating a message; producing a verbal response. Oral encoding, therefore, means the same as talking, and graphic encoding means the same as writing. Decoding, on the other hand, is extracting a message from a set of verbal symbols. Thus, auditory decoding is the same as listening to and comprehending a spoken utterance, whereas visual decoding means reading.

Eisenson (1954) divides his test into the two major dimensions of "productive" and "evaluative disturbances" which correspond to expressive (encoding) and receptive (decoding) impairments. The Minnesota Test for Differential Diagnosis of Aphasia (Schuell, 1965) has four major and one minor sections. The major subtests are: auditory disturbances, visual and reading disturbances, speech and language disturbances, and visuomotor and writing disturbances.

Although there are some apparent differences in the construction of tests of aphasia, they all have certain features in common. Stimuli or tasks are presented to the patient and the examiner evaluates the nature of the patient's verbal responses to these tasks. Basically, the examiner is probing the patient's ability in each of four processes: speaking, writing, reading, and listening.

The decision about which test of aphasia clinicians might use depends on a number of considerations. There are some practical matters, such as cost of the test and the length of time needed to administer the test. For example, the Minnesota Test for Differential Diagnosis of Aphasia (Schuell, 1965) requires from 2 to 6 hours to administer completely, whereas the Aphasia Language Performance Scales (Keenan and Brassell, 1975) can be administered in 20 to 30 minutes. Examining for Aphasia (Eisenson, 1954) was published almost 30 years ago and some clinicians might wish to use a test which is based upon more modern clinical constructs. The Boston Diagnostic Aphasia Examination (Goodglass and Kaplan, 1972) is a good test to use for classifying patients on the basis of probable site of brain lesion. A test which provides prognostic information about recovery from aphasia is the Minnesota Test for Differential Diagnosis of Aphasia. The Porch Index of Communicative Ability (Porch, 1981) has a very complicated system of scoring patients' verbal responses. In order to become proficient at administering the Porch Index, clinicians need to undertake an extensive (40 hour) course of instruction. On the other hand, because of the detailed scoring system used in the Porch Index, this test is very useful for showing subtle changes in speech and language skills over time.

The examiner does not always have to administer a commercially available test of aphasia to make some judgments about patients' speech and language abilities. Clinicians can devise a number of informal procedures. We will describe several approaches which can be used in the examination of aphasic patients. Many of these ideas are taken directly from *A Procedure Manual in Speech Pathology with Brain-Damaged Adults*, by Joseph Keenan (1975).

A series of listening, reading, writing, and speaking tasks characterized by various levels of difficulty can be presented to the patient. The purpose is to progressively increase the difficulty of the tasks until the patient experiences failure. This procedure is used to define the patient's "score" or ceiling in each task.

Before beginning the examination, the clinician should set the stage for the patient by describing what tasks are being given and why they are used. The clinician might say something like this:

> I'm going to ask you to do some things which involve talking, listening, reading, and writing. The reason is that many people who have had a stroke often find that they're having trouble with those things. I simply want to find out what

sort of things you have trouble with and what ones are pretty easy for you. You'll probably find that some of the things I'll ask you to do will be difficult. But there will also be some which should cause you no difficulty whatsoever. As a matter of fact, you may think they're awful silly. But try as best you can. OK?

The examiner will want to determine the severity of the patient's impairment in each of the four speech-language modalities: listening, talking, reading, and writing. If one of the formal tests of aphasia was administered, it may be possible to derive a severity ranking from the patient's numerical score in each of the sections of the test. Such is the case with the ALPS (Keenan and Brassell, 1975) and the Sklar Aphasia Scale (Sklar, 1973). The examiner can also estimate severity on the basis of informal observations of the patient's verbal abilities. A few general things to look for at different levels of impairment are summarized in Table 7.1. This material is drawn from the work of Keenan (1975) and from my own clinical experiences with aphasic patients. The information summarized in Table 7.1, together with the procedures outlined below should enable you to obtain a fairly good description of the nature of an aphasic patient's verbal functions.

Many brain-damaged adults have problems with recent memory. Consequently, when assessing a patient's speech and language functions, one typically should avoid using verbal tasks which pertain to things that have recently happened to the patient. For example, do not be surprised if patients are unable to tell you what they had for breakfast or what they watched on television last night. A better set of questions would be to have them tell you about their job, how they became ill, or where they went to school. Remote past memory is usually better than memory for recent events.

One of the first things the examiner must do is determine whether the patient has a hearing loss. If a patient has difficulty hearing, he or she may also have difficulty understanding what is said. Thus, clinicians must determine that the patient can hear adequately for speech purposes. They must rule out hearing loss as the reason for a patient's difficulty in auditory verbal comprehension (see Chapter 2 for details).

Examination of Auditory Verbal Comprehension

Patients with aphasia often have problems understanding spoken messages. The patient with severe or profound comprehension difficulties may only be able to follow simple, single-word responses and some short phrases. One examination approach is to say the patient's name with a rising intonation as in a question, and observe how the patient reacts. You might also try the same intonational pattern but produce the wrong name. Does the patient respond appropriately and consistently? It is prudent to avoid yes-no questions, such as asking the patient, "Is your name Mr. Jones?" Some patients with severe comprehension disturbance have difficulty responding correctly on a yes-no basis even though they may know the correct answer.

Table 7.1   Levels of impairment

Listening

Mild follows radio and TV programs and general discussion and ordinary conversation with only minimal difficulty; accurately performs three instructions in sequence, e.g., "Point to the floor, the window in the room, and your chair."

Moderate follows most conversation but sometimes fails to grasp essentials or requires repetition; can perform one- or two-step commands with simple noun plus verb construction, e.g., "Point to the ceiling and the mirror," or "Loosen your tie."

Severe follows only brief statements and may need considerable repetition; often responds inappropriately because he or she does not always understand what is being said; inconsistently points to objects named by single spoken words, e.g., bed, chair, lamp, pen

Profound may understand situations in general and may respond appropriately to tone of voice; may recognize own name when it is spoken; typically does not follow spoken instructions unless they are routine, or unless they are supplemented by gesture, demonstrations, or assistive actions

Talking

Mild converses on many topics easily with only occasional word finding errors or difficulty expressing ideas; uses whole sentences with only minor errors of articulation and syntax; can describe a rather complex action performed by the examiner

Moderate uses short sentences or phrases to describe fairly simple functions, actions, or relationships; some conversational speech but marked difficulty in expressing long or complex ideas; frequent occurrences of word finding errors and some jargon; scattered instances of unintelligible words or phrases

Severe expresses needs and wishes in a limited or defective manner; uses single words to indicate site of pain or discomfort, to ask for assistance, or to name desired objects; much difficulty in retrieving specific words, especially on command

Profound messages limited to gestures, unintelligible attempts to speak; an occasional automatic word or common expression; no voluntary use of words to name objects or actions; serial responses, such as counting, days of the week, etc., may be partially retained

Reading

Mild reads and comprehends average adult materials with only minimal difficulty; can read a newspaper and short magazine articles

Moderate reads phrases, simple sentences, and short paragraphs with some errors; may need occasional assist on recognition of some words

Severe can match words to pictures and some spoken to printed words; may be able to match cursive and printed words or capital and lower case letters; patient has no functional reading abilities

Profound may be able to match identical letters or words; may recognize some words, such as own name, *stop*, *men*, etc.

Writing

Mild can write an acceptable personal letter with minimal errors; spontaneous writing is present with only slight impairment of spelling and word formulation; uses whole sentences

Table 7.1   *(Continued)*

Moderate can write short, easy sentences spontaneously and to dictation; spelling vocabulary of 100 or more words; can write some phrases and sentences to describe simple functions, actions, or relationships

Severe can write own name unassisted and a few simple single words to dictation, but has no functional writing abilities

Profound can copy or trace simple words or numbers (1 to 10), and may need some guidance of the patient's hand by the examiner

Of course, other patients who do not know the answer but can respond with a "yes" or "no," may answer correctly on the basis of chance alone.

Patients can also be required to identify objects placed in front of them after they have been named. For patients with severe comprehension disturbance, only 2, 3, or 4 objects should be presented during initial testing. Do not confuse patients with a large array of objects. Only simple objects familiar to adults should be used, and objects should have easy names (e.g., *spoon*, *pen*, *match*, etc.). Body parts, clothing, or objects available in the examining room can often be used. Some patients have difficulty with the concept of "pointing." Therefore, rather than saying, "Point to the pen," it is often better to say, "Where are your glasses," "Show me your bed," "Let me see your tongue." Pictures of objects can be used instead of the actual objects. However, pictures are more abstract than objects. If the patient does not do well with pictures, real objects might be used to determine whether performance improves.

Many aphasic patients have visual field deficits because of the damage to the central nervous system. In these cases, the patient may have a restricted field of view. If objects are placed outside the effective field of view, the patient will not see the objects and, therefore, cannot identify them when named by the examiner. Because of the location of the visual pathways in the brain and the probable site of lesion in aphasia, many of these patients have a right visual field deficit. That is, they see things to their left, but not to their right. Clinicians should generally sit on the patient's left and place objects, pictures, and other stimuli in the patient's left visual field.

Patients who have a moderate to severe deficit of auditory verbal comprehension may be able to perform simple two to four word commands. Here, clinicians ask the patient to do more than indicate, show or point to things. We want them to do something with the objects. For example, we might ask the patient to do the following: "Turn on your light," "Unlock your wheelchair," "Lift up the cup." To perform at this level, the patient has to comprehend both the object and the action. Clinicians also ask patients to complete two-step commands. A two-step command requires the patient to be able to comprehend two different objects or tasks, such as "Point to the ceiling and the chair." Clinicians can get more complicated. For example, "Show me the ceiling and then point to my coat." Many patients are confused by the pronoun "my" (or "mine") versus "yours." Also, this command requires a sequence of pointing to the ceiling first and then to the coat. Additional activities can be called forth using sequential relationships, elicited by such words as "after," "first," "before," "next," and so on. Clinicians can also examine the comprehension of prepositions, ("beside," "on top," "underneath," etc.). This can be accomplished with two or more objects, as in the command, "Put the spoon in the cup." If use of objects is impractical, try something like, "Put your hand behind your head."

Many aphasic patients are not able to manage auditory comprehension at levels more difficult than two-step commands, seven- or eight-word sentences, and simple sequential and prepositional relationships. For patients who are less impaired, however, the next level to examine would be 10- to 14-word sentences, three-step commands, and some relatively abstract concepts the patient must follow. You might say, "Point to the floor, the window in the room, and your chair," "Show me your left foot, the wooden table, and the TV." An interesting test example that Keenan (1975) suggests is, "If you lost one ear, how many would you have left?" You can have patients identify objects by function: "Pick up the one you use with your hair." In testing at still higher levels of auditory verbal comprehension, one must be aware that some normal, nonaphasic individuals might have difficulty retaining commands such as "Turn the spoon upside-down and cover the dime with it, but first put the dime on the napkin" (Keenan, 1975).

Some aphasic patients, regardless of the severity of their disturbance, seem able to follow conversation and comprehend spoken language at levels which are higher than their "test" performance would indicate (Keenan, 1975). In those instances, the patient may be relying on factors such as facial expressions, gestures, context, and visual cues. Also, the speaker may be repeating much of what is said and providing some redundancies in the message.

Examination of Talking

It is likely that during your examination of auditory verbal comprehension the patient has made some attempts at oral expression. The intelligibility of those utterances should be judged. The examiner must estimate the percentage of responses that would be understood by a listener not familiar with the patient or the topic. Finally, the amount of stimulation needed to elicit oral responses from the patient must be determined.

You will probably want to begin examination of talking with some automatic social responses, for example, "hi," "how are you," "OK," or "fine." Then, you should try some easy questions that can be answered with short, common words. Most clinicians will have patients attempt to produce some overlearned, serial responses, such as counting, days of the week, and so on. This approach can be varied by having the patient tell you how many fingers you are holding up, how many buttons are on your shirt, or what day comes before Wednesday. These answers require the ability to select a response and not just utter a string of automatisms.

As we have seen, confrontation naming is a commonly used technique. This refers to having the patient name various pictures or objects as you point to each one. Most aphasic patients have some degree of difficulty with confrontation naming. The terms *anomia* and *dysnomia* specifically refer to word-finding problems. As Keenan (1975) points out, anomia is what we all experience when we are groping for words or cannot remember someone's name.

Some patients have great difficulty producing words spontaneously. It is important to determine whether performance improves if the patient is given some assistance. For example, the patient may not be able to name such objects or pictures as a pen, door, or thumb. The patient might say the words, however, if you provide an incomplete sentence: "You write with a _____," "There is someone at the _____," "The baby sucks his _____." Another helpful technique is to provide visual information. If the patient is trying to say the word *pen*, you could position your lips for the /p/ sound. The patient might speak if you describe and show how to move the articulators to produce the word being attempted. Sometimes, having the patients watch you and themselves in a mirror is helpful, although with other patients, this approach may be upsetting and make speaking more difficult. Writing the word, in addition to the approaches just discussed, may help the patient to retrieve words.

Latency of response is another important dimension to consider. How long does the patient take after the stimulus is presented before an utterance is produced? Is the response immediate, or is there a long delay time? During the delay, is the patient struggling and apparently making a conscious attempt to speak, or is there just empty silence, as though the patient is not responding?

If the patient is making errors naming, you should analyze the nature of the errors. Sometimes the intended word is not produced, but the word spoken may be related in meaning to the intended word. We refer to these errors as semantic, in-class errors (e.g., stimulus word is *pen* but the patient says *pencil*; stimulus is *cup* but the patient says *saucer*). A semantic out-of-class error is a response that has no apparent meaningful association to the target (e.g., saying *paper* in response to the stimulus *comb*).

What about the patient who is producing a lot of jargon or unintelligible responses? Do the responses have some phonetic resemblance to the intended word? Is there some differentiation in response? That is, are the various responses different from one another? Does the patient demonstrate perseveration? All of these observations are important in an examination of talking.

Most of the procedures discussed are designed to examine the patient's use of nouns. You will want to examine the use of other parts of speech as well. One technique is to ask questions, such as, "What do you do with a watch?" You can ask the patient to describe an action you are doing, like putting something in your pocket. Prepositional responses can be elicited by asking the patient, "Where is the dime?" (under the paper).

For the patient who is performing at higher linguistic levels, you must note whether most of the patient's oral responses are complete, grammatically accurate sentences. Can the patient verbally explain concepts, such as explaining what a newspaper is or describing a TV show?

Of course, you will want to engage patients in some informal conversation. If they are in the hospital, ask them about the people from whom flowers and cards were received. Do not just ask for their names. Have patients talk about themselves. You will want to find out about their jobs. Have patients talk about their families. It is important to sound genuinely interested. Do not just give a series of questions but create a real dialogue. If this kind of open-ended conversation is not successful in eliciting connected speech, you might use situational pictures obtained from magazines or other sources to elicit speech. Use pictures in which things are happening. The patient should be encouraged to talk about what is going on in the pictures and not simply name things or objects shown in the pictures.

Examination of Reading

Evaluation of abilities in reading and writing parallel those described for listening and talking, respectively. Talking is oral verbal output and writing is graphic verbal output. The specific techniques used to examine listening and talking can be easily modified for reading and writing, respectively.

The adult patient who was illiterate before the stroke creates a particular problem in diagnosis. Through interviewing the patient or a relative, you should try to determine whether the patient had any reading and writing deficits before the stroke. If the patient could not read and write before the stroke, then there really is not much that can be done. You still might want to determine if the patient can recognize some simple words. Words on road signs or trade names (Coca Cola, etc.) are useful. In addition, you may wish to determine whether the patient can copy designs, letters, and words which you present. Porch (1971) indicates that literate patients usually will attempt the tasks of reading and writing even though they have lost these abilities. On the other hand, illiterate patients are aware that they cannot read or write and, therefore, quickly reject these tasks. For the rest of this section, we will assume the patient had reasonably adequate reading and writing skills before becoming aphasic.

In the examination of reading skills, clinicians are not interested in the quality of patients' oral responses, but rather in silent reading comprehension. Thus, reading aloud is typically not the best approach. The examiner should not read the material aloud to the patient, because then it becomes a listening, rather than a silent reading task.

For patients with severe disturbance, tasks more simple than reading can be used to examine visual recognition. Various identical matching tasks would be appropriate. Can the patient match a picture to an object? If shown a series of identical geometric shapes, letters, or single words, can he or she locate the same ones in another series?

In any reading task, you will want to make the letters quite large, ½ to ¾ inch high. Whether you use block letters or script will depend upon the patient's level of performance and preference. Reading materials should be presented at increasing stages of difficulty, not unlike what was described for listening tasks. Single-word stimuli might consist of showing the patient's name or identifying objects. Written sentence commands of increasing length can also be presented to the patient. A short paragraph with printed questions is a good way to examine complex reading skills. Some patients may have difficulty when there are several lines of material. In these cases, you may want to isolate each line with some blank paper.

Some patients do markedly better on reading than on listening tasks. The visual stimulus is permanent and can be repeatedly scanned or reviewed by the patient. The auditory stimulus is transitory and fleeting, and cannot be repeatedly scanned or reviewed.

Examination of Writing

Many, if not most, aphasic patients will have some degree of paralysis of one hand and arm, usually the preferred hand. When examining writing, you will want to determine whether the patient is able to use the preferred hand for writing or whether you need to encourage the patient to use the non-preferred hand. In either case, there is awkward motor control which needs to be taken into account. A basic reason for examining writing is to determine the level at which the patient is functioning in graphic language processing.

Here are some ways to assist the patient in writing. A large-diameter (elementary school) wooden pencil or a felt-tip pen can be used to assist the patient to attain better grasp. Some support for the arm may also be helpful. You should, at a minimum, provide the patient with a writing tablet which has a stiff backing. Many patients will be writing left-handed; therefore, position the paper at a convenient angle so that it lines up with the left, not the right arm.

In examining the writing abilities of severely impaired patients, you will need to start at a very simple level. For instance, have the patient copy a design, such as a circle or a square. Sometimes patients who cannot copy these simple designs can trace over them. Keenan (1975) has suggested that patients sometimes are helped when you tell them what to do while you guide their hand.

As in the examination of listening, talking, and reading, writing tasks are presented at progressively more difficult levels. If the patient can do some paragraph writing, there are a variety of things that can be tried. Provide a situational picture and have the patient write about what is happening in the picture. A more difficult task would have the patient explain in writing how to fix a flat tire on a car, or to explain the differences between a magazine and a newspaper, or a watch and a clock. After patients have written something, it is important to determine whether they can then look at what was written and identify errors. Some patients may be able to correct errors if the examiner simply indicates where one exists. These are useful observations to make in determining the patient's writing abilities.

Integration of Clinical Findings

Let us review what we have covered. We began by describing the four levels of oral communication: ideation, symbolization, translation, and execution. It was suggested that impairment due to neurological damage can exist at any one of these levels. The effects would be mental-verbal dysfunction, aphasia, apraxia of speech, and dysarthria, corresponding, respectively, to each of these four levels. One purpose of diagnosis is to determine whether the patient has any or all of the four types of neurogenically based communication problems, realizing that the patient may well have multiple speech-language disorders. Thus, a primary outcome of the examination process is a differential diagnosis. Here, our concern is to determine the disorder: aphasia, dysarthria, apraxia of speech, mental-verbal dysfunction. In addition, another principle goal is to specify the severity of disturbance(s). Specification of type(s) of communication disturbance can actually contribute to neurological diagnosis.

In this chapter we have dealt with mental-verbal dysfunction and aphasia. The first of these (mental-verbal dysfunction) is a breakdown of cognitive functions and can be recognized in the language of confusion and dementia. As we have learned, these patients are usually managed through programs of social interaction and reality orientation. Aphasia was defined as an impairment of symbolic formulation, comprehension, and expression due to specific brain damage, usually in the left hemisphere. A number of linguistic impairments might be observed in an aphasic patient. We have learned that patients with aphasia can be grouped into categories, in part, on the basis of certain speech and language characteristics. The verbal parameters of fluency, auditory comprehension, and ability to repeat have been found to be most useful in classifying patients into categories (for example, Broca's, Wernicke's, etc.). Classification information is extremely useful in formulating therapy plans, another important facet of diagnosis. The general approach to therapy for aphasic patients is to provide specific program(s) of language stimulation to facilitate language performance. Classification enables the clinician to develop profiles or descriptions of a patient's relative language strengths and liabilities. Therapy must take into account those profiles and descriptions. Clinicians develop therapy programs to strengthen areas of liability and/or to enhance areas of relative strength.

Finally, we consider prognosis. Darley (1982) has provided a thorough review of published research on prognostic variables which influence recovery of language functions among aphasic patients. His conclusions are that "initial severity of the aphasia (more severe deficits eventuating in less complete recovery), the etiology of the aphasia and the extent and site(s) of the lesion are the most important determinants of outcome" (p. 140). In terms of etiology, Darley noted that patients with aphasias resulting from direct head injuries (trauma) tend to have a better prognosis for improvement than patients with aphasia resulting from stroke. As one would expect, the greater the extent of damaged brain tissue, the poorer the prognosis. In terms of site of lesion, Darley (1982) suggested that recovery is poorest when the pathology encroaches upon the cortical region surrounding the Sylvian fissure of the dominant hemisphere. Patients with aphasia occurring from sites more distant from the Sylvian fissure show faster and more complete recovery. Darley goes on to conclude that poor general health, presence of additional sensory and motor deficits, advanced age, low intelligence, and emotional problems all may have negative influences on recovery. These latter factors are not as important as initial severity, etiology, and extent and site of lesion.

Study Guide

1. Briefly define and differentiate among aphasia, apraxia of speech and dysarthria.

2. In order to talk, the speaker goes through a sequential series of steps. There are four distinct steps, or levels, of activity. What are they?

3. Define and differentiate between speech and language.

4. Describe some major clinical features confused patients exhibit.

5. a. Describe some major features of communication demented patients exhibit.
   b. What assessment procedures can be used with the patient suspected of having intellectual deterioration?

6. Identify and describe the major forms of linguistic impairment observed among aphasic patients.

7. Why would a speech-language pathologist want to classify aphasia into various groups?

8. What type of aphasic patient is being described in each of the following?
   a. Patient A has difficulty understanding what people say. Perhaps because of that, A has trouble repeating a sentence when it is spoken to him. Nevertheless, A's speech tends to be quite fluent.
   b. The speech of patient B is very disruptive and nonfluent; yet B comprehends spoken language rather well. If someone says a sentence or two, and asks B to say it back, however, B has a difficult time doing that.
   c. Patient C's speech has good prosodic features with adequate rate and fluency and no real difficulty in understanding spoken language. The interesting thing is that she is unable to repeat much of anything that she hears when instructed to do so.
   d. Patient D has severe impairment in all language functions, that is, all output and input modalities.
   e. Patient E has nonfluent speech, but can comprehend spoken language and can repeat things after the examiner.
   f. Patient F speaks fluently but occasionally has a few pauses in speech as he searches for an elusive word. Furthermore, comprehension, repetition, reading, and writing are relatively intact.
   g. Patient G has paraphasic, fluent speech; impaired comprehension and naming; impaired reading; but she can repeat things said to her.

9. Assume you are testing an aphasic patient for auditory verbal comprehension abilities. When you have three simple, familiar objects on the table (e.g., cup, pencil, and book), and you say slowly, "Show me the cup," the patient gets essentially 100% of the commands correct. On the other hand, if you read a short paragraph from the newspaper aloud to the patient, and then ask some yes-no questions about what you read, the answers are no better than chance. Based upon these observations, what can you say about the patient's auditory verbal comprehension abilities? What explanation can you give for the discrepancy in performance between these two tasks?

10. In testing a patient, how might you distinguish between intellectual deterioration (dementia) and aphasia? That is, what kinds of test responses might you observe that would be different with a patient having intellectual deterioration as contrasted to an aphasic patient? Conversely, what kinds of test responses might be the same for both types of patients?

11. Succinctly define each of the following terms or concepts:

anomia	syntax
association fibers	encode
decode	reality orientation
primary auditory cortex	jargon
circumlocution	paraphasia (literal and verbal)
Wernicke's area	Broca's area
confabulation	confrontation naming
latency of response	disorientation
agrammatism	paragrammatism
perseveration	diffuse brain damage
focal brain damage	echolalia

REFERENCES

Benson, D. F. 1979. Aphasia, Alexia, and Agraphia. Churchill Livingstone, New York.

Bloom, L., and Lahey, M. 1978. Language Development and Language Disorders. John Wiley and Sons, New York.

Brookshire, R. H. 1978. An Introduction to Aphasia 2nd Ed. BRK Publishers, Minneapolis, MN.

Brown, J. W. 1972. Aphasia, Apraxia and Agnosia. Charles C Thomas, Publishers, Springfield, IL.

Canter, G. J. 1979. Syndromes of Aphasia in Relation to Cerebral Connectionism. Short course presented to the Indiana Speech and Hearing Association, South Bend, IN.

Darley, F. L. 1982. Aphasia. W. B. Saunders Co., Philadelphia.

Darley, F. L., Aronson, A. E., and Brown, J. R. 1975. Motor Speech Disorders. W. B. Saunders Co., Philadelphia.

Eisenson, J. 1954. Examining For Aphasia (Revised) The Psychological Corp., New York.

Eisenson, J. 1973. Adult Aphasia: Assessment and Treatment. Appleton-Century-Crofts, New York.

Espir, M. L. E. and Rose, F. C. 1970. The Basic Neurology of Speech. Davis, Philadelphia.

Folsom, J. C. 1968. Reality orientation for the elderly mental patient. J. Geriatric Psych. 1:291–300.

Geschwind, N. 1970. The organization of language and the brain. Science 170:940–944.

Geschwind, N., Quadfasel, F. A., and Segarra, J. M. 1968. Isolation of the speech area. Neuropsychologia 327–340.

Goodglass, H., and Kaplan, E. F. 1972. The Assessment of Aphasia and Related Disorders. Lea & Febiger, Philadelphia.

Halpern, H. 1972. Adult Aphasia. The Bobbs-Merrill Co., Indianapolis.

Halpern, H., Darley, F. L. and Brown, J. R. 1973. Differential language and neurological characteristics in cerebral involvement. J. Speech Hear. Disord. 38:162–173.

Holland, A. L. 1980. Communicative Abilities in Daily Living. University Park Press, Baltimore.

Horenstein, S. 1971. Amnestic, agnostic, apractic, and aphasic features in dementing illness. In: C. E. Wells (ed.), Dementia, Contemporary Neurology Service No. 9. Davis, Philadelphia.

Hutchinson, J. M., and Beasley, D. S. 1976. Speech and language functioning among the aging. In: H. J. Oyer and E. J. Oyer (eds.), Aging and Communication. University Park Press, Baltimore.

Jackson, H. 1978. On affections of speech from disease of the brain. Brain 1:304–330.

Keenan, J. S. 1975. A Procedure Manual In Speech Pathology With Brain-Damaged Adults. The Interstate Printers and Publishers, Danville, IL.

Keenan, J. S. and Brassell, E. G. 1975. Aphasia Language Performance Scales. Pinnacle Press, Murfreesboro, TN.

Perkins, W. H. 1977. Speech Pathology: An Applied Behavioral Science 2nd Ed. The C. V. Mosby Co., St. Louis, MO.

Phillips, D. F. 1973. Reality orientation. J. Am. Hospital Assoc. 47:191–200.

Porch, B. E. 1971. Porch Index of Communicative Ability (Revised) Consulting Psychologists Press, Palo Alto, CA.

Porch, B. E. 1981. Porch Index of Communicative Ability 3rd Ed. Consulting Psychologists Press, Palo Alto, CA.

Schow, R. L., Christensen, J. M., Hutchinson, J. M., and Nerbonne, M. A. 1978. Communication Disorders of the Aged: A Guide for Health Professionals. University Park Press, Baltimore.

Schuell, H. 1965. Minnesota Test for Differential Diagnosis of Aphasia. University of Minnesota Press, Minneapolis, MN.

Sies, L. F. (ed.). 1974. Aphasia Theory and Therapy: Selected Lectures and Papers of Hildred Schuell. University Park Press, Baltimore.

Sklar, M. 1973. Sklar Aphasia Scale (Revised). Western Psychological Services, Los Angeles.

United States Public Health Service. 1966. Verbal Impairment Associated with Brain Damage. Film produced for Institute of Physical Medicine and Rehabilitation, New York University Medical Center, New York.

Wells, B. B. 1969. The long-term implications of reality orientation. In: The Hospital and Community Psychiatric Service, Reality Orientation. American Psychiatric Association, Washington, DC.

Wertz, R. T. 1978. Neuropathologies of speech and language: An introduction to patient management. In: D. F. Johns (ed.), Clinical Management of Neurogenic Communicative Disorders. Little Brown and Co., Boston.

Whitaker, H. A. 1976. Disorders of speech production mechanisms. In: E. C. Carterette, and M. P. Friedman (eds.), Handbook of Perception, Volume VII, Language and Speech. Academic Press, Inc., New York.

8

Diagnosis of Speech and Language Disorders Associated with Acquired Neuropathologies: Apraxia of Speech and the Dysarthrias

J. Douglas Noll

Outline

Educational Aims

1. *To define the acquired motor disorders of speech: apraxia of speech and the dysarthrias;*
2. *To describe the process of speech-language diagnosis used for patients with acquired motor speech disorders.*

In this chapter we are concerned with the acquired motor disorders of speech, that is, apraxia of speech and the dysarthrias. In both of these disorders, basic language processes are relatively intact; but because of nervous system damage, the mechanical production of speech is impaired. *Apraxia of speech* is a disruption of the capacity to program the skilled oral movements necessary for speech. *Dysarthria*, on the other hand, is an impairment of actual neuromuscular execution resulting from damage to the motor neural pathways. In dysarthria, precision of movements of the articulators is deficient because of defective neural innervation.

Chapters 7 and 8 should be read together, because they were prepared to complement one another. At a minimum, students using this chapter as part of coursework dealing with motor disorders of speech should read the section entitled "A Neurological Model of Oral Communication" in Chapter 7 before reading this chapter.

APRAXIA OF SPEECH

In terms of the neurological model of oral communication described in Chapter 7, apraxia of speech represents an impairment of Level III activity (translation). The patient with apraxia of speech has difficulty voluntarily programming articulatory positions and movements needed to produce the desired speech sounds. These patients do not have inherent muscle paralysis or weakness; there is no impairment of muscle innervation. Muscle function and muscle tone, per se, are intact. The problem is one of motor coordination associated with incorrect neural commands at higher, more central levels. It is as though the patient has forgotten or cannot recall the motor instructions needed to make the necessary articulatory movements to produce words. For some reason, motor programming difficulty is most apparent in attempts at voluntary, purposeful, connected speech. Automatic or emotional utterances may be error free, and many reflexive and vegetative movements of the articulators are accomplished easily, as in chewing, eating, licking food off the lips, and so on.

Speech Characteristics

A large number of studies have been completed to specify the speech symptoms noted in patients with apraxia of speech (Deal and Darley, 1972; DiSimoni and Darley, 1977; Johns and Darley, 1970; LaPointe, 1969; LaPointe and Johns, 1975; Shankweiler and Harris, 1966; Trost, 1970). We begin by listing the articulatory characteristics of this disorder. Much of this material comes from the work of Darley (1978), who along with Aronson and Brown of the Mayo Clinic, have made significant contributions to our understanding of apraxia of speech (see, for example, Darley et al., 1975).

1. Patients with apraxia of speech struggle to avoid errors or to correct articulatory positioning. This may result in equalization of syllabic stress patterns, slow rate of speech, and other prosodic alterations.

2. Sound substitution errors predominate, although additions, prolongations, and repetitions do occur. Phonemic distortions and omissions are less frequent.

3. Sound or syllable transpositions may be present. For example, for the word "bicycle" the patient with apraxia might say "tise, sicycle, licycle, sprykle, sprickle, . . . spicycle" (LaPointe, 1982, p. 384).

4. Occasionally, articulatory errors are complications rather than simplifications. For example, the error may be physiologically more difficult than the intended sound, such as a consonant cluster being substituted for a singleton.

5. Inconsistent off-target approximations, variability in type of articulatory errors, and instances of error-free fluent speech on some words, phrases, or even whole sentences are noted. LaPointe (1982) offered the example of a patient who said the following while attempting to say "refrigerator": "Refrig . . . ridgerator, ridgefrigerator, frigerator, frefridgerator, refrigerator, regrigerator, ridgerator."

6. Anticipatory errors may be present. The patient with apraxia of speech may anticipate a speech sound which will occur later in the word or sentence, for example, "glean glass" for "green glass" (Dabul and Bollier, 1976).

7. Difficulty in initiating speech may be present. This difficulty can be noted by the presence of hesitations and nonfluencies, visible searching, or groping movements of the articulators prior to or during speech attempts. Numerous trials and false starts are common. For example, when asked "Where do you live?" one patient responded, "(pause) Coneve . . . Goneve . . . Jah . . . Jake (silent visible tongue movements) . . . L . . . Lakel . . . LLLake Geneva . . . *whew*" (LaPointe, 1982, p. 384).

8. Speech perception/comprehension and word recognition abilities are often disproportionately better than speech production abilities.

9. Patients recognize their articulatory errors. This recognition often causes numerous retrials or attempts to correct word productions.

10. Number of errors and articulatory struggle increases as a function of word length.

11. More errors occur on consonants and on those sounds which require more precise articulatory adjustments, for example, fricatives and affricates.

12. Greater articulatory difficulty is noted during volitional or purposeful speech than during the production of automatic, reactive, emotional, or nonpropositional speech.

Consider the following speech sample from a patient at Mayo Clinic diagnosed as having apraxia of speech (Darley et al., 1975). The portions within the brackets are phonetic transcriptions of this patient's speech attempts, whereas the words within the parentheses are the target words. The patient is describing a picture of a farm scene with a tornado visible in the distance, moving toward the farm. The people in the picture are obviously quite frightened as they anticipate the arrival of the tornado.

> I am looking on a ['drɔrɪŋ] (drawing) of a [pɛk-] (false start) picture of what is apparently a [tɔrnetijəd] (tornado) [blu-] (false start) brewing in the [kʌ-] (false start) country-side. This is having [ənənə'midiət] (an immediate) and frightening [ə'fɛkʰ] (effect) on a farm ['fæmərli] (family) numbering six humans and [ə' sɔšt'sɔrtəd] (assorted) farm animals. There (they) are ['kwɪkəli] (quickly) going into a [šɔrm] (storm) cellar with fright in their [ar-] (false start) eyes and their every movement.

The patient was then asked to repeat the word "tornado." He made a number of attempts to produce this word.

> "[tɔːr'netəjo] Excuse me. [tɔr'neti — tɔr'nedi] I mean [tɔr'nɔjt'tʰo] I don't know: I seem to be getting further from it, but what really mean to say that it's a [tɔr'nɔjt'tʰɔj — tɔr'net'tʰɔːr — tɔr'nedo — tɔr'netejo] It was a [tɔr'nɒd͵tɒj — tɔr'nəto]."

The transcription does not adequately reflect the hesitant, disruptive character of the patient's speech output. Nevertheless, several things are noteworthy. First, he seems to have intact language competence, reflected in auditory verbal comprehension, vocabulary usage, and grammatical skills. Articulatory errors are evident. There are many sound substitutions, omissions, and distortions. The patient certainly was aware of his problems, tried to correct them, but usually was not very successful. Thus, this patient demonstrates several of the characteristics of apraxia of speech enumerated earlier.

Several terms other than apraxia of speech are used to refer to the type of distinctive articulatory impairment from cerebral damage we have been describing. These include aphemia, speechlessness, pseudo-dysarthria, subcortical motor aphasia, peripheral motor aphasia, phonetic disintegration, articulatory dyspraxia, poor verbal agility, phonemic-articulatory disorder, anarthria, and cortical dysarthria (cited in Johns and Darley, 1970; Trost, 1970). One reason there are so many different terms is that there is much disagreement about the basic nature of the disorder. Some believe apraxia is not a distinct entity. They believe apraxia should be included as part of other existing diagnostic categories. For example, in Chapter 7 we described the speech output of patients with Broca's aphasia. These patients are often relatively nonfluent, exhibit effortful and awkward articulation, produce short utterances, and may transpose some sounds. This description of Broca's aphasia seems very much like apraxia of speech. The controversy is

Controversial Views

not simply a semantic one. The disagreement is more fundamental. Those who use the term apraxia of speech generally believe the problem is a unique motor programming disorder. Those who refer to such patients as having Broca's aphasia, motor aphasia, and so on, would characterize the problem as language based, because, as we have seen in Chapter 7, the term aphasia implies a language or linguistic impairment.

In an article entitled, "Some Objections to the Term Apraxia of Speech," Martin (1974) questions the appropriateness of the term apraxia from both the descriptive and classification points of view. Martin states that apraxia of speech reflects early views of language as a simplistic receptive/expressive dichotomy. According to Martin, the existence of the disorder depends on the ability to separate phonological processes from other processes involved in higher language functions. Martin claims that if apraxia of speech is a pure articulatory motor programming problem, the grammatical class of words should cause no change in articulatory abilities. Grammatical class, being a higher language function, should have no significant influence on speech performance if the two processes are separable. Yet semantic components such as grammatical class do, indeed, cause articulatory accuracy of patients to change. Increased errors are found in the production of nouns, verbs, adjectives, and adverbs (Deal and Darley, 1972). When the patient is asked to repeat meaningful versus nonsense stimuli, articulatory accuracy increased with the meaningful stimuli. Hardison et al. (1977) found that the linguistic variables of noun phrase position and level of word abstraction influenced the ability to program movements for speech production. Chapey (1981) pointed out that the context of the utterance and the nature of the task being performed influenced the speech output of such patients. That is, fewer errors are produced during unstructured spontaneous language than in word repetition or imitation tasks. Increased effort tends to aggravate the problem so that difficulty is encountered when the individual attempts to produce specific responses on request.

All of these observations would imply to Martin (1974) that the phonological problems which these patients exhibit are not a result of a discrete motor impairment. Rather, they seem to reflect a disruption of the language system and should, therefore, more appropriately be included under the label of aphasia. He proposes the diagnostic term, aphasic phonological impairment.

There is yet another possible interpretation. We noted in Chapter 7 that the various processes involved in oral communication are not completely independent. Intellectualization, symbolization, translation, and execution have complex interactions; they influence and are influenced by each other. Thus, it is not surprising that motor programming is influenced by certain higher level language variables. One would expect it to be this way even though the programming of the movements of the articulators can, in part, be considered from a motor control perspective, per se. Phonological behavior may well be influenced by higher level linguistic processes, but it does not necessarily follow that phonology is an intrinsic part of, or is brought about by these linguistic processes.

The evidence suggests to this writer that there is a separate process in oral communication which programs the neural events necessary for motor movement sequences of the articulators during speech. When this process is disordered, a predictable result occurs: apraxia of speech. For this reason, the concept of apraxia of speech is used here as a useful diagnostic entity.

Although there is some disagreement, it is generally thought that apraxia of speech results from damage to the inferior frontal convolution of the dominant hemisphere. You recall from our earlier discussion (see Chapter 7) that this is the region of Broca's area, which is probably involved in the motor programming of movements of the articulators for speech. As La-Pointe (1982) suggests, however, the same brain lesion which disturbs motor programming for speech movements can also impinge upon areas which influence language skills. Frequently, the disorders of aphasia and apraxia of speech do coexist (Wertz et al., 1970). The speech-language pathologist must sort out the nature of the patient's communication problem and determine which aspect contributes most to the disorder.

Diagnosis

The primary diagnostic methods available to the speech-language clinician are listening to the patient's speech and observing oral motor movements. Speech-language pathologists will want to present a series of speech tasks to the patient and determine whether articulatory characteristics of apraxia of speech are present. Impairment of skilled motor movements by patients with apraxia of speech may also be noted during attempts to produce non-speech activities as well. The patient might do well in performing involuntary, reflexive oral movements, although these same movements may be quite defective when the patient consciously tries to do them on command. Some types of oral movements that may be examined (Darley, 1978; De Renzi et al., 1966), are listed:

Stick out your tongue
Puff or blow
Show me your teeth
Pucker up your lips
Try to touch your nose with the tip of your tongue
Bite your lower lip
Whistle
Lick your lips
Clear your throat
Move your tongue in and out of your mouth
Click your teeth together once
Smile
Click your tongue as if imitating the sound of a galloping horse

Chatter your teeth, as if you are cold
Try to touch your chin with the tip of your tongue
Cough
Puff out your cheeks
Wiggle your tongue from side to side
Show how you would kiss someone
Alternately pucker and smile
Yawn
Give a "Bronx cheer" or "raspberry"

Initially, the clinician should use single instruction when asking the patient to perform each task. If the patient is unsuccessful, the clinician should demonstrate these tasks and observe the patient's performance on imitation.

It is not sufficient to determine whether each task was done correctly or not. A careful examination should be made of the qualitative nature of the patient's movement patterns. To examine the qualitative nature of movement patterns the clinician should consider the presence of:

accurate movement patterns preceded by trial and error
searching movements of the tongue or lips
accurate movement preceded by pauses
crude, awkward, erratic, or extraneous oro-facial movements
overall gesture patterns which are grossly acceptable, but defective in terms
    of amplitude, accuracy, or speed
perseverated movement

As we have indicated, diagnosis of patients with apraxia of speech is accomplished largely on the basis of informal evaluation. Currently, there is one commercially available test for apraxia of speech. This is the Apraxia Battery for Adults (ABA) by Barbara Dabul (1979). In this battery, several subtests are used to identify the presence of apraxia of speech and to obtain severity estimates. One of the subtests deals with nonspeech oral motor movements. Tasks similar to those discussed earlier are used. The clinician notes whether the movements are made accurately, promptly, and completely, or whether the movements are ambiguous, crude and defective. In another subtest of the ABA the patient is instructed to produce two sets of disyllables (/p ʌ t ʌ/ and /t ʌ k ʌ/) as rapidly as possible for three seconds, and one trisyllable (/p ʌ t ʌ k ʌ/) for five seconds. Dabul (1979) reported that moderately involved patients with apraxia of speech were only able to produce one or two trisyllables in each 5-second trial, whereas those with severe involvement could not produce a single trisyllable in a given 5-second trial. Langenhorst (1981) found that 11 of 25 subjects with apraxia of speech could not produce a single combination of /p ʌ t ʌ k ʌ/, whereas no normal subject produced less than eight trisyllables per trial.

An examination technique frequently used with patients having apraxia of speech is the production of words of progressively increasing length (e.g., thick-thicker-thickening, hope-hopeful-hopefully). Aten et al. (1971), Dabul (1979), Deal and Darley (1972), Johns and Darley (1970), and Langenhorst (1981) have shown that the articulatory performance of patients with apraxia of speech tends to deteriorate as the length of words increases.

Another subtest of this battery requires patients to say several poly-syllabic words three times, for example, butterfly-butterfly-butterfly. The rationale for inclusion of this type of task is that some patients with apraxia of speech may reduce the number of articulatory errors during repeated utterances of a particular word (Johns and Darley, 1970). On the other hand, Dabul (1979) found that patients with apraxia of speech were highly incon-sistent. In some patients performance improved, whereas for others, per-formance deteriorated as a function of repetition. Langenhorst (1981) noted that mildly involved patients improved from the first to the third production. She stated that these patients seem "... to take advantage of errors on early trials." The performance of more severely involved patients deterio-rated. Finally, the ABA includes an action picture designed to elicit spon-taneous speech.

Thus, one purpose of diagnosis is to identify the cluster of speech and nonspeech characteristics generally associated with apraxia of speech. If a patient exhibits these characteristics, the clinician can be reasonably certain that apraxia of speech is present. Another primary reason for arriving at a diagnosis is to give some direction to what might be done in therapy. If the patient has apraxia of speech, treatment would emphasize motor commands, movement sequencing of the articulators, voluntary neuromotor control, and so on.

THE DYSARTHRIAS

Now we consider the other major form of impaired motor control of speech, namely, the dysarthrias. Darley et al. (1975) provide a complete definition of dysarthria, which slightly modified, reads as follows:

> Dysarthria refers to a collection of speech disorders resulting from defects in the mechanical or muscular control of the vocal structures used in speaking. There may be abnormalities of muscular strength, range, speed, tone, or ac-curacy. Dysarthria arises from damage to those neuromotor pathways of the central or peripheral nervous system which directly or indirectly innervate the larynx, soft palate, tongue, etc. Any or all of the basic processes involved in speech production may be impaired: respiration, phonation, resonance, artic-ulation, and prosody.

This is a fairly involved definition. Let us consider some of the major points. First, dysarthria is an organic disorder of speech caused by some damage to specific motor pathways of the nervous system. The pathways are those which control movements of the structures involved in speech production. In other words, dysarthria is a collection of speech disorders represented by breakdown of motor execution noted in speech production, not a higher-level language or cognitive impairment. The effects of the motor deficits are reflected in a variety of neuromuscular symptoms and depend upon which pathways are damaged and on the severity of the pathology. For example, there may be weakness or reduced range of movement. Muscle tone may be exaggerated (hypertonicity), or tone may be diminished (hypotonicity). Motor control may be impaired in terms of accuracy or precision of movement. Any of these forms of impairment may cause problems in the speed and timing of neuromuscular movements. The speech-language pathologist will want to carefully examine patients' motor control of the speech articulators to detect whether these forms of neuromotor impairment or symptoms are present.

The term dysarthria and articulation both include the root *art*. Dysarthric patients may have problems which go beyond articulation. As the definition suggests, and as we will discuss later, breath support, voice quality, rate of speaking, and prosodic features may also be disturbed in quite predictable ways. This is why the definition begins by emphasizing that dysarthria is "a collection of speech disorders."

As we said, dysarthrias result from some type of damage to the nervous system. The specific etiology of dysarthrias varies from patient to patient. A stroke can cause dysarthria. Also, several different diseases often have dysarthria as one of their chief symptoms, (for example, Parkinson's disease, multiple sclerosis, etc.). Children with cerebral palsy are usually dysarthric because cerebral palsy occurs from congenital damage to the motor pathways of the brain.

Thus, we can see that abnormalities of motor control for speech can be a part of several diverse neurological problems. It has been shown that different diseases may involve different regions of the nervous system. For example, myasthenia gravis is a disease in which there is a defect in the conduction of impulses at the juncture between the nerve fiber and the muscle. Another condition, called Bell's Palsy, results from damage to specific cranial nerves. There are several other serious disorders that result from degenerative changes within parts of deep, internal aspects of the brain, such as, multiple sclerosis, Parkinson's disease, and amyotrophic lateral sclerosis ("Lou Gehrig disease"). We will not describe these disorders. Those interested in learning more about them can read clinical neurology texts (e.g., Chusid, 1979). Patients with these conditions or diseases can have some degree of dysarthria, because the motor nerve pathways which innervate structures that subserve speech production are impaired. Different neurological diseases will have different effects upon speech. For example, a patient with myasthenia gravis will have a different kind of dysarthria than a patient with Parkinson's disease for the simple reason that different parts of the nervous system are affected by these two distinct diseases.

We will now consider general strategies clinicians use to examine dysarthric patients, adults or children. Many of the suggestions offered come from the reading by LaPointe (1982).

Medical Examination

The speech pathologist will want to obtain a report of the medical examination. In this report, the physician will probably explain the nature of the disorder, the symptoms of motor dysfunction, the neurological history, and the results of specific medical tests. There may be some indication as to what part of the motor system is involved, and a statement about the patient's prognosis for improvement of motor function. The patient may be under an active program of medical care, and this should be described as well.

Examination of the Speech Mechanism

The clinician will want to complete a careful examination of the speech mechanism (see Chapter 2 for details). The physician might have made observations about the adequacy of the speech mechanism as part of the medical examination, but speech-language pathologists should also make their own observations. Our definition of dysarthria emphasized that patients with dysarthria may have abnormalities of muscle strength, range, speed, tone, and/or accuracy. How does one determine whether these neuromotor problems are present and estimate their severity?

Clinicians can obtain much information about the neuromotor system by examining oral-facial posture and nonspeech movements. These postures and movements can be examined in terms of the strength, range, speed, tone, and accuracy attributes. *Tone* refers to the degree of background muscle tension. Some neurological diseases result in increased muscle tone, referred to as *hypertonicity* or *spasticity*; whereas, some other diseases result in just the opposite—decreased tone, referred to as *hypotonicity* or *flaccidity*. Usually, the physician's report will indicate whether there is impaired muscle tone and if it is hyper- or hypotonic. Some inference can be made about the state of muscle tone by watching patients faces while they are at rest and during various voluntary movements. Adjectives used to describe what clinicians generally note in association with hypotonicity are: flabby, lax, limp, droopy, saggy, and so on. On the other hand, adjectives used to describe hypertonicity are: tense, tight, rigid, taut, and so on.

Another characteristic mentioned in the definition is strength. *Reduced strength* or muscle weakness is a frequent symptom of neurological disease. Bach-y-Rita, et al. (1981) have described fourteen different procedures to use when there is suspected weakness of the facial musculature:

Raise eyebrows and wrinkle forehead
Frown and draw eyebrows downward
Close eyes tightly and wink with one and then the other eye
Open eyes widely
Sniff strongly
Curl upper lip and raise and protrude upper lip
Curl lower lip down (pout)
Pucker lips and attempt to whistle
Blow air into cheeks, attempting to keep mouth closed
Compress lips
Smile without showing teeth
Smile showing teeth
Wrinkle nose
Draw angle of mouth upward so as to deepen furrow from side of nose to
    side of mouth

How well can the patient move the lips and tongue against resistance? To test the strength of the lip musculature, a button can be tied to a length of string. The patient can attempt to hold the button behind closed lips while the patient or the clinician pulls on the string. The presence of tongue weakness can be detected by instructing patients to place the tongue-tip against the inside of the cheek, while the examiner pushes on the outside of the cheek with a finger. The patient should try to resist by pressing the inside of the cheek with the tongue. Strength of tongue protrusion and lateralization may be determined by resisting the tongue movements with a wooden tongue blade.

As mentioned in our definition of dysarthria, range of movement may be affected. *Range of movement* refers to the ability to move a part of the body from one extreme to the other, first in one direction and then in the opposite direction. Several dysarthric conditions cause a restricted (reduced) range of lip and tongue movement. These types of restrictions can be evaluated by asking the patient to lateralize the tongue as far as possible from one side to the other, and to elevate and depress the tongue outside the mouth. How well does the patient move the lips from a drawn-back smile to a rounded pursing posture (for example, back from an exaggerated /i/ to an /u/ position)? Patients with limited range of lip and tongue movements tend to speak with a monotonous pattern and often speak at a slow rate. Their speech may be somewhat reduced in intelligibility because of articulatory slurring and speech sound distortions.

Speed of motor movements is another important variable to examine. A relatively simple way to assess this function is to instruct patients to move their lips or tongue as rapidly as possible. A useful way to examine rate of movement is to instruct the patient to take a deep breath and repeat the syllables /p ʌ/, /t ʌ/ and/or /k ʌ/ as rapidly as possible. This form of examination is called diadochokinetic testing. Darley et al. (1975) have suggested that clinicians do not need to obtain an accurate count of the number of times patients repeat each syllable, provided that they have an approximate knowledge of normal diadochokinetic responses. Patients who can not produce more than three or four repetitions in a 5-second interval clearly exhibit reduced rate of muscular movement. On the other hand, patients with Parkinson's disease may have accelerating and excessively rapid movements. The movements of these patients may become so rapid that during speech individual sounds and syllables become undifferentiated.

It is important to note whether there is independent movement among or between articulators. For example, in some patients movements of the lower jaw parallel movements of the lips or tongue during repetitions of /p ʌ/, /t ʌ/, and /k ʌ/. The jaw, lips, and tongue move as a single unit. One method to examine independent movement is to stabilize the jaw by placing a bite block or wooden pencil between the back teeth and to ask the patient to bite down on the stabilizer. The patient should then repeat /p ʌ/, /t ʌ/, and /k ʌ/. Does stabilizing the jaw improve rate of movement or lead to further rate reduction?

The last neuromotor abnormality mentioned in our definition of dysarthria is *accuracy*. This refers to the precision of motor movements. As the patient is tested for rate and range of movement, observations can also be made to determine whether the movements of the tongue and lips are made in a precise manner. There are some simple nonspeech tasks to try. With the mouth slightly open, ask the patient to move the tongue-tip very carefully around the upper and lower red margin of the lips without going off. This requires fine control of tongue-tip movement. Can patients track the movement any better when they view themselves in a mirror? Another technique involves stimulation. Here, patients are instructed to close their eyes and open the mouth. Using a sharp instrument, the lips and the mouth are stimulated. The patient is instructed to put the tongue tip on the spot(s) which were stimulated. We have found this technique to be a simple, yet effective method clinicians can use to identify errors in direction or placement of tongue movements.

Examination of Speech Processes

We have indicated that the dysarthric patient may exhibit impaired respiration, phonation, articulation, resonance, and prosody. We now consider how each of these processes can be examined as patients complete a variety of speech tasks.

Respiration-Phonation

The respiratory mechanism provides the basic driving force for speech production. LaPointe (1982) has pointed out that when respiratory adequacy for speech is impaired, patients with dysarthria may exhibit reduced loudness and may produce fewer syllables per breath group, resulting in short phrases. Phonation refers to the process of producing sound at the level of the larynx or vocal folds. As we learned in Chapter 5, phonation and respiration are intimately related. Review the material dealing with voice assessment offered in Chapter 5, because the principles of examination explained in that chapter are applicable to individuals with neurological problems.

A number of perceptual judgments relating to vocal adequacy can be made simply by asking the patient to prolong the vowel /ɑ/ as long and as steadily as possible. First, judgments about maximum phonation duration can be made. Abnormally short vowel prolongation is often caused by excessive air wastage as a product of inefficient laryngeal valving and rapid depletion of the lung volume (Darley et al., 1975). Second, judgments can be made about voice quality. Dysarthric patients with neuromuscular problems characterized by weakness and hypotonia tend to have breathy voices which result from incomplete approximation (adduction) of the vocal folds. Also, if these patients are asked to produce a voluntary cough, they may not be able to produce a cough characterized by a sharp, abrupt onset. Rather, they often produce what is termed a "weak cough" (see Appendix B, Chapter 5). During vowel prolongation, dysarthric patients with spasticity (hypertonicity), may exhibit voice qualities characterized by harsh, strained, and effortful attributes. Third, judgments can be made about laryngeal control. For example, clinicians can evaluate the constancy of vocal production during the sustained production of vowels and discourse. Are pitch and loudness held constant, or are there variations in pitch and loudness? Is voice tremor present? Intermittent arrests or voice breaks and periodic waxing and waning of vocal loudness are frequently noted in dysarthric patients (Darley et al., 1975).

Articulation

An essential part of diagnosis is an examination of the precision of speech sound production. Sound production should be tested in single words, short sentences, and connected discourse, because the patient's skill may vary as a function of task complexity. Emphasis in this chapter is with the adult patient, therefore written word lists and sentence forms of various articulation tests (e.g., Templin-Darley Tests of Articulation, 1960) can be used.

Sound substitutions are not common among dysarthric speakers. However, distortion and omission errors occur quite frequently. There may be a pattern in which sounds and syllables at the end of words are omitted. Some patients may omit some of the elements of consonant clusters. For example, instead of "spray," they might say "spay" or even "say." Speech sound distortions generally result from imprecision due to weakened or light articulatory contacts (LaPointe, 1982). Patients may "undershoot" target gestures. These problems may be most evident during the production of stops, fricatives, and affricates, in which there is a need to obstruct or form narrow constrictions. Some of the vowels may tend to be neutralized, that is, may resemble a central, nondescript /ʌ/ or /ə/. Here, the vowels lose their distinct phonetic character.

Perceptual testing of speech sound production should be undertaken to determine whether breakdown is constant or whether it varies. If variation is present, is there some pattern to the dispersion? Do errors occur on certain sounds but not on others? Are the errors most noticeable for certain places of articulation (bilabial, lingualveolar, linguapalatal, etc.)? If they are, such observations might suggest a specific locus of neuromuscular problem. Clinicians must also determine whether muscle fatigue influences the patient's articulatory abilities. This aspect of speech performance can be evaluated by instructing the patient to repetitively read a paragraph aloud or to count aloud vigorously for several minutes. Significant progressive deterioration of function with muscle use is common in patients with some neurological diseases. In these patients, recovery of muscle function is likely to occur after a period of rest.

Not only should the production of individual speech sounds be examined, but analysis of the patient's movements from one sound position to the next should also be completed. Are the tongue movements clumsy, awkward? Are they slow? Having patients produce both symmetrical consonant-vowel-consonant nonsense syllables (e.g., /sus, pip, kuk/) and asymmetrical syllables (e.g., /tus, pik, sup/) are useful for the examination of these abilities. Are movements easier when the initial and final consonants are the same? Is there a difference in motor skill depending on the vowel? Do movements become more abnormal as the stimuli are increased to two- and three-syllable utterances?

An estimation of the patient's speech intelligibility should be made. If the listener does not know the context, what percentage of the speech is understandable to the listener? If the clinician is very familiar with the patient's speech pattern, someone who does not know the speaker should be asked to make this judgment. The references by Tikofsky (1970) and Yorkston and Beukelman (1980) describe more systematic methods to determine the intelligibility of dysarthric speakers.

Resonance

Resonance is, in part, concerned with the oral-nasal balance in the person's voice. In normal speech the /m, n, ŋ/ sounds are produced with nasal coupling because the soft palate is away from the pharyngeal wall, allowing the nasal cavities to be coupled into the vocal tract. For all other English speech sounds, however, there is a closure or near complete closure of the velopharyngeal port, active movement of several muscles of the palate and pharynx, and no or minimal nasal coupling. If the motor pathways to the muscles of the soft palate and pharynx are impaired, function of the soft palate and pharynx will often be affected (Noll, 1982). In patients with severe forms of dysarthria, the soft palate may be completely paralyzed with virtually no movement at all. Lesser degrees of impairment may result in slow or sluggish movements of the soft palate. Movements of the soft palate may also be improperly timed, so that closing and opening of the velopharyngeal port occurs at inappropriate moments during speech.

When there is severe neuromotor involvement of the soft palate, the patient may be nasal and hypernasality is usually quite obvious. The listener can rather easily detect excessive nasal voice quality in these situations and this attribute of speech is probably very consistent. However, if the impairment is marginal or inconsistent, then the perceptual impressions about hypernasality may be less evident and considerably more difficult to make (see Chapter 2, "Evaluation of Velopharyngeal Function in Relation to Speech"). We are not always sure what we hear in the patient's speech. A technique some clinicians use is the cul-de-sac resonance test (LaPointe, 1982). In this test, the patient is asked to sustain a vowel sound or to repeatedly say some syllables which do not contain nasal consonants. The patient may also be requested to produce some short sentences that do not have nasal consonants. For example:

We see three geese at the beach.
His father likes apple sauce.
Where is the back door?

The examiner should alternately occlude and release the patient's nostrils while the person is speaking these sentences. If the speaker achieves velopharyngeal closure, speech would sound the same during both the pinched and nonpinched conditions. On the other hand, if there were significant opening in the velopharyngeal port, there may be a definite change in voice quality.

Sequencing between nasal and non-nasal consonant sounds requires rapid adjustments of the soft palate. Dysarthric patients may have difficulty timing palatal movements to produce such combinations (for example, Bambi, handy, hamburger, bumble bee, etc.).

Rate and Prosody   Speech rate can be measured in a variety of ways. One of the easiest is in terms of words per minute. Rate can be determined by simply asking the patient to read a passage aloud and timing the duration. The rate in words per minute is calculated by multiplying the number of words in the passage by 60 and dividing by the speaking time (in seconds). If a patient reads a 200-word passage in 2 minutes, speaking rate would be 100 words per minute ($200 \times 60 \div 120 = 100$). Most dysarthric patients demonstrate an abnormally slow speech rate because of sluggish movements of the articulators and increased pause time. However, some patients (such as those with Parkinson's disease) may speak at a faster than average rate or demonstrate instances of accelerated speech separated by pauses (Darley et al., 1975).

Rate of speech and articulatory proficiency may interact. Adult dysarthric patients will frequently try to speak at a rate which approximates that used before the illness. Because the articulators may not now be capable of being moved at the same speed, the result may be that articulatory gestures become incomplete and speech intelligibility is reduced. In some cases, if the patient is told to speak at a slower rate the speech becomes more intelligible. In other cases, speech intelligibility does not change as a function of altering speech rate. Clinicians should determine whether the patient can voluntarily change rate of talking and if so, whether articulatory accuracy and intelligibility are altered as a result of these rate changes.

In Chapter 5 we learned that control and regulation of voice pitch (fundamental frequency), vocal loudness (intensity), together with control over durational aspects of speech, in large part, determine how efficiently a speaker realizes prosody. Netsell (1973) has commented that "a host of terms has been applied to the prosodic (or suprasegmental) features; including pitch, intonation, loudness, intensity, stress, duration, rhythm, juncture, tempo, and voice quality" (p. 224). Prosodic aspects of speech reflect events which extend beyond the level of individual sound segments; hence, the terms suprasegmental or prosodic features. Patients with dysarthria often exhibit altered prosodic features. For example, they may exhibit altered stress patterns, deviant intonational patterns, etc.

In connected speech, *stress* refers to the relative emphasis given to words and syllables. Alterations in stress occur as a result of changes in fundamental frequency ("pitch"), vocal intensity, and/or duration. Stressed words or syllables generally have longer duration, higher pitch, and greater intensity than unstressed words or syllables. There is evidence which suggests that in order for a speaker to stress a word or syllable there has to be a momentary increase in neural signal strength to the entire speech musculature in order to effect these changes (Netsell, 1973; Ohman, 1967). By definition, the dysarthric patient has abnormal neuromotor functions, therefore, it can be expected that there might be disturbances in stress patterns during speech.

Patients can be asked to read aloud a series of sentences or a paragraph. The clinician should listen critically to the patterns of syllabic and word stress. Are these patterns normal? Does the speaker realize stress? Remember, in general, auxiliaries, some pronouns, prepositions, conjunctions, and articles in sentences are given little stress. The patient might also be asked to produce some multisyllabic words (for example, constabulary, encyclopedia, fundamental, introduction, and correspondent). Finally, the patient might be asked to produce sets of stress contrasts (e.g., INsult versus inSULT, DIgest versus diGEST, WHITE house versus White HOUSE, etc.). Is the patient able to realize these contrasts?

Intonation refers to pitch changes that occur during a sentence. In English, differences in intonational patterns or pitch changes distinguish statements from questions. For example, consider the following sentences: Bev loves Bob. versus Bev loves Bob?; Joe went downtown. versus Joe went downtown?; Today is Sunday. versus Today is Sunday?

All questions do not terminate with a rising intonation. For example, if the question is not answerable with yes or no and begins with a wh- word (what, why, where, etc.), the question is generally terminated with a falling intonation pattern (What day is this?, How do you make coffee?, Why did she fall down?)

Patients with dysarthria may exhibit altered stress and intonational patterns. These alterations in prosodic features of speech reflect diminished control or impoverished regulation of voice fundamental frequency and intensity and speech timing and duration. Alteration in speech prosody may cause problems conveying meaning, highlight abnormality, and contribute to the perception of speech deviance. Hence, identification of altered prosody in patients with dysarthrias is essential. Identification of such problems is important to the formulation of therapy plans. Identification is also important in differential diagnosis, because patients with some form of dysarthria have distinctive forms of prosody alteration. For example, cerebellar ataxia and parkinsonism are characterized by specific forms of stress alteration (Darley et al., 1975; Kent and Rosenbek, 1982).

CONTRASTING APRAXIA OF SPEECH AND THE DYSARTHRIAS

In this chapter we have considered the motor disorders of speech: apraxia of speech and the dysarthrias. We have learned that apraxia of speech is a disturbance of the programming or motor commands to the articulators. Dysarthrias, on the other hand, are the result of damage to the specific motor pathways. As we have learned, apraxia of speech and dysarthria often co-exist. Hence, a fundamental diagnostic problem is to differentiate and estimate the severity of each of these two broad types of motor disorders of speech. A summary of some of the salient speech characteristics which contrast apraxia of speech with the dysarthrias is presented in Table 8.1. This information is useful in differential diagnosis and treatment planning.

INTEGRATION OF CLINICAL FINDINGS

A major purpose of this chapter is to define the acquired motor disorders of speech. An important part of differential diagnosis for patients with acquired neuropathologies is to determine whether motor disorders of speech exist. In addition, clinicians must define the type (apraxia of speech versus the dysarthrias) and severity of motor disorders of speech present. This must often be accomplished in the presence of coexisting language disturbance (aphasia).

Table 8.1.   Characteristic features of dysarthria and speech apraxia

Dysarthrias	Apraxia of speech
Very little difference in articulatory accuracy between automatic-reactive and volitional purposive speech (no error-free production).	Articulatory accuracy is better for automatic-reactive speech than for volitional-purposive speech (moments of error-free production).
Substitution errors are infrequent. Speech is characterized more by phonetic distortions and omissions.	Substitution errors are more frequent than other error types.
Except occasionally in hypokinetic dysarthria, no difficulty with initiation of speech.	Initiation difficulty is frequent; characterized by pauses, restarts, repetition of initial sounds, syllables, or words.
Consonant clusters are frequently simplified; speech sound additions are rare.	Consonant clusters may be simplified but more frequently the intrusive schwa /ə/ is inserted within clusters ("puhlease" for "please").
Audible and silent groping of the articulators to locate target articulatory placements is rare or nonexistent.	Audible or silent groping and articulatory posturing to locate target articulatory placements is common.
Quality of production and error type is consistent when asked to repeat the same utterance; some improvement may be noted under conditions of extreme effort or motivation.	Variability in production of repeated utterances is common. Error type may change or production may vary off and on target, particularly on repeated utterances of polysyllabic words.

Reprinted from LaPointe (1982, p. 375).

Definition of the type of motor disorders of speech is critical to the formulation of therapy plans. For example, we have learned that apraxia of speech involves disruption of higher level programming or planning of motor movements. Dysarthria involves deviant neuromuscular execution due to impaired motor innervation to the speech mechanism. Hence, remediation of therapy for these two types of motor speech disorders is fundamentally different. For example, therapy for patients with apraxia of speech emphasizes the completion of motor commands, improvement in movement sequencing of the articulators, and maximizing voluntary neuromotor control. Therapy for patients with dysarthria highlights more direct drill. Here, patients are often directed to reduce their rate of speaking, exercise more direct control of articulatory movements, "overarticulate" consonant sounds, increase muscle strength, tone, accuracy, and so on, and control phrasing, prosody, and so on. Darley et al. (1975) have provided detailed descriptions of speech therapy techniques used for patients with dysarthria and apraxia of speech.

The work of Darley et al. (1975) indicates that it is possible to identify several different types of dysarthria: flaccid, spastic, ataxic, hypokinetic, hyperkinetic, and mixed. Determination of the type(s) of dysarthria is based upon knowledge about the neuromotor pathways which are impaired and upon identification of specific clusters of speech symptoms. We will not delineate the specific features of each of these types of dysarthria. Rather, students are encouraged to study the detailed descriptions of these features in Darley et al. (1975) and Wertz (1978). Differential diagnosis of dysarthria may also involve specification of the type (flaccid, spastic, ataxic, etc.) of dysarthria.

Finally, there is the issue of prognosis. Little has been written about prognosis for apraxia of speech per se, although as we have learned (see Chapter 7), considerably more has been written about prognosis for recovery of aphasia. Presumably, prognosis for patients with apraxia of speech depends upon those factors (initial severity, etiology, and extent and site of lesion) which influence prognosis for recovery from aphasia.

We have also learned that dysarthria can result from a large number of neurological problems. The prognosis for recovery of dysarthric symptoms clearly depends upon the nature and severity of the underlying disease. If the disease is reversible or can be controlled by drugs or other forms of medical treatment, the prognosis for dysarthria is generally more favorable. Conversely, if the severity of disease progresses rapidly and/or if the patient's condition reflects severe disturbance, then the prognosis is generally less favorable. The therapy goals and expectations established by speech-language pathologists should be formulated in terms of the natural course of the neurological problem.

Study Guide

1. What are the similarities and differences among aphasia, apraxia of speech, and dysarthria? There are several things to consider in your answer. First, you should state the basic definitions and briefly describe each of these three communication disorders. Then, list the salient speech and language characteristics of these patients. Third, identify the probable neurological sites of lesion associated with these communication disorders.

2. In terms of the neurological model of communication described in Chapter 7, what distinct step or level of activity is impaired when apraxia of speech is evident? What level of activity is impaired when dysarthria is present?

3. Describe some major speech symptoms noted in patients with apraxia of speech.

4. Describe the primary diagnostic methods speech-language pathologists use to evaluate speech in patients with apraxia of speech. Do the same for the dysarthrias.

5. Succinctly define each of the following terms or concepts:
   myasthenia gravis
   intonation
   stress
   range, rate and strength of movement
   cul-de-sac resonance test
   prosody
   muscle tone

REFERENCES

Aten, J., Johns, D., and Darley, F. 1971. Auditory perception of sequenced words in apraxia of speech. J. Speech Hear. Res. 14:131–143.

Bach-y-Rita, P., Balliet, R., Arieta, J. et al. 1981. Rehabilitation medicine management in aphasia. Sem. Speech Lang. Hear. 2:259–267.

Chapey, R. 1981. The assessment of language disorders in adults. In: R. Chapey, (ed.), Language Intervention Strategies in Adult Aphasia. Williams & Wilkins, Baltimore.

Chusid, J. 1979. Correlative Neuroanatomy and Functional Neurology 17th Ed. Lange Medical Publications, Los Altos, CA.

Dabul, B. 1979. Apraxia Battery for Adults. C. C. Publications, Inc., Tigard, OR.

Dabul, B. and Bollier, B. 1976. Therapeutic approaches to apraxia. J. Speech Hear. Disord. 41:268–276.

Darley, F. 1978. Differential diagnosis of acquired motor speech disorders. In: F. L. Darley and D. C. Spriestersbach, (eds.), Diagnostic Methods in Speech Pathology. 2-nd Ed. Harper & Row, New York.

Darley F., Aronson, A., and Brown, J. 1975. Motor Speech Disorders. W. B. Saunders Co., Philadelphia.

Deal, J., and Darley, F. 1972. The influence of linguistic and situational variables on phonemic accuracy in apraxia of speech. J. Speech Hear. Res. 15:639–653.

De Renzi, E., Pieczuro, A., and Vignolo, L. 1966. Oral apraxia and aphasia. Cortex 2:50–73.

DiSimoni, F., and Darley, F. 1977. Effect on phoneme duration control of three utterance-length conditions in an apractic patient. J. Speech Hear. Disord. 42:257–264.

Hardison, D., Marquardt, T., and Peterson, H. 1977. Effects of selected linguistic variables on apraxia of speech. J. Speech Hear. Res. 20:334–343.

Johns, D., and Darley, F. 1970. Phonemic variability in apraxia of speech. J. Speech Hear. Res. 13:556–583.

Kent, R., and Rosenbek, J. 1982., Prosodic disturbance and neurologic lesion. Brain Lang. 15:259–291.

Langenhorst, V. 1981. Performance of apraxic and Non-Apraxic Subjects on The Apraxia Battery For Adults. Masters Thesis, University of LaVerne, LaVerne, CA.

LaPointe, L. 1969. An investigation of isolated oral movements, oral sequencing motor abilities and articulation of brain-injured adults. Doctoral dissertation, University of Colorado, Boulder.

LaPointe, L. 1982. Neurogenic disorders of speech. In: G. Shames and E. Wiig (eds.), Human Communication Disorders. Charles E. Merrill Publ. Co., Columbus, OH.

LaPointe, L. L., and Johns, D. 1975. Some phonemic characteristics in apraxia of speech. J. Commun. Disord. 8:259–269.

Martin, A. 1974. Some objections to the term apraxia of speech. J. Speech Hear. Disord. 39:53–64.

Netsell, R. 1973. Speech physiology. In: F. Minifie, T. Hixon, and F. Williams (eds.), Normal Aspects of Speech, Hearing, and Language. Prentice-Hall, Inc., Englewood Cliffs, NJ.

Noll, J. 1982. Remediation of impaired resonance among patients with neuropathologies of speech. In: N. Lass, L. McReynolds, J. Northern, and D. Yoder (eds.), Speech, Language and Hearing. W. B. Saunders Co., Philadelphia.

Ohman, S. 1967. Word and sentence intonation: A quantitative model. Quarterly Progress Status Report, 2–3: 20–54. Speech Transmission Lab, Royal Institute of Technology, Stockholm.

Shankweiler, D., and Harris, K. 1966. An experimental approach to the problem of articulation in aphasia. Cortex 2:277–292.

Templin, M., and Darley, F. 1960. The Templin-Darley Tests of Articulation. Bureau of Education Research and Service, Extension Division, Iowa City, IA.

Tikofsky, R. 1970. A revised list for the estimation of dysarthric single word intelligibility. J. Speech Hear. Res. 13:59–64.

Trost, J. 1970. A descriptive study of verbal apraxia in patients with broca's aphasia. Doctoral dissertation, Northwestern University, Evanston, IL.

Wertz, R. 1978. Neuropathologies of speech and language. In: D. Johns (ed.), Management of Neurogenic Communication Disorder. Little Brown and Co., Boston.

Wertz, R., Rosenbek, J., and Deal, J. 1970. A review of 228 cases of apraxia of speech: classification, etiology, and localization. Paper presented to the American Speech and Hearing Association, New York.

Yorkston, K., and Beukelman, D. 1980. Assessment of Intelligibility of Dysarthric Speech. C. C. Publications, Inc., Tigard, OR.

Clinical Report and Letter Writing
Irv J. Meitus

Outline

In this chapter, we present information about the organization of clinical reports and professional letters. After completing an examination and formulating a diagnosis, the clinician must document what has taken place. A written summary is used to provide a permanent record and a basis for future contact with the patient. Diagnostic information is usually recorded in the form of a clinical report. Essential parts of this report are often transmitted to professionals in allied disciplines in the form of a summary letter.

THE CLINICAL REPORT: INTRODUCTORY CONCEPTS

Purpose of Report

The clinical report serves several basic functions. First, the report is an official record of the meeting with a patient (and possibly the family) and of the findings, diagnosis, and recommendations made during that meeting. For patients, the clinical report also represents a formal point of entry into the clinical service delivery system. Information accumulated during the diagnostic evaluation is often referred to as *base-line data*, a record of the conditions preceding the onset of therapeutic contact. Speech-language pathologists cannot place themselves in a position of accountability unless they carefully prepare clinical records.

Accountability requires that decisions be made on the basis of accurate information and necessitates that future judgments concerning changes in patient behavior be made on the basis of comparison to reference (base-line) points. Without careful documentation of these reference points, clinicians will have considerable difficulty accounting for the changes in speech patterns produced by patients over the course of examination and treatment. Accountability is sometimes more difficult to achieve when patients are seen over time by more than one clinician. In this situation, continuity of clinical reporting represents the only means by which long-term accountability can be achieved.

The clinical report also serves as an internal or "in-house" document. In this function, the clinical report represents a working document that is meant to be read by fellow speech, language, and hearing professionals. The language of clinical reports typically contains technical or specialized terminology. For example, terms like velopharyngeal, diadochokinesis, pragmatics, and allophones, are regularly used in the preparation of clinical reports, although they may not be used in reports sent to other professional workers. Clinical records often contain data. For example, data about the response rates of a patient over a number of trials are often included in such reports. Moreover, this type of data is often characterized on a phonetic basis. Clinical terminology associated with the use of specialized tests and inventories also represents a natural part of the report. Because patients or parents have the right of access to such information, we cannot insure that clinical reports will remain exclusively in house.

Finally, the clinical report represents the clinician's "face to the world." Fellow professionals will come to know and establish confidence in a clinician, in part, on the basis of what is committed to paper. Regardless of how proficient the clinician is as an interviewer, examiner, or a diagnostician, failure to organize a well-written and appropriately structured report will serve to diminish clinical effectiveness. A common error is to write for oneself. In this situation, the clinician may write in an abbreviated style and assume that no one else will read the record. Although this approach may appear helpful, eventually the shortcomings of poorly written and organized clinical reporting will catch up with the writer. The policy we suggest is to always prepare clinical reports using accepted grammatical practices, as though every report will be read by several fellow professional workers (Strunk and White, 1959). This policy will maximize personal accountability and help to maintain the prestige of the agency for which the clinician works.

The Time Perspective

Information contained within a clinical report, be it history, examination findings, impressions, or recommendations, represents a view of a patient obtained over a specific interval of time. The reader of a report must understand that the contents of such reports apply to a report date which is typically specified at the beginning of the writing. Although this may seem obvious, it is appropriate to highlight the fact that behaviors, test scores, physical traits, and so on may change over time. Human characteristics and behaviors are dynamic and clinicians should not fall into a pattern of writing and reading reports as though they are considering static events. What is placed into clinical reports often summarizes observations made over relatively short periods of time. When reviewed consecutively, the observations made in various reports will act as links which should assist clinicians in identifying patterns of change that occur in patients with speech and language disturbance.

Writing about Facts and Assumptions

The language of fact and assumption is used regularly in the writing of clinical records. Clinical fact refers to statements made about events which actually take place and which can be directly observed by the clinician or examiner. Statements of clinical assumption refer to what clinicians judge to be true, although they may not observe or measure attributes related to these events on a direct basis. This basic concept was first presented in Chapter 1. It is important for the clinician to use fact and assumption appropriately because the way in which these concepts are used (or misused) gives the reader information about the competence of the examiner.

A few examples may prove helpful:

Patient 1

    A.   Johnny consistently distorted /s/ during the production of all words spoken within a spontaneous language sample.

(This is a statement of clinical fact based on observed events. This type of statement is typically found in the examination section of clinical reports).

B. The misarticulation of /s/ is the primary cause for the diminished intelligibility of Johnny's speech.

(This is a statement of clinical assumption reflecting what the clinician judges to be true. This type of statement is typically found in the clinical impression section of clinical reports).

Patient 2

A. Lingual movement is labored and generally inaccurate in terms of the direction of movement.

(Again, this is a factual statement based on observed behavior; an examination finding).

B. Labored lingual movement results in imprecise articulation.

(Assumption based on clinical evidence; stated as part of the diagnosis).

Patient 3

A. Twenty percent of the patient's attempted productions of words consisted of off-target approximations.

(Fact based on analysis of data after the administration of a test of aphasia).

B. The language disorder of this 68-year-old post-CVA male is classified as Broca's aphasia.

(Judgment of the examiner based on experience with use of aphasia classification systems).

Although these examples suggest a clear-cut distinction between fact and assumption, many statements cannot readily be distinguished on the basis of this dichotomy. Descriptions about psychological states provide good examples of the problems incurred in differentiating between fact and assumption. For example, a clinician can accurately report that a child cried, avoided eye contact, failed to separate from the parent, failed to stay seated during testing, and so on. These are all facts based upon directly observable events. The factors responsible for these behaviors are varied and may be extremely difficult to specify. Such behaviors may result from chronic alterations in emotional state, immediate reactions to the testing or general clinical situation, the effects of parenting practices, or other unspecified factors. When a child is described as "shy," "withdrawn," "hyperactive," or "immature," the clinician must realize that these descriptors represent assumptions made by the observer. Refusal to speak is a fact. Shyness is a behavioral construct which can only be validated by "entering the mind of the patient." In general, the more a patient can reveal about emotional states, the more accurate clinicians can become as reporters.

Reporting historical information merits special attention. Information dealing with past events (developmental milestones, results of past diagnostic and therapeutic services, opinions of other professionals, etc.) should be reported differently from the reporting of observed behaviors. Although retrospective historical information is often critical to the formulation of a diagnosis, the accuracy (reliability and validity) of this type of information must be carefully assessed. For this reason, language such as "It was reported that _____," "Mrs. Jones described her daughter as being _____," or "The patient described her earlier therapy at the Downtown Clinic as consisting of _____," is often used to emphasize how the type of information was obtained. Where historical data has come to the clinician in the form of referral letters or reports, the reporting of such information is indeed factual.

Written Language: A Reflection on Professional Competence

When writing the clinical report, speech-language pathologists should use language commensurate with their professional competence and experience. Speech-language pathology is an interdisciplinary profession. We frequently share information with physicians, educators, psychologists, vocational rehabilitation workers, and so on. Members of these allied fields often refer patients with disorders of communication for examination and diagnosis. Conversely, speech-language pathologists often refer patients to members of these allied fields for examination and diagnosis. The language used in these types of communication must reflect the reciprocal interactions between these allied fields if professional credibility is to be maintained.

Examples of this reciprocity are common in clinical practice. One specific area of written language which reflects professional competence relates to the need to distinguish between the making of physical observations and the formulation of a medical diagnosis. For example, speech-language clinicians should be able to make detailed observations of the structure and function of the oral-facial area. They should be trained to recognize such physical functions as facial asymmetry and muscular weakness. They should be able to determine when the faucial tonsils are hypertrophic and when lingual movements are poorly coordinated. They should recognize abnormalities and differences in palatal structure and function. This is all part of speech-language pathology examination and diagnosis. On the other hand, the diagnosis of certain types of physical problems (e.g., oral cancer, vocal nodules, etc.) is part of medical practice. The written language used in the preparation of clinical reports should reflect this distinction. Hence, report language which "suggests the presence of" such physical conditions represents a prudent approach to clinical writing, in that this approach serves to maintain professional competence and preserve the disciplinary distinctions addressed.

Additional examples of the need to maintain professional respect and preserve professional competence are prevalant in clinical practice. For example, clinical psychologists make diagnoses of cognitive, intellectual, emotional, and social disorders. Educators have expertise in school placement issues. Vocational rehabilitation personnel are competent to deal with adult patients in relation to their placement in a productive work environment. Speech-language pathologists diagnose and treat disorders of human communication. The more fully our written reports reflect this competence, the more our interdisciplinary relationships will flourish.

CLINICAL REPORT STRUCTURE

Clinical reports require a structure or format to be effective. This structure should provide the reader with pertinent information and should incorporate a logical sequencing of information. Various formats and section headings used in the preparation of reports have been suggested (Darley and Spriestersbach, 1978; Emerick and Hatten, 1979; King and Berger, 1971; Knepflar, 1976; Nation and Aram, 1977; Peterson and Marquardt, 1981). This writer suggests a general format to be used in the preparation of clinical reports that can be adapted to a variety of clinical settings (see Appendix A).

Identifying Information

All clinical reports must provide a small number of readily retrievable pieces of information. These types of information are summarized in Appendix A and require no additional comment. Some clinicians or clinic administrators prefer to add a disorder classification entry in this section. This entry is often useful in clinical census taking and permits rapid identification of the final diagnostic classification of the patient.

Statement of the Problem

Every clinical report should specify the person being interviewed. If this person is not the patient, the relationship of this person to the patient should be specified. In addition, each report should contain a statement of the problem and the rationale for requesting the examination at this particular time. It is helpful to use the specific words of the person being interviewed if their language would assist the reader in understanding that person's perception of the problem. If appropriate, identification of a referral source and a statement of the reason for the referral should also be provided.

History

Historical information represents an essential and often critical part of the examination process. Hence, a summary of historical data is needed in every clinical report. The areas outlined in Chapter 2 (see ''Gathering the History'') can be used to provide structure to this phase of the examination and to assure adequacy of topical coverage.

Two rather divergent styles of historical reporting are used in clinical writing. One style is characterized by reporting all facts relating to specific events, developmental milestones, physical observations, and so on. In this style, information about both normal and abnormal findings is summarized. This approach tends to produce a fairly long report, because the writer systematically presents everything that was explored in the interview. The alternate approach is to focus only on the abnormal findings, designating areas where no problems are found as "unremarkable". Here, the philosophy seems to be that the professional who reads the report will assume normality unless it is otherwise stated. This approach leads to a more truncated style of writing, yielding comparatively shorter clinical histories.

The determination of which style is used depends upon a number of variables: writer preference, clinical environment (agency, hospital, school), time constraints, and whether a pre-evaluation questionnaire has been used. Experience suggests that most clinicians prepare reports which incorporate a style reflecting balance between these two stylistic extremes. Clearly, commenting on every detail is unnecessary. This approach burdens the reader with more information than is needed and often fails to clearly distinguish what is important from that which is trivial, unrelated, or removed from the core of the existing problem. On the other hand, a very brief history may fail to give the reader enough information. Ultimately clinicians must find the proper balance between these two stylistic extremes as they prepare clinical reports.

Examination Findings   In this section, the clinician summarizes the findings of the examination process. Here, specific test results should be detailed. These findings should be reported in a systematic fashion, using subtopical designations to assist the reader in rapidly locating areas of particular interest.

The results of the clinical examination can be categorized or subdivided. Although the need to develop each category will depend upon the particular diagnostic problem, each clinical report should deal with several common areas discussed in Chapters 1 and 2. These areas are listed below.

General behavior observations
Examination of the speech mechanism
Evaluation of respiratory function
Linguistic characteristics
Speech sound production behavior
Voice production
Fluency characteristics
Nonverbal aspects of communication
Audition and auditory perceptual skills
General developmental characteristics
Cognitive and intellectual functioning
Emotional and social status

As discussed in the previous section, the clinician must determine the amount of information needed to provide adequate coverage of each of these areas. Where it is immediately apparent that certain functions are not disordered (e.g., a child with a speech sound disorder who exhibits normal conversational language and fluency characteristics for his age), formal testing might not be performed in those areas, and the statement that language and fluency are "within normal limits on the basis of informal probes" can be used.

The reporting of observations and specific test results requires objectivity. In particular, empirical measures and normative comparisons must be distinguished from diagnostic statements or clinical impressions. Peterson and Marquardt (1981) give consideration to this subject:

> When writing reports . . . it is also important to separate test results from interpretation. . . . The data collected and their significance are a function of the measurement device used. For example, you may well report that "Henry obtained a vocabulary recognition age-score of 6–3 (C.A. 5–7) on the Peabody Picture Vocabulary Test." This system immediately does two things: It shows where the data came from, and it provides a comparison by your inclusion of the child's chronological age. . . . In the summary or impressions section you would report the vocabulary recognition score was within normal limits for his age. . . . The point to be emphasized is that your examination data are to be reported as specific to a test, with necessary descriptive or normative comparisons, and that test results are separated from the interpretive summary. Your data, with the necessary comparisons and qualifications, are shown as examination results. Your interpretation of the significance of the total results, included in the clinical impressions or summary section, is then your professional judgment. It should be possible for another professional reader to accept your data and make a different interpretation of their overall significance (pp. 318–320).

Clinical Impressions

In Chapter 1, we discussed the formulation of a diagnosis, or what is referred to by many as the *clinical impression*. The point was made that this formulation is considered to be the most complex part of the evaluation process. This is true because it requires the clinician to integrate information obtained through historical interviewing and direct examination with knowledge of communication pathology and human behavior. This synthesis is accomplished against a background of clinical experience. The terms *synthesis* and *integration* are used to underscore the need to discuss interrelationships among observations or variables, and to emphasize the meaning of data. This process differs from summarizing what has been uncovered in the clinical history and noted during examination phases of the diagnostic process. The diagnostician takes a position about the patient, bringing data or information to bear upon the formulation of an opinion, impression or diagnostic category. In setting opinions down on paper, both writer and reader must recognize that clinical judgments are often not formulated solely on the basis of objective measures or observations. Interpretations of the same data or information may vary from clinician to clinician. We seldom deal in absolutes. One process is common to all forms of examination and diagnosis: the clinician must formulate an impression or opinion and commit it to writing in such a way that the rationale for this impression is clear.

The written diagnostic statement should consist of a disorder classification, a specification of the severity of the symptoms, a statement of the etiologic and contributing factors, a compilation of both the positive and the negative factors that are expected to influence intervention, an opinion about the relevance of a particular intervention approach, including referrals, and a prognostic statement. When this has been accomplished, the clinician has stated a position with respect to the patient and the problem and only a brief summary of specific recommendations remain.

Recommendations

The final section of each clinical report should provide a statement of the specific recommendation(s). Typically, this is a rather brief part of the clinical report. Recommendations are usually presented in a structured format so that the reader can clearly and quickly identify what has been suggested. There may be recommendations for speech and/or language therapy, for parent education or counseling, for referral to allied professionals, for a follow-up appointment, for re-evaluation at some future date, and so on. In some instances, the recommendation may simply be a statement that no further contact is necessary.

It is this writer's opinion that a step-by-step listing of therapeutic suggestions is not suitable to efficient clinical reporting. If it is necessary to describe a therapeutic approach in detail, it would be appropriate to attach this information to the report as an appendix, thereby keeping the thrust of the report focused upon the diagnostic findings.

A final comment regarding recommendations. It is desirable to include information about the final arrangements that were made with the patient. For administrative purposes, it is often helpful to add a statement indicating whether the patient or family members plan to follow through with the recommendations. In most instances, there will be full compliance and statements such as, "Mr. and Mrs. Jones accepted the above recommendations and have agreed to place Jane in speech therapy early in September, 1982," or "Mr. Smith agreed to see his laryngologist at the earliest possible date and requested that a report be sent to _____" are all that is needed. Statements such as, "Mr. White agreed to consider our recommendations and asked that we contact him by telephone in one week," provide the reader with information that clinical contact with this patient has not terminated. Statements such as "Mr. Black declined to begin voice therapy until some later date, when he will contact us," are helpful to include as part of the clinical record, and for accountability purposes.

Signatures

The final stage of clinical reporting requires the signature of the responsible clinician, identified by name, title and professional qualifications. The title of the responsible clinician (Speech-Language Clinician, Speech Pathologist, Graduate Clinician, etc.) might be dictated by the policies of the institution in which one works. The use of the Certificate of Clinical Competence in Speech Pathology (CCC-SP) may be used if one is a professionally certified worker.

A sample clinical report which incorporates the format described is provided in Appendix B.

PROFESSIONAL WRITING STYLE

In this instance, *style* refers to the manner by which one expresses thought in written language. We would expect each clinician to write in a distinctive style which, in part, reflects former training and experience. Clinical writing, although substantially different from creative writing, adheres to the traditional rules of English grammar and to the attributes found in technical reporting. It is this writer's opinion that the best way to learn clinical writing is to first have a sound foundation in English composition, then read many samples of reports written by experienced professionals, and finally, begin to write reports, subjecting them to the criticism of experienced workers in the field.

Within the scope of this chapter, it is not possible to give detailed information or provide extensive examples of appropriate writing styles. The sample report in Appendix B represents a common pattern of appropriate style. There are a number of references that address this topic particularly well. The booklet on report writing sponsored by the National Student Speech-Language-Hearing Association (Knepflar, 1976) is particularly helpful. In his chapter on writing style, Knepflar makes the following points.

1. Use specific language. Avoid ambiguous terms (p. 29).
2. Use nontechnical language that can be understood by the reader. Define terms that might not be universally comprehended. Avoid jargon. (p. 30).
3. Use complete words, which may be clearly understood by readers. Avoid abbreviations. (p. 31).
4. Use a variety of language styles and word selections, according to the needs of the report. Avoid stereotype. (p. 32).
5. Use specific, accurate, brief sentences. Avoid verbosity and needless words. (p. 33).
6. Convey a sincere, serious professional attitude in your writing. Avoid flippancy. (p. 34).
7. Use complete verb forms and correct punctuation. Avoid contractions and hyphens. (p. 35).
8. Use positive statements that show what testing or observations have revealed. Avoid qualifiers and noncommittal language. (p. 36).

9. Use personal pronouns when they are a natural way to make a clear statement. Avoid awkward circumlocutions. (p. 37).
10. Use accurate, descriptive language that can be supported by fact. Avoid exaggeration and overstatement. (p. 39).
11. Select the exact words you need to express a specific concept or idea. Avoid misusing words. (p. 39).
12. Use active-verb construction whenever possible. Avoid passive-verb forms. (p. 40).

In addition, Darley and Spriestersbach (1978), Emerick and Hatten (1979), Haynes and Hartman (1975), Hutchinson et al. (1979), Moore (1969), Pannbacker (1975), Peterson and Marquardt (1981), and Strunk and White (1959) provide information that can assist the beginning student to learn efficient and appropriate styles of writing.

CLINICAL LETTER WRITING

After completing the examination and formulating the diagnosis, frequently, the clinician writes clinical letters to convey the findings to 1) professionals in allied disciplines; and 2) individuals responsible for the care of the patient, for example, parent, spouse, or guardian. Letters are also written for the purpose of referring the patient to another professional, from which additional services or information may be needed. When writing such letters, it is important for the clinician to recognize how much information will be useful. It is easy to assume that persons outside our profession will find all of the information in our clinical reports equally useful. This is usually not the case. The amount of information needed is usually less than that typically offered in our clinical reports. In addition, the language used in letters should be relatively free of professional jargon.

Letters Conveying Clinical Findings

Letters to professionals in allied disciplines and responsible caregivers should contain concisely stated accounts of our evaluations. These accounts can generally be divided into three basic areas:

1. An opening statement relating who was examined, when, and for what purpose (brief statement of the problem)
2. A summary of pertinent historical and examination findings
3. A statement of clinical impressions (diagnosis) and recommendations

A summary letter is presented in Appendix C. This letter summarizes the results of the clinical report offered in Appendix B.

Referral Letters

As stated earlier, referral letters are usually written to allied professionals. They are used to request specific diagnostic information which the speech-language clinician may not be trained to collect, and/or are initiated to determine the need for additional forms of management. These letters are typically brief. They should provide the usual identifying information, a statement of your professional relationship with the patient, diagnostic findings that would be pertinent to a consulting professional, and a specific statement concerning why the referral has been made. This last point is of particular importance. Consultants can be more efficient in their examination of the patient when they know why the patient has been sent to them. Precise statements concerning why referrals are made will also assist in obtaining direct answers to our specific questions and needs.

A sample of a referral letter is provided in Appendix D. The referral letter is also based on the patient presented in Appendix B. An alternative way of contacting the consulting laryngologist would be to use the laryngology counsult form presented in Table 5.1.

CONFIDENTIALITY OF WRITTEN INFORMATION

Clinical data, written reports and summary letters all contain confidential information. The original copy of the reports and the copies of summary letters are typically kept in the clinical folder as part of hospital, school, or clinic records. Under normal circumstances this information cannot be released to unauthorized persons without the written consent of the patient or a responsible adult (see, for example The Code of Ethics of the American Speech-Language-Hearing Association, January 1977 Revision Section A, No. 2C).

An example of a consent form used for securing an authorization to release clinical information is provided in Appendix E. Contemporary privacy laws are responsible for insuring specificity in the language used in clinical consent forms. Examination of Appendix E will reveal the manner by which the patient is protected. It should be noted, that once information is released to another individual or agency, speech-language clinicians have no control over how that information will be used. This fact highlights the need to ensure that any piece of clinical writing represents a well-founded, objectively prepared document that places its writer in a fully accountable position.

Study Guide

1. Identify the major purposes served by clinical reports and professional letters.

2. Distinguish between the language of fact and assumption and make clear why it is important for the clinician to use these two forms of written language appropriately in the preparation of clinical reports and letters.

3. Identify the major sections to be included in the preparation of clinical reports.

4. Identify the major sections or issues to be included in the preparation of professional letters.

REFERENCES

American National Standards Institute. 1970. American National Standards Specifications for Audiometers, ANSI-S3.6-1969. American National Standards Institute, Inc., New York.

Darley, F., and Spriestersbach, D. 1978. Diagnostic Methods in Speech Pathology. 2nd Ed. Harper & Row, New York.

Emerick, L., and Hatten, J. 1979. Diagnosis and Evaluation in Speech Pathology. Prentice-Hall, Inc., Englewood Cliffs, NJ.

Haynes, W., and Hartman, D. 1975. The agony of report writing: A new look at an old problem. J. Natl. Student Speech Lang. Hear. Assoc. 3:7–15.

Hutchinson, B., Hanson, M., and Mecham, M. 1979. Diagnostic Handbook of Speech Pathology. Williams & Wilkins Co., Baltimore.

King, R., and Berger, K. 1971. Diagnostic Assessment and Counseling Techniques for Speech Pathologists and Audiologists. Stanwix House, Inc., Pittsburgh.

Knepflar, K. 1976. Report Writing in the Field of Communication Disorders. The Interstate Printers and Publishers, Inc., Danville, IL.

Moore, M. 1969. Pathological writing. Asha 11:535–538.

Nation, J., and Aram, D. 1977. Diagnosis of Speech and Language Disorders. The C. V. Mosby Company, St. Louis, MO.

Pannbacker, M. 1975. Diagnostic report writing. J. Speech Hear. Disord. 40:367–379.

Peterson, H., and Marquardt, T. 1981. Appraisal and Diagnosis of Speech and Language Disorders. Prentice-Hall, Inc., Englewood Cliffs, NJ.

Smitheran, J. R., and Hixon, T. J. 1981. A clinical method for estimating laryngeal airway resistance during vowel production. J. Speech Hear. Disord. 46:138–146.

Strunk, W., and White, E. 1959. The Elements of Style. MacMillan, New York.

APPENDICES

A. Clinical Report Format

Clinic Identification

Report of Speech-Language Examination

Identifying Information

Name: _____ Birthdate: _____ Age at Examination: ___

Address: _____ Date of Examination: _____

Telephone: _____ Clinic Number: _____

Parents or Guardian: _____ Examiner(s): _____

Statement of the Problem

Patient or parental complaint

History

Pre-examination information

Examination Findings

Results of testing and observation

Clinical Impressions

The diagnostic statement

Recommendations

Suggested course of action

Signatures

B.   Sample Clinical Report

Purdue University Speech and Hearing Clinic
West Lafayette, IN 47907

Report of Speech-Language Examination

Name: _____ Jones, David M. _____   Birthdate: ___ 10/23/70 ___   Age at Examination: 11;9

Address: _____ 123 East Street _____   Date of Examination: ___ 7/15/82 ___

_____ Lafayette, IN 47909 _____   PUSHC Number: ___ 82-999 ___

Telephone: ___ 456-7890 ___   Examiner(s): _____ J. D. Williams _____

Parents or Guardian: John and Mary Jones _____

Statement of the Problem:

David M. Jones, an 11-year, 9-month-old boy was seen on July 15, 1980 for a speech-language examination. Mrs. Jones, David's mother, accompanied David to the examination and provided information during the interview. She was referred to this clinic by Robert L. Black, M.D., the family pediatrician who indicated that David's voice "does not sound normal." The mother's concern was that "David's voice sounds husky."

History:

Mrs. Jones reported that David's voice disturbance began "about 1 year ago." At that time, David's teacher indicated to Mrs. Jones that she felt "David's voice was not normal." Mrs. Jones reportedly chose to wait until David's next annual pediatric examination to discuss his voice problem with the family pediatrician. Dr. Black encouraged Mrs. Jones to obtain further professional assistance through referral to the Purdue University Speech and Hearing Clinic. There is no history of previous examination or treatment of David's voice problem.

Mrs. Jones completed a comprehensive historical questionnaire (Child Form-Voice History Questionnaire) prior to the examination. The information provided in this questionnaire, together with information offered by David's pediatrician and his mother, revealed that David's development was unremarkable and that he had a history of excellent health. School progress has been excellent. David's most recent (January 1982) screening examination for hearing conducted at school was also unremarkable. Mrs. Jones reported that David did not use any prescription or nonprescription medication during the past year.

David's family consists of his father, a 38-year-old university professor, his mother, a 38-year-old woman currently working on a doctoral degree, and a 20-month-old sister. Mrs. Jones reported that "our family is a close-knit group, is highly verbal, and very affectionate." She also indicated that "our family has been under no unusual stress or tension." She reported that no one in the family has had a history of speech or voice disturbance.

During the course of direct interviewing with David, he indicated that "I have a voice problem. My voice sounds hoarse." David reported that he felt his voice problem was mild and that it did not have a significant negative effect on his school achievement or social relationships. He indicated that he was unaware of why he has a problem.

303

Both David and his mother agreed that his voice sounded "better" when he was rested, when he was not in school, when he was not participating in sports, and in the mornings. They also agreed that David often engaged in "shouting" and that he spoke "excessively."

Examination Findings

General Behavioral Observations

David cooperated fully in all phases of the examination. He appeared to be a mature and capable 11-year-old, willing to express his feelings freely. Formal behavioral testing (motoric, cognitive-intellectual, etc.) was not undertaken.

Speech Mechanism Examination

The results of our examination of structural and functional aspects of David's speech mechanism were unremarkable.

Phonatory Behavior

A thorough perceptual examination of David's voice production was completed. During the production of conversational speech and reading, David's voice had a consistent breathy component. Vocal pitch characteristics were judged to be normal. Analysis of the sustained production of three vowels (/i,a,u/) indicated fundamental frequency levels ranging between 220 and 230 Hz. David's phonational range was 25 semitones. His loudness characteristics during conversation and reading were unremarkable. No pitch breaks or interruptions of the voice were noted during the examination.

David was able to sustain vowels (/i,a,u/) consistently for durations in excess of 10 seconds. He did not use hard glottal attacks to initiate either sustained vowel productions or vowel-initiated utterances associated with verbal discourse or reading. His cough was unremarkable. David's intonation and stress patterns appeared normal and he exhibited no difficulty producing voicing distinctions.

Significant changes in David's voice were not apparent during the examination. Several episodes of throat clearing occurred during all phases of the examination. David was not able to modify, minimize, or eliminate the breathy component to his voice in association with the use of several facilitative techniques (e.g. modification of pitch and loudness and variation in method of glottal attack) that were attempted.

Respiratory Examination

Various types of respiratory testing were completed. First, estimations were made of glottal airflow rate using a face mask and pneumotachographic instrumentation. These estimations were obtained as David sustained vowels /i,a,u/ on an isolated basis and produced vowels in words spoken within sentences. During the production of vowels produced in speech or on a sustained basis, airflow rate through David's larynx ranged between 0.25 and 0.35 LPS. These airflow rates were outside the normal range. Second, estimations were made of glottal or laryngeal airway resistance using procedures described by Smitheran and Hixon (1981). David's laryngeal airway resistance was about 34 cm H_2O LPS, a value well within the range of normal limits. Analysis of the pressure and flow functions used in the calculation of David's laryngeal airway resistance indicated that he was able to supply adequate pressures to the larynx during voice production. Third, informal observations indicated that David's air volume adequacy and chest wall movements used during voice production were unremarkable.

Audition

David responded positively to pure tone audiometric screening conducted at 20 dB HL (re: ANSI, 1969) for 1000 and 2000 Hz, and at 25 dB for 4000 Hz, bilaterally. The results of tympanometry and acoustic reflex testing were unremarkable.

Speech-Language Behavior

David's language and fluency characteristics were judged to be normal on the basis of his performance on various examination activities. During conversation and oral reading, David consistently interdentalized /s/. This interdentalization was present in all productions of /s/ and gave rise to a mild distortion or allophonic change in the this sound. David was able to produce acceptable /s/ sounds simply by instructing him to keep his back teeth together when producing /s/. No other speech sound errors were noted.

Clinical Impressions:

David has a mild voice disorder characterized by the consistent presence of breathy voice quality. A definitive statement of the etiology and of factors operating to sustain this problem cannot be made on the basis of this examination. A laryngological examination is needed to determine whether there is a need for medical treatment, to identify factors that might limit the production of normal voice or influence behavioral treatment, and to clarify the etiology of David's vocal disturbance. No factors were identified in our examination that would be expected to negatively influence management of David's voice problem. On the other hand, David's awareness of his problem, his level of cooperation, and his willingness to attempt voice modification were interpreted as positive influences toward possible future intervention. A definitive statement concerning David's ability to eliminate or minimize the breathy component in his voice cannot be made until the laryngoscopic examination has been completed.

In addition to verifying the presenting complaint of vocal disturbance, David consistently interdentalized the /s/ sound. This isolated speech sound error, although consistently present, represents a mild disturbance which does not influence intelligibility. The etiology of this isolated error is unknown and has not been of concern to David or his family. David's ability to modify this pattern by simply instructing him to keep his back teeth together when producing /s/ was interpreted to represent a positive indication toward recommended future intervention.

Recommendations:

The following recommendations were made and accepted by David and his mother:

1. A laryngology examination was scheduled with George B. Wilson, M.D. on July 23, 1982.
2. A return visit was scheduled August 15, 1982, to discuss laryngological findings and a possible program of voice remediation.
3. Initiate therapy program to modify interdentalization of /s/. Therapy to begin on the August 15, 1982 visit.

John D. Williams, CCC-SP
Speech Pathologist

C. Sample Clinical Summary Letter

Purdue University Speech and Hearing Clinic
West Lafayette, IN 47907

July 17, 1982

Robert L. Black, M.D.
2901 Reading Road
Lafayette, IN 47905

Re: JONES, David M.
D.O.B.: 10-23-70
PUSHC #: 82-999

Dear Doctor Black:

This is a summary report on David M. Jones, an 11-year, 9-month-old boy you referred to our clinic because "his voice did not sound normal." David was examined on July 15, 1982. He was accompanied by his mother who felt that David's primary problem was "huskiness" of the voice.

Significant historical information included Mrs. Jones' report that David's voice disturbance began "about 1 year ago." David received no prior examination or treatment for this problem. His development has been unremarkable and his health history is excellent. David's school progress has been outstanding. Mrs. Jones reported that their family is a "close-knit group", is "highly verbal," and is "very affectionate." There is a negative familial history of speech or voice disturbance.

During the course of the direct interview with David, he acknowledged that he has a voice problem. He correctly indicated that his voice problem is mild and that it does not have a significant negative influence on his school achievement or his social relationships. He was unaware of why his voice problem exists. Both David and his mother agreed that there are times when his voice sounds "better" (e.g., when rested, when not in school, when not participating in sports, and in the morning). They agreed that David often engages in "shouting" and that he speaks excessively.

David cooperated fully in all phases of the examination. He appeared to us to be a capable 11-year-old who freely expresses his feelings. The results of our examination of David's speech and hearing mechanism were unremarkable. A comprehensive examination of various aspects of David's voice production was completed. His voice had a consistent breathy component. Vocal pitch and loudness characteristics were perceptually unremarkable, and no pitch breaks or interruptions of the voice were noted during the examination. Significant changes in David's voice were not apparent during the examination. He was not able to modify the breathy component to his voice in response to several facilitative techniques we attempted.

Various types of respiratory testing were also completed. The results of these forms of testing revealed that: 1) airflow rate through David's larynx (0.25–0.35 LPS) was higher than normal; 2) laryngeal airway resistance (about 34 cm H_2O LPS) was well within normal limits; 3) he was able to supply adequate pressure to the larynx during voice production; and 4) his chest wall movements and air volume characteristics associated with voice production were unremarkable.

With one exception, David's speech and language function was judged to be normal. The exception was that he consistently distorted the /s/ sound, but was able to produce acceptable /s/ sounds with limited instruction.

Our impression is that David has a mild voice disorder characterized by the consistent presence of breathy voice quality. Statements about the etiology of this problem and plans to initiate voice therapy must await laryngological examination. The etiology of David's isolated speech sound error is also unknown and has not been of concern to David and his family. David's ability to modify this isolated error was an indication that speech therapy would be productive.

The following recommendations were made and accepted by David and his mother:

1.   A laryngological examination was scheduled (July 23, 1982) with George B. Wilson, M.D.

2.   A return visit was scheduled with us for August 15, 1982. During this visit we expect to discuss the laryngological findings and possible voice remediation, and initiate a therapy program for the /s/ sound.

We appreciate your referral of the Jones family and urge you to contact us if further information concerning David is needed.

Sincerely yours,

_____

John D. Williams, CCC-SP
Speech Pathologist

D. Sample Clinical Referral Letter

Purdue University Speech and Hearing Clinic
West Lafayette, IN 47907

July 17, 1982

George B. Wilson, M.D.
3075 West Bend Road
Lafayette, IN 47908

Re: JONES, David M.
D.O.B.: 10-23-70
PUSHC #: 82-999

Dear Doctor Wilson:

David M. Jones, an 11-year, 9-month-old boy is referred to you for a laryngological examination following our examination on July 15, 1982. Mrs. John Jones brought David to our clinic on the recommendation of his pediatrician, Robert L. Black, M.D. The primary concern about David is that his voice has a consistent breathy component. His voice disturbance has existed for about 1 year and there is some information to suggest that he abuses his vocal mechanism.

The results of our examination of David's speech mechanism were unremarkable. Perceptual evaluations indicated that David's vocal pitch and loudness characteristics were normal. He did not exhibit any pitch breaks or voice interruptions and did not use hard glottal attack. David did exhibit several episodes of throat clearing during our examination. He does have excessive (0.25–0.35 LPS) airflow rate through the larynx during the production of vowels. His laryngeal airway resistance (about 34 cm H_2O LPS), air volume adequacy, and chestwall movements were all unremarkable. In addition, David passed a pure tone audiometric screening test. With the exception of a consistent distortion of the /s/ sound, David's language and speech characteristics were judged to be normal.

We have recommended a laryngological examination to determine the need for medical treatment, to identify factors that might influence voice modification, and to clarify the etiology of David's vocal disturbance. Please call me if there is a need to discuss this request or to clarify the results of your examination.

Sincerely yours,

_____

John D. Williams, CCC-SP
Speech Pathologist

E. Sample Consent Form for Release of Information

Purdue University Speech and Hearing Clinic
West Lafayette, IN 47907

CONSENT TO RELEASE INFORMATION

TO: _____

I hereby request and authorize you to release to _____

_____

information you may have concerning: _____

with respect to any evaluation, consultation, clinical or educational contact pertaining to medical, physical, psychological, educational status and behavior during the period of _____ to _____,

for the purpose of _____

_____
(State exact purpose. DO NOT generalize)

I understand that I may phone or write the above agency to request that specific portions of my records not be released or referred to in the course of taking action upon this request.

The following portions of my record shall be released: (The statement "Any and all records" is no longer acceptable by law.)

_____

_____

I understand that this consent is subject to revocation by me at any time except to the extent that action has been taken in reliance thereon. In the absence of such revocation, it will expire upon fulfillment of the above purpose.

I, the undersigned, have read this consent and understand it. All blanks were filled in prior to my signing.

Dated and signed this _____ day of _____, 19_____.

_____   _____
Client/Parent/Guardian   (Birthdate of concerned person)

10

Talking with Patients and Their Families

Irv J. Meitus

Outline

Educational Aims

1. *To underscore the importance of interviewing and counseling as an essential part of speech-language clinical practice*
2. *To identify the major roles speech-language pathologists assume as they interview and counsel patients and their families*
3. *To clarify how speech-language pathologists can learn to communicate effectively with patients and their families.*

In this concluding chapter, we provide information about how speech-language pathologists can effectively talk with patients and their families. This information is needed to understand the role interpersonal communication plays in establishing helping relationships. Students in speech-language pathology are typically consumed with learning about the nature of various evaluative tests and with the procedures used in their administration. Students are also immersed in learning to execute various types of clinical examinations and becoming skillful at using various types of instrumentation. As we have seen, report writing represents another skill that commands considerable time of both student and clinical instructor.

Unfortunately, learning about interpersonal communication in professional relationships is typically approached on an experiential basis (Emerick and Hatten, 1979). Stated differently, problems in interpersonal communication which may occur between clinicians and patients or their families are typically dealt with as they occur within the students' direct clinical experiences. This approach contrasts markedly with taking a direct, a priori look at the various functions assumed by an interviewer and at the basic concepts related to the realization of efficient interviewing. In keeping with the latter approach, we offer information about important aspects of interpersonal communication and the influence these aspects exert upon the establishment of professional relationships.

We will discuss various functions clinicians assume as they conduct evaluations of patients with speech-language problems. For example, we discuss the roles clinicians assume in the early stages of the examination process (history taking) and those assumed in later stages which generally require the examiner to assume an interpretive or counseling role. At all stages, we stress 1) the need for clinician sensitivity to patient needs; 2) the meaning of efficiency in relation to effective communication; and 3) the potential impact the clinician may have upon patients and their families. Our main concern is with the manner and style of the interaction that should take place in the interview process. We will use typical clinical problems as examples where appropriate, but will not provide in-depth discussion of special problem areas. Thus, the concepts and suggestions offered transcend those associated with managing special problems (e.g., counseling children with cleft palate and their families, the family of a patient with aphasia, the patient who stutters, the child with a behavior problem, etc.). Rather, emphasis will be directed toward describing broader aspects of communication relationships, for it is upon these relationships that our professional credibility will eventually rest.

THE INTERVIEWER-COUNSELOR CONTINUUM

As we have learned, talking with patients and their families requires the development of skills in gathering historical information and interpreting clinical findings. The term *interviewing* refers to types of communication used when clinicians collect historical information about patients and their problems. In this context, interviewing functions are more prevalent in the initial stages of speech-language evaluations. On the other hand, *counseling* more often refers to communication directed toward the interpretation of clinical findings and toward the offering of specific therapeutic recommendations. Counseling functions are more prevalent in later stages of the speech-language evaluations.

Clinicians must learn to move flexibly between these two phases of the interviewer-counselor continuum. The functions clinicians assume within this continuum are largely determined by the immediate, situational needs of the patient. These needs highlight the fact that the patient is the central object of the examination. Thus, the patient's, not the clinician's, needs are paramount. Clinicians-in-training often assume one specific function as they execute given phases of the evaluation process. The adherence to the assumption of a specific role (e.g., gathering information) is appealing, because it offers a firm sense of direction. Unfortunately, such rigidity often undermines the efficiency of communication between the clinician and the patient and fails to meet the primary needs of the patient.

Two examples illustrate the necessity for clinicians to remain flexible in the roles they adopt during the conduct of diagnostic evaluations. During the history taking part of the evaluation, a parent might be moved to tears, thereby expressing deep concern about the condition and welfare of the child. At this point, pressing forward to obtain additional information about the child's development may become secondary to providing immediate emotional support to that parent. This example emphasizes the fact that the assumption of specific functions (e.g., offering support, exploring feelings and attitudes, etc.) cannot be rigidly allocated to a particular time in the evaluation.

As indicated earlier, it is more usual to counsel parents during interpretive phases of the evaluation. Although this is the case, we find that it is not uncommon for parents to offer the clinician new information at this stage of the evaluative process. This information is no less important because it was revealed late in the evaluation. In some cases, information which was withheld and revealed later may take on added significance. This occurred in an interview between a clinician and parents of a child seen by us. The child clearly required more consistent behavioral management. It was not until late in the evaluation that the clinician learned that the parents of this child were in counseling at another agency for precisely this problem. One might argue that a perceptive and efficient interviewer might have elicited such information during earlier stages of the evaluation process. The more important lesson, however, is that information emerges at various times, in various ways, and for various reasons. More often than not, people tell us things about themselves when they, rather than we, are ready (Garrett, 1972).

INTERVIEWER-COUNSELOR FUNCTIONS

In this section we discuss specific behaviors in which speech-language clinicians engage as they interview and counsel. These behaviors mark the basic functions clinicians assume during interviewing and counseling. Specification of these functions also provides operational definitions of interviewing and counseling. The reader must realize that the process of specifying functions introduces certain difficulties. First, categorical descriptions of functions can impart various meanings to different people, depending upon their experiences and their use of language. What one person perceives as motivation, another might view as support. Functions are also overlapping. For example, motivation of patients is generally viewed as a supportive behavior, whereas supportive behaviors are generally motivating. The semantic pitfalls associated with description of functions can be avoided if focus is directed toward specifying the clinical goals we seek to accomplish. Finally, the order in which functions are discussed is not intended to reflect any particular hierarchy. In general, the functions discussed early are those associated with interviewing, whereas those discussed later are typically used in fulfilling counseling functions.

Rapport Building

In this context, *rapport* is defined as the establishment of a positive relationship between a patient and a clinician. Certainly all clinical interactions are based upon attaining this rather general goal. In this instance, we should be a bit more specific. In addition to providing an understanding atmosphere, the clinician should spend time building readiness for the patient's acceptance of what is to come during the clinical relationship. Although there are some educational aspects to this function, we are emphasizing emotional perspectives. For example, clinicians often say: "We know this situation may be difficult for you . . . We are here to help you . . . You'll need to look at your (child's, spouse's) behavior . . . We'll explore the possible changes together." In these ways, clinicians introduce and consistently restate the message that they are building a relationship within an environment conducive to the welfare of the patient and family.

Collecting Information

A large part of establishing relationships with patients and their families is initiated by assembling information that is needed to make a responsible clinical diagnosis. The information may come to the clinician in the form of completed questionnaires or the history-taking interview. Items such as names, dates, places, significant events and milestones are all types of factual information vital to understanding the nature and history of the problem. Attitudinal information is also collected. Eliciting and interpreting this type of information is often a more difficult process, particularly for inexperienced clinicians and students-in-training.

Although the collection of information is necessary, it is important to point out that the clinician must constantly evaluate the quality of the information gathered. For example, the accuracy (reliability and validity) of the information reported merits continual appraisal. Reported facts must be viewed within the context of the overall history and never viewed as isolated events. What is not said by a patient or family member may be as significant as what is said. Lack of attention to certain details about a problem, or the avoidance of discussion of particular topics often gives the clinician insight into the manner patients and their families deal with difficulties. Useful information is also obtained by observing nonverbal behaviors (e.g., body language) of the person being interviewed (Birdwhistle, 1970; Knapp, 1978). Although the significance of nonverbal types of information is more subject to the interpretations of the interviewer, nonverbal language provides definite clues to the emotional states of individuals and aids the clinician in adjusting communication strategies to the patient's more immediate needs.

Facilitating Communication

Much of what workers do in helping relationships can be described as facilitating communication. Using various approaches, the aim of this function is to make it easier for the patient or parent to provide necessary information and to express emotional concerns. Facilitation can be accomplished by using various forms of questioning (see Table 10.1) and by carefully relating questions and statements to the antecedent responses of the person being interviewed (see Table 10.2). In this way, a feeling of continuity in exchange is promoted (Benjamin, 1981; Richardson et al., 1965).

Categorizing the interviewer's questions and statements provide assistance in the early learning of interviewing skills. Students interested in developing efficient interviewing skills will find it useful to analyze the types of statements and questions made by interviewers and respondents as they conduct diagnostic evaluations. By using post-session analyses of tape recorded clinical interactions, the student and clinical instructor can categorize the types of statements and questions used, determine the variety of approaches used, and determine how appropriate the nature of questioning was in light of the responses made by the patient. Students can use this technique to study interviewing and counseling techniques of others and to assess their own skills as an interviewer and counselor. Over time, each clinician will develop a characteristic style of communication. This style emerges, in part, as a product of the clinician's personality and the demands of the clinical situation. Clinicians should avoid developing a style that is characterized by limited variation in question and response forms, because this limitation generally causes the interview to become stilted or redundant.

Another important consideration is silence. Silence can be facilitating. The clinician must learn to listen to the verbal cues that preceed silences and to assess nonverbal cues present during silent intervals to determine whether waiting for a response is productive (Enelow and Swisher, 1972).

Table 10.1. Question types used in interviewing

Question type	Definition	Clinical example
Closed Question	A question which can be answered adequately in a few words	
Identification type	A question calling for the identification of person, place, group, time, number, etc., by asking *who, where, when, how many,* or *which*	What is the name of the psychologist and who tested David? When was this done?
Selection type	Fixed-alternative question, in which the respondent is asked to select one from the two or more possible responses offered	Do you recall Mary using specific words in communicating around her first birthday, or was it much later than that?
Yes-no type	A question that can be adequately answered *yes* or *no*, possibly supplemented by a redundant phrase such as, *I think so*, or *I doubt it*.	Were you annoyed at the other students laughing at your difficulty?
Open question	A question that may require more than a few words for an adequate response.	How do you usually respond to him when he behaves that way?

Based upon a format and categories presented in Richardson et al. (1965).

A distinction should be made between patients or parents who are silent because they do not have the requested information or do not understand the question, and individuals who are just taking time putting their thoughts and feelings together. In the former instance, the interviewer needs to intercede with a facilitating question or statement. In the latter, an interruption by the interviewer can be felt as a personal intrusion which might be counterproductive to communication. Beginning students have a tendency to fill silences with talk. They feel that silence is interpreted as nonproductive behavior. On the contrary, we encourage the students to use silence productively, both by allowing the patient to think and organize responses and by allowing themselves to do the same.

Listening

Anyone who has been burdened with a problem has probably experienced the good feelings associated with telling someone about their distress. We are often able to identify persons as "good listeners" even though we are not always certain what they do that makes them good at listening. It is likely that such persons are able to give us their full attention, are relaxed, and convey feelings of acceptance and understanding. The literature on interviewing and counseling often emphasizes the value of ventilation, or *ca-tharsis*. The prospect of getting a problem "off your chest" is often regarded as therapeutic (Garrett, 1972; Kahn and Cannell, 1957). Helping professionals do alot of listening. Knowledge about when communication should

Table 10.2.   Relationships between statements/questions and antecedent responses of the interviewee

Relationship type	Definition	Clinical example[a]	
Extension	A request for new information related to something already said	RSP:	We noticed he was beginning to react to the teasing of his playmates.
		IER:	In what ways did he react?
Echo	An exact or nearly exact repetition by the interviewer of the respondent's words (prompts the respondent to continue, expand, reflect, etc.)	RSP:	I was really disturbed with the outcome of the IEP conference this semester.
		IER:	Disturbed
		RSP:	Yeh, I don't think they consider all of Joey's problems.
Clarification			
Direct	A direct request for information on a vague or ambiguous prior part	IER:	So you're not getting home till nearly eight o'clock each evening.
		RSP:	No, I'm not working the second job during the summer.
		IER:	Oh, you're not? I'm not quite clear on that.
Inferential	An explicit inquiry about information implicit in a prior part of the interview	RSP:	She was last examined by Dr. Smith, last May I believe.
		IER:	When she was still in the county speech and hearing clinic program?
Summary	A question or statement which summarizes information previously stated explicitly, and explicitly or implicitly requests confirmation	RSP:	When he began wearing the speech appliance and began the therapy, it made a world of difference . . . and his friends reacted so differently to him . . . and it was obvious that he felt better about himself.
		IER:	This new approach was a real turning point for Joey.

Table 10.2.   *(Continued)*

Relationship type	Definition	Clinical example[a]	
Confrontation	A question or statement in which the interviewer presents the respondent with an inconsistency between two or more of the respondent's statements	RSP:	. . . and we agree that Jimmy shouldn't get what he wants without asking for it . . .
		RSP:	. . . then he'll take us by hand to the refrigerator and point to the juice jar and I'll give him some.
		IER:	You seem to be saying that you do not consistently practice what you consider to be best for Jimmy in helping him learn to use words.
Repetition	A question which merely repeats a question previously asked	IER:	What was the purpose in keeping Suzie in preschool an additional year?
		RSP:	Well, we just felt it was best for her.
		IER:	Yes, I understand . . . but what did you hope to accomplish by keeping her in preschool?

Based upon a format and categories presented in Richardson et al. (1965).
[a] RSP, Respondent; IER, interviewer.

and should not be interrupted with questions or suggestions is a vital clinical skill students must learn. Sometimes, just listening to someone provides the best help a clinician can offer.

The gathering of factual information (e.g., birth history, developmental mile- **Exploring Feelings** stones, physical problems, etc.) is typically easier to obtain than information **and Attitudes** about feelings and attitudes. There are several reasons for this situation. One reason is that the clinical interview might represent the first time a respondent has been asked to verbalize feelings or attitudes about a problem. For some individuals, talking openly and accurately about one's feelings and attitudes is difficult. Some respondents are simply not accustomed to expressing feelings or attitudes. Although these people may feel or experience emotions, the particular style of communication they have developed is not characterized by open sharing of feelings laden with high emotional content. The point to remember is that different communication styles are adopted by and are appropriate for different people. This discussion emphasizes the fact that we must sometimes work harder to obtain information about emotional or attitudinal factors that are part of certain disorders of human communication.

Finally, some parents find it emotionally painful or embarrassing to discuss negative feelings they may have about themselves or their children. It is natural to want to be seen as a good parent, especially to a professional worker who is carefully examining the dimensions of their child's problem. Most parents engage in behaviors with their children that are helpful. Some use approaches that are clearly counterproductive. Usually parents do both at one time or another. Helping parents to discuss these areas of concern and to permit information to emerge freely in the interview is an important first step toward determining how parents can best assist in a therapeutic program (Webster, 1977).

Motivating

We would like to assume that every new patient or family comes to us ready and willing to tackle their own problems. We would like to believe that they are ready to freely provide accurate information and use the suggestions we offer to them. When this is the case, our motivation usually takes the form of positive verbal reinforcement, designed to let patients know they are on the right track and to inform them that we recognize they are doing a good job. Our experience reveals that these conditions are not always present. For example, some patients are resistive. When this occurs, we must seek to determine the basis of their resistance by exploring their feelings and attitudes. We can also motivate by citing the rewards of cooperation, by discussing the probabilities for a favorable outcome, by explaining the altruistic values of helping other people, and by proclaiming our faith in people's ability to change their own behavior. Whatever the approach, the function is to help a person move toward the goal of establishing a mutually rewarding professional relationship.

Offering Support

There are some patients who come to the interview in clear need of emotional support. They are looking for reassurance in the words and behaviors of the clinician. The wife or husband whose spouse has just suffered a stroke, the laryngectomized patient, the person who stutters, and the parents of a neurologically impaired child are examples of patients and families which bear heavy emotional burdens and need support. In these situations, the professional must neither "paint a rosey picture" of the future nor promote dependency upon the clinician. Rather, the clinician should communicate such concepts and feelings as "We understand . . . We are here to help . . . We will work with you to do the best we can under the circumstances . . . I will be here when you need me."

The function of providing patients and their families with information is **Educating**
important. The dissemination of information will enable patients and their
families to understand the results of the diagnostic examination, the general
features of the disorder and its implications for management, and so on.
There is credence to the view that giving respondents specific information
generally fosters increased understanding of problems.

The beginning student must not turn an explanation into an academic
exercise. Questions from parents such as "What does cause stuttering?"
require careful responses. To answer this question fully, the various theories
of the causes of stuttering, together with supporting and opposing arguments
for each, would have to be discussed. Naturally, time does not permit this
form of answer as part of routine clinical practice. Hence, the response "Let
us examine Johnny and discuss the possible causes with you afterwards,"
puts the question into proper perspective and allows the clinician to shift
from an academic focus to a more relevant personal one. Indeed, this is
really what most parents want.

A few words about the language used in interviewing. As a general rule,
keep the language simple and speak directly to the point. Although a few
well educated parents might be able to decipher what a "phonological disorder" is, or what "velopharyngeal deficit" means, most parents are better
able to handle language that addresses "problems in forming speech sounds"
or "an inability to close off the nose from the mouth during speech." Likewise, statements such as "we need to interface structured learning with
functional communication in the home environment" place an inappropriate
burden of interpretation on the parent. A paraphrase of the above might be:
"We're trying to get Jimmy to use the language at home that he's been using
in therapy." It is easy to deceive ourselves by thinking we can display our
professional competence by using clinical jargon. The clinician must always
be aware of what is lost by doing this.

Often more than one approach can be used to modify communication be- **Examining Behavioral**
haviors in patients served by speech-language pathologists. There may also **Alternatives**
be a variety of changes of parental behavior suggested to assist in the resolution of problems related to communication and parent-child interaction.
Thus, speech-language clinicians must often evaluate a set of behavioral
alternatives and help patients or parents choose from among these alternatives. When possible, the clinician should involve the patient or parents
directly in the process of choosing between these alternatives, because their
direct involvement fosters increased responsibility for decisions made about
rehabilitation.

A clinical example which illustrates the need to examine behavioral
alternatives was provided by a senior-level high school youth evaluated for

a fluency disorder. One outcome of the diagnostic process was to recommend speech therapy. However, choices had to be made. For example: should therapy be given in a community speech clinic, the school system, or in a university clinic? To what extent should the parents of this youth be involved in this program of therapy? Insuring that the patient was actively involved in the consideration of these alternatives made it possible for him to take an active role in the decision process and provided him with a greater sense of satisfaction about his program of management. It is also important to provide patients with an opportunity to express their feelings about the alternatives suggested and to consider the advantages and disadvantages of these alternatives. This opportunity will also facilitate the establishment of sound clinical relationships and enhance personal responsibility, both of which are essential to effective speech-language management.

From the clinician's point of view, certain alternatives may be more attractive than others. Although this is true, patients and parents sometimes select less attractive or productive alternatives for remediating a problem. In this situation, the clinician must counsel the patient about their choices. Clinicians may sometimes have to acknowledge honest differences of opinion. Finally, clinicians must weigh the value of involving patients and parents directly in decision making against the sometimes more efficient process of merely offering a direct set of recommendations. Experienced clinicians often use skillfull counseling techniques to assist patients and parents to choose the most effective courses of clinical action.

Evaluating Information

Interviewing and counseling require the clinician to evaluate information. The verbal and nonverbal behaviors of patients and their family members represent the fabric upon which professional relationships are established and nurtured. Data and information are sorted, classified, and compared and then stored for use. The clinician must constantly assess the accuracy of information offered by patients and their families. Inaccuracies can result from several factors: faulty memory, diminished perception, lack of interest, fabrication, and so on. Inaccuracy may also be reflected in discrepant or inconsistent comments made by the respondent at various times during the interview. The interviewer must look for patterns of consistency or congruence in the communication of patients. When a consistent pattern does not appear, exploration should continue until there is reasonable certainty (i.e., adequate reliability and validity) about the clinical history provided.

Confrontation may be helpful in bringing discrepant information into congruence. An example of how confrontation may be used to clarify the difference between what a parent feels he should do with a child and what is actually done is summarized in Table 10.2. Confrontation is not meant to be interpreted as an aggressive (''showdown'') type of exchange between the interviewer and the respondent. Rather, confrontation may be used as a facilitating strategy and this strategy may, in fact, help a person deal with attitudes that conflict with actual behaviors.

Clinicians often make recommendations to patients and families. We have seen that the making of recommendations represents an essential part of the interpretive phase of the diagnostic process. Some recommendations are fairly general and are designed to initiate or continue therapeutic services of one type or another. For example, "We recommend that Johnny be seen for language therapy. . . , That Johnny continue therapy during the summer. . . , That Johnny be examined by an otologist," and so on, are recommendations often used for this purpose. Another type of recommendation is one which has as its objective the changing of someone's behavior. For example, "It would be helpful for you to read with Johnny each evening" is a recommendation offered to assist in a child's therapy. On the other hand, a recommendation may take the form of a request to stop some specific behavior. In either instance, the clinician has decided that it is better to make a direct suggestion than to have the parent or client discover the new behavior on their own.

Making Recommendations

FACTORS INFLUENCING COMMUNICATION STYLE

There are a number of factors which place limitations upon the interviewing process. There is no constraint-free situation. In this section, we will examine some major constraining factors: 1) time; 2) demands imposed by specific clinical settings; 3) designated clinical roles; 4) the physical setting; and 5) personal stylistic preferences. As in the previous section, this listing of constraints is not meant to be exhaustive, but merely identifies representative factors which influence what takes place in the interviewing process.

The clock is always running. From the moment we introduce ourselves to the patient or family to the time we finalize our recommendations, we are forced to carry out our duties within the constraints of a running clock. The amount of time we allow for a given patient will be a function of how we structure our day. This structure is likely to be different in various institutions. We will discuss this later. In every case, we are obligated to take a history, administer an examination, and offer our recommendations and counseling, all within a fixed period of time. How the clinician chooses to utilize time will be a product of choices made as the interview progresses. Each of these choices necessitates choosing between moving ahead in the interview and exploring more deeply issues which surface during the inter-

Time Constraints

view. A schematic representation of these choices is illustrated in Figure 10.1. It is evident that there is always a trade-off between the need of the interviewer to move laterally (broad coverage) and the need to move vertically (in-depth coverage). As with most choices in life, we usually gain something at the expense of losing something else. The clinician must choose, and the choice to move laterally or vertically will be based primarily upon a decision about what is more important (i.e., broad versus in-depth coverage of issues).

In clinical practice, the experienced interviewer learns when to explore in-depth and when to move ahead. This skill can only be developed on an empirical basis. The clinician comes to recognize important pieces of information and behaviors and learns to proceed to significant issues quickly and thoroughly. The ability to recognize individual patient differences is learned through clinical experience. Learning to conduct an interview efficiently is an important skill which requires balancing the need to be comprehensive with the need for pursuing more major issues on an in-depth basis.

Demands within Specific Clinical Settings

The professional setting in which the clinician works may impose certain restrictions upon the structure of the diagnostic evaluation. These restrictions can be viewed in terms of organizational characteristics or stylistic constraints. The organizational structure in which most speech-language clinicians work typically differs from the structure under which clinicians are trained.

The university speech and hearing clinic will frequently provide a setting with liberal constraints on the allotment of time for counseling and interviewing. Because students are at various levels of training and are practicing newly learned interviewing techniques, there is a tendency to allow the student clinician ample time for these purposes. In some cases, opportunities are provided for the student to confer with a supervisor during the evaluation to insure that nothing is overlooked. Students in later stages of their training program may be given greater responsibility and more restrictions, one of which may be a specific amount of time to complete the interview. In many educational settings, there will be organizational variations such as dividing students into diagnostic teams and assigning specific evaluation tasks to each student.

The community clinic represents a setting in which there is a high degree of concern for fiscal accountability. Therefore, the clinician often needs to see a specified number of patients over a given period of time. The community agency is usually dependent upon at least two types of funds: 1) money collected in the form of fees from patients; and 2) money received from local or regional health service agencies or federations. The latter identifies the clinic as an agency receiving funds from community drives such

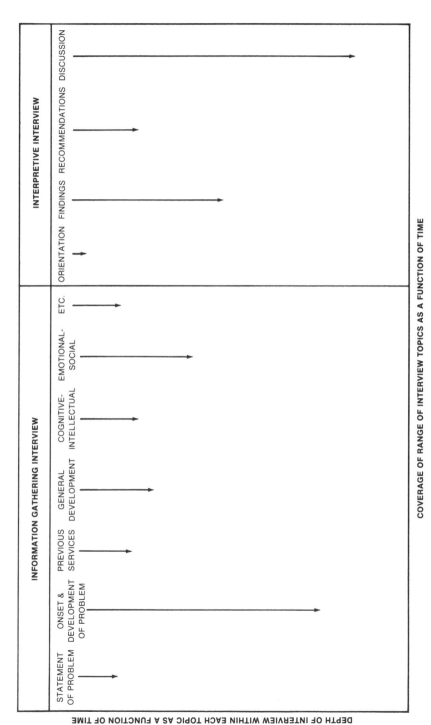

COVERAGE OF RANGE OF INTERVIEW TOPICS AS A FUNCTION OF TIME

Figure 10.1. Clinical diagnostic interviewing as a function of time.

as United Way. Because the community clinic is usually a free-standing service unit, there is little opportunity to offset financial deficits by reallocating funds from other service units, a mechanism often used in hospital settings. As a result, diagnostic scheduling is often based upon the need to serve a maximum number of patients on a daily basis balanced against the need to preserve the quality of diagnostic contacts.

This arrangement is a difficult one, for it leaves little room for flexibility within the interview. In this situation, appointments are usually arranged well in advance and there is often a need to adhere to a fairly rigid schedule. The need for expanded interview time might result in the scheduling of additional appointments which may serve the clinician's needs, but which may impair continuity of communication. Naturally, experienced clinicians working in such settings save valuable time by identifying major problems early in the interview and by spending the major portions of their time discussing matters of significance. It is not unusual for several professionals in a community clinic to specialize in diagnostic undertakings in an attempt to maximize the efficiency with which patients are evaluated.

The hospital setting presents still another set of circumstances that will influence talking with patients and their families. In this setting, the clinician often needs to deal with individuals who are acutely ill. For purposes of discussion, we will not consider out-patient services that are provided in many hospital settings. In hospital settings, clinical interviewing performed by the speech pathologist may, of necessity, become subordinate to the medical treatments offered to the patient. Scheduled medical tests and treatments, nursing concerns, levels of comfort and alertness of the patient, and so on represent constraints around which the clinician must work.

Likewise, contact with families in this setting may be different from that made in other settings. In a hospital, the clinician may not know when or if a family member will be present. In the best of circumstances, an interested family member will be present when requested and will be eager to talk with the clinician. On the other hand, the clinician may find that some hospitalized persons are without family assistance or that information about a patient often comes from other professionals (e.g., the nurse, the social worker, etc.). Finally, because the general medical facility may serve the acutely ill, patients frequently do not stay in the hospital long enough for the examiner to accumulate comprehensive diagnostic information. Patients are often moved to a less restrictive setting (skilled nursing facility, residential rehabilitation center, home, etc.) after their condition stabilizes.

A school-clinic setting offers yet another set of conditions that require adjustments in communication strategy. School children are often referred to the speech-language clinician by classroom teachers or are identified by the clinician through screening procedures. Children may be seen for evaluation before any historical information has been obtained from the parent. It may be difficult to obtain access to parents and even then, contact may be brief. The caseloads of clinicians in the schools may be sufficiently large to limit the time clinicians can spend with each parent. In practice, more time is typically spent interviewing parents of children with more complicated problems, less time with others. Once again, it is essential that the interviewer identify and focus upon the more significant features of the disorder so that contact time can be used efficiently.

The manner in which one conducts the diagnostic interview may be influenced by the professional role(s) the clinician has been assigned. Some diagnosticians are strictly that; they engage in diagnostic work only. They may make recommendations for therapy, but therapeutic management is administered by another staff member. In this role, the clinician views the diagnostic evaluation as a finite event. There may be no opportunities to expand the interview through later meetings with the patient or family. This arrangement may lead to the use of more rigidly structured interviewing strategies. The interviewer might be less inclined toward a rigid structure if both the role of examiner and therapist are assumed. Under this arrangement, the examiner can conduct the diagnostic evaluation, make recommendations, and initiate therapy. When there is insufficient time for in-depth interviewing, the clinician can use portions of therapy sessions to expand upon areas needing further clarification.

Designated Clinical Roles

Finally, clinicians find themselves assuming the role of a therapist, accepting a patient from another agency. Here, the clinician will probably want to conduct an interview before beginning therapy to confirm findings uncovered during the patient's initial evaluation. Many clinicians report the need to hear certain information for themselves, rather than rely solely upon information provided in the written reports of other examiners. In this situation, the nature of the interview will depend upon the clinician's need for verifying the original recommendations.

The places where interviews are conducted and the physical circumstances surrounding the interview can have profound effects upon the outcome (Benjamin, 1981; Fenlason et al., 1962). Consider the effects of physical comfort within the interview room. Austere and impersonal examining room settings can influence communication profoundly. As a general rule, examining room settings that are nicely furnished and appealing to the respondent will enhance communication and bring about a professional atmosphere. Noise represents another factor that can influence the quality of the interview. The placement of interview rooms adjacent to busy corridors, the clatter of typewriters, and so on can detract from the completion of effective interviewing. Such factors may make concentration difficult for both interviewer and respondent.

Physical Setting

Privacy is vital to the conduct of many clinical interviews. Interruptions not only break continuity, but make the respondent feel that the interviewer is not giving full attention to the problems at hand. Precautions must be taken to eliminate interruptions. An additional constraint may be present when young children accompany parents who are being interviewed. Although the presence of young children may interfere with interviewing parents, it can be said that the arrangement provides the clinician with an opportunity to observe parent-child interactions, providing insight into the social communication styles used.

Personal Constraints

Personal constraints influence the clinical process. Here, we are addressing the dominant characteristics of the interviewer (e.g., warmth, openness, empathy, etc.). This is not to say that the clinician who does not exhibit these characteristics cannot be effective in a helping relationship. It is, however, important to understand how you are perceived by patients and their families. Objective perception of the response of patients and families in relation to the clinician's own personality traits is difficult. Where there is a clear message that clinician behaviors inhibit communication, adjustments are necessary.

Clinician attributes are often present in subtle ways. How the clinician wishes to be referred to (first name versus title + last name), the presence or absence of credentials on the office walls, and the manner of dress all reflect the self-image of the clinician (Enelow and Swisher, 1972). Although the counseling literature is filled with arguments about interviewer "neutrality" versus doing what the interviewer feels "natural," our aim is to emphasize that both of these extremes will introduce constraints (Richardson et al., 1965).

COMMENTS ON TAKING THE CLINICAL HISTORY

Basic to obtaining a clinical history is the necessity for control. In the context of interviewing, *control* can be defined as the ability to move forward or to move from the surface level to deeper levels of discussion. Control can be achieved in a variety of ways. One method is to vary the questioning strategy from a closed question approach to methods that use open ended questions or statements (see Tables 10.1 and 10.2). The latter approach embraces client-centered methods. Although there has been a tendency to look upon the use of open ended questions or statements as manifestations of unstructured communication, client-centered approaches afford much control, allowing the clinician to lead the respondent from topic to topic in an efficient manner. In this case, control is exercised in a more subtle manner than when using direct questioning.

Client-centered approaches value the concept of "starting where the patient is" (Garrett, 1972; Rogers 1951, 1961). This means that the patient, spouse, or parent begins the interview by telling us what is important to them. We follow their leads and pick up information about developmental, physical, emotional, and social aspects of the problem at varying points in the evaluative process. This approach contrasts with the highly structured approach in which a clinician announces "I would like to discuss the development of your child's problem." Although it represents a legitimate alternative and may be effective under some circumstances, there is an underlying danger in this approach. The danger is that it is easy to become totally interested in soliciting specific types of information, rather than learning about significant aspects of the patients behavior or problem. This writer has often observed beginning students struggling to get a parent to answer precisely ordered questions and has heard clinicians ask questions that appear next on their precisely ordered list which have already been answered at an earlier point in the interview. Of course, these are extreme examples of reliance upon structure. Such reliance seriously handicaps effective communication. Attaining structure in the interviewing process is certainly attractive to the beginning clinician. Structure provides a well-defined path, and on the surface gives the appearance of efficiency. One danger is that the clinician may fail to experiment adequately with alternative forms of interviewing which ensure that flexibility is achieved.

We have seen that clinicians need to be flexible. Variations in the communication styles of patients or family members may require further adjustment by the interviewer. Some respondents come to us filled with information which they are ready to share. Others are tentative and need help, direction, or encouragement. Still others come under pressure and may not want to be in this situation. Such patients may signal resistance. Clearly, no single style can meet the needs of all patients. The clinician might consider beginning with a more open-ended approach, encouraging the patient or family member to relate their concerns in their own particular manner, keeping track of specific information through note taking as the interview progresses. Leads, probes, reflections, and so on will keep the respondent moving along. Where movement begins to break down, communication can become more focal. The clinician may guide the respondent with specific questions and may suggest alternative choice answers in situations in which the respondent needs assistance. Clinicians should be encouraged to begin experimenting with interviewing techniques using role-playing activities and should begin using varied approaches early in their clinical contacts.

Another important topic is note taking. The persons we serve expect clinical workers to take notes. The taking of notes signals to the patient that the clinician is listening and is interested in what is being said. The interviewer needs to become proficient at note taking. The use of the tape recorder has spurred the notion that note taking may not be needed. There are a number of problems associated with tape recording an interview. Tape recorders are mechanical devices. They do not always work properly. Although audio recordings provide an acoustic record, they do not permit recording of significant nonverbal pieces of information. Tape recordings usually require a complete second listening. Finally, tape recording is not always welcomed by the respondent. Use of audio or video tapes can certainly be helpful as an adjunct to listening. Recording of interviews provide a robust record useful in assessing the interviewing skills of clinicians. In the clinical training setting, tape recording is indispensable. Its use in this context should be separated from the clinician's need to become a proficient note taker.

Before leaving this topic, consideration should be given to talking with children. It is desirable and frequently helpful to talk directly to young children about their speech and language related problems. This assumes that the child can understand the questions of the examiner and has sufficient skills to make the responses interpretable. The clinician must realize that children have feelings and attitudes. These feelings relate to themselves, their problems, and their relationship with significant others. Clinicians must not ignore these feelings and attitudes and should not depend solely upon what a parent tells them about the child. This form of omission may introduce significant bias into the interview. There may be discrepancy between the way a parent thinks a child feels and the way the child actually reports he or she feels about a problem. There may also be a discrepancy between the child's perception of the reason for his or her being brought to a speech-language clinician and the actual reason for the referral. Contemporary practice dictates that we communicate directly with children about issues that bear upon our final diagnosis and recommendations. The clinician will need to be honest with children. The clinician should use language that facilitates understanding, and needs to recognize the feelings and attitudes children bring to the evaluative process.

COMMENTS ON THE INTERPRETIVE INTERVIEW

A common task undertaken during the interpretive phase of clinical interviewing is to present a diagnosis to the patient or responsible adult(s). As discussed in Chapter 1, the diagnosis or clinical impression can be divided into several parts. To review, the diagnostic statement usually contains:

1. Information specifying the classification of the disorder and its severity
2. A statement of the etiologic and/or behavioral factors that precipitate or sustain the problem
3. A presentation of factors that may influence intervention

4. Information concerning the relevance of particular forms of treatment and/or referrals
5. A prognostic statement

These classes of information are often useful to the clinician because of the need to synthesize clinical findings and present these findings in a formal written report. It is doubtful that the patient or family member would welcome an interpretation of the findings in this form. Although these classes of information are useful to them, their immediate need to understand the problem can best be served by addressing the following:

1. What was done (or measured) today?
2. What were the findings in relation to norms or standards?
3. What is the outlook for improvement?
4. What is recommended to be done?

Clinicians should use language that the respondent can understand. Answering these four basic questions during the interpretive phase of the interview will leave the patient or family in a better position to comprehend what the problem is and what can or cannot be done to minimize or resolve this problem. Naturally, there must be time to answer additional questions. The offer to answer questions is particularly helpful. The technique of providing a brief summary before proceeding to new topical areas is also helpful.

After recommendations have been made, the clinician should secure a verbal response from the patient or family member to determine whether the recommendations have been accepted or rejected. Where speech or language therapy has been recommended, rejection is rare. This situation occurs occasionally when persons have been sent for an evaluation against their wishes. There are instances in which therapy is not recommended. In some situations, parent education is recommended or referral for other types of evaluation and treatment (medical, psychological, family counseling, etc.) have been made. In these cases, the recommendations may be received with resistance or outright rejection. The clinician is obligated to fully explore the respondent's feelings about the recommendations and patients and family members should not leave with unexpressed negative reactions. Once a patient or family member leaves the professional's office, clarification of problem areas and resolution of disagreements are more difficult to achieve.

A concluding step in the interpretive diagnostic interview is for the clinician to secure confirmation of the patient's or parent's intent to carry out the recommendation(s). Most cases will simply require immediate, positive administrative action (enrollment in therapy as soon as possible; send a referral report to Dr. Jones, etc.). In other cases, the patient or parent may want time to consider what they want to do ("I'll call you Monday to get your decision," or "Please call me when you have decided."). The clinician may encourage the patient or parent to get a second opinion. In any case, it is important to conclude the interview with a clear understanding of what is to be done, who will do it, and when it is to be done. In this manner, the diagnostician will be in a better position to bring closure to each evaluation.

THE CLINICIAN AS COUNSELOR

Before bringing this chapter on talking with patients to a close, we shall consider the clinician's role as a counselor. This role will be discussed in relation to 1) patient and family needs; 2) academic training; 3) clinical experience; and 4) institutional policy. There is general agreement that speech-language clinicians need to become competent counselors. The counseling function begins in the diagnostic setting and extends across the therapeutic relationship. The criteria used to determine whether a speech-language clinician should undertake a specific counseling problem have not been well defined. The writer will attempt to provide more specific criteria within this section and within the context of Figure 10.2.

Patient and Family Needs

The range of problems which come to the attention of the speech-language clinician is extensive. Behavioral management of children, problems of self-concept associated with physically handicapping conditions, emotional-social problems associated with stuttering, and adjustment problems of patients and spouses of persons with aphasia represent just a few areas in which counseling may play a significant role. Usually, problems arise as a result

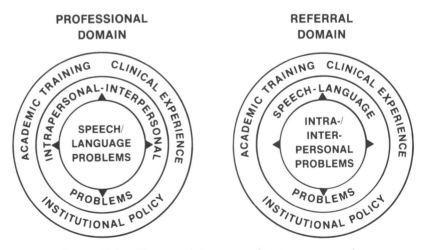

Figure 10.2. The speech-language clinician as counselor.

of the patient's inability to communicate effectively. These problems can generate additional negative feelings about one's self (intrapersonal attitudes) and about others (interpersonal attitudes). In the case of children, communication problems can generate feelings of frustration, inadequacy, and hostility. In this context, the communication disorder may become responsible for maladaptive behavior on the part of the patient or parent.

In other cases, the speech and language disability may not represent the core of the problem. Here, the communication impairment can be viewed as a symptom of some underlying intrapersonal and/or interpersonal difficulty. The loss of voice in the face of stressful situations or disturbances in the quality of the voice as a product of personality attributes are examples of this situation. The inability to effectively manage children's behavior represents another broad problem. This problem influences parent relationships with all siblings, including children with speech-language disorders.

In situations in which speech-language disability is the central or core problem, the counseling role generally falls within the responsibility of the speech-language clinician. In this situation, understanding concommitant behaviors cannot be achieved without understanding the nature of the communication impairment. Furthermore, treatment may need to embrace both physical and attitudinal perspectives. In the situation in which long-term emotional components are central to the problem, the decision about who should provide counseling is not easily answered on a categorical basis.

Academic Training

The ability to carry out effective counseling should be included as part of the academic training of speech-language clinicians. Professional training programs vary widely in their ability and interest in carrying out this training function. In some programs, information is presented in a single course format within the curriculum. At others, parts of individual disorder-oriented courses are given over to discussion of counseling needs. There is usually an option for a student to take courses in counseling in other departments of the university (e.g., psychology, educational counseling, social work, etc.). Few programs require specific coursework in counseling, leaving the student to choose between various elective courses.

The ability to counsel effectively requires an interest in understanding people and a desire to become knowledgeable about this important facet of clinical intervention. Understanding the dynamics of human behavior is certainly critical to the development of helping relationships. Knowledge about the diverse approaches used in counseling are often helpful in considering the alternative choices that the clinician faces in clinical practice. The same is true for more specific techniques used in counseling. These areas of knowledge and skill represent prerequisites. They allow a clinician to develop a philosophy about counseling, plan courses of action with patients, and execute a clinical style which incorporates dynamic interplay between one's personal qualities and clinical effectiveness.

The clinician's academic experiences provide one form of assistance that will help determine how counseling needs will be met. Hopefully, the clinician will meet some minimum standard. Academic experiences in counseling should be broad in scope, current in content, and realistically linked to clinical experience.

Clinical Experience

The old saying, "There is no substitute for experience," has reasonable validity, particularly in relation to the question of the extent to which a clinician should serve as counselor. Experience alone does not breed competence. Experience must be subjected to quantitative and qualitative analysis to insure that growth and skills are enhanced. Few clinicians can expect to experience all types of counseling problems. It is important for clinicians to come to terms with clinical process and with themselves as helping professionals (Rogers, 1961). Process and self cut across all types of problems. Success with one type of clinical problem will often foster success in other situations. Experience is collected through clinical opportunities, through supervisory encouragement, and on the basis of taking personal risk. All things being equal, successful clinical experiences as a counselor will serve to help the clinician meet this criterion in the future.

Institutional Policy

Finally, the clinician may need to deal with institutional policy regarding counseling. Policy is present in many forms in clinical institutions. Policy may be manifested in the form of explicitly written regulations or it may be transmitted in the form of subtle cues. Some institutions will encourage and provide time for speech-language clinicians to do their own counseling. Other institutions will hire personnel in psychology or social work to perform this role. Still other settings may foster group counseling programs. Both time and money are important factors which cannot be ignored. The provision of sessions for counseling which necessitates use of clinician time may be costly. These sessions consume time that could be spent in other activities. For this reason, charges are usually necessary and these expenses may tend to limit the extent of counseling activity offered.

In closing, this writer is reminded of a personal clinical situation. This situation concerned a young patient who both stuttered and was also acting out aggressively. His aggressive behavior occasioned several contacts with the local police. The relationship between the young man and the clinician was favorable. Rapport was excellent and trust had been established over a number of years. On the surface, it seemed unlikely that a speech clinician should work on the problem that arose when the young boy poured paint remover on automobiles of friends of his parents who came to visit at his home. When the psychiatrist who worked with the family was consulted about the situation, he advised that work with the patient should be approached by a single person. This recommendation was made because the psychiatrist knew that the speech-language clinician was capable of providing counseling. In addition, he knew that the speech clinician had a well-established personal relationship with the boy, had regular access to him, and understood how these issues might be interwoven. The psychiatrist also knew that the speech clinician would ask for interpretation and assistance when it was needed. In this case, the speech clinician ventured out of his traditional domain and did some risk taking. He did this with the understanding and support of a member of the medical profession. This, of course, could only be done in an institution in which policy, be it subtle or explicit, would permit.

Study Guide

1. Identify the major roles speech-language clinicians assume as they interview and counsel patients and their families.

2. Describe some major techniques you may use to enhance the efficiency of your interviewing skills.

3. Why is the gathering of factual information generally less difficult than gathering information about feelings and attitudes?

4. Identify some major factors which influence communication style and place constraints upon the interviewing process. Make clear precisely how the factors you have identified influence communication style and constrain the interview process.

REFERENCES

Benjamin, A. 1981. The Helping Interview. 3rd Ed. Houghton Mifflin Company, Boston.

Birdwhistle, R. 1970. Kinesics and Context. University of Pennsylvania Press, Philadelphia.

Emerick, L., and Hatten, J. 1979. Diagnosis and Evaluation in Speech Pathology. Prentice-Hall, Inc., Englewood Cliffs, NJ.

Enelow, A., and Swisher, S. 1972. Interviewing and Patient Care. Oxford University Press, New York.

Fenlason, A., Ferguson, G., and Abrahamson, A. 1962. Essentials in Interviewing, (Revised). Harper & Row, New York.

Garrett, A. 1972. Interviewing: Its Principles and Methods. 2nd Ed. Basic Books, Inc., New York.

Kahn, R., and Cannell, C. 1957. The Dynamics of Interviewing. John Wiley, New York.

Knapp, M. 1978. Nonverbal Communication in Human Interaction. 2nd Ed. Holt, Rinehart and Winston, New York.

Richardson, S., Dohrenwend, B., and Klein, D. 1965. Interviewing: Its Forms and Functions. Basic Books, Inc., New York.

Rogers, C. 1951. Client-Centered Therapy. Houghton Mifflin Co., Boston.

Rogers, C. 1961. On Becoming a Person. Houghton Mifflin Co., Boston.

Webster, E. 1977. Counseling with Parents of Handicapped Children. Grune & Stratton, New York.

Author Index

Subject Index